FEMINIST PHENOMENOLOGY AND MEDICINE

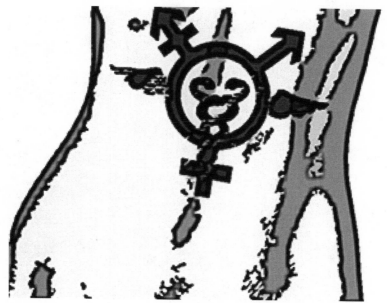

Image by Anders Lind. Reprinted with permission.

FEMINIST PHENOMENOLOGY AND MEDICINE

Edited by
Kristin Zeiler
and
Lisa Folkmarson Käll

Published by State University of New York Press, Albany

For information, contact State University of New York Press, Albany, NY
www.sunypress.edu

Production by Diane Ganeles
Marketing by Michael Campochiaro

Library of Congress Cataloging-in-Publication Data

Feminist phenomenology and medicine / edited by Kristin Zeiler and
  Lisa Folkmarson Käll.
    pages cm
  Includes bibliographical references and index.
  ISBN 978-1-4384-5007-0 (hardcover : alk. paper)
  ISBN 978-1-4384-5006-3 (pbk.: alk. paper) 1. Women—Health
and hygiene—Social aspects. 2. Medicine—Philosophy. 3. Feminist theory.
4. Feminism—Health aspects. 5. Medical care—Sex differences. 6. Phenomeno-
logical psychology. I. Zeiler, Kristin, 1973– editor of compilation. II. Käll, Lisa
Folkmarson, editor of compilation.
  RA564.85.F467 2014
  613'.04244—dc23

                                    2013012779

            10   9   8   7   6   5   4   3   2   1

CONTENTS

WHY FEMINIST PHENOMENOLOGY AND MEDICINE?

LISA FOLKMARSON KÄLL AND KRISTIN ZEILER

Feminist Phenomenology and Medicine brings together two strands in phenomenological research. First, a growing number of feminist, queer, and critical race scholars have shown that the philosophical tradition of phenomenology offers valuable resources for approaching issues concerning the lived experience of marginalization, invisibility, nonnormativity, and oppression. Particularly phenomenological accounts of embodiment, focusing on the lived experience of the body, have provided a useful starting point in examinations of how the singular body, that is, the body as unique and different from other bodies, with a particular sex, of a particular age, race, ethnicity, and ability can form and inform our embodied selves and influence our ways of interacting with others and the world (see Alcoff 1999; Weiss 1999; Fisher 2000; Diprose 2002; Heinämaa 2003; Young 2005; Ahmed 2006; 2007; Käll 2009a; 2010; Al-Saji 2010; Heinämaa and Rodemeyer 2010, Zeiler 2013a). This research points at the value of bringing together phenomenology and feminist theory: both unveil and scrutinize taken-for-granted and in this sense 'hidden' assumptions, beliefs and norms that we live by, that we strengthen by repeated actions and that we also resist, challenge and question. Furthermore, and beyond a feminist application of phenomenology, feminist phenomenology provides ways of deepening the phenomenological framework by asking questions of how experiences of, for instance, sexuality, sexual difference, pregnancy, birth, race, ethnicity, etc. inform phenomenology as a philosophical project (Schües 1997; Alcoff 2000; Oksala 2004, 2006; Heinämaa 2012). Second, phenomenological studies have offered pertinent analysis of relevance for medical practice, such as analysis of experiences of illness, pain, and bodily alienation (e.g., Zaner 1981; Leder 1990, Toombs 2001; Svenaeus 2009, Carel 2008; Bullington 2009), offered analysis of clinical encounters (Toombs 1993, 2001), and the meaning of health (Svenaeus 2001), to mention but a few examples.

Whereas there is a growing area of feminist phenomenology dealing with concrete issues of embodiment and situatedness and whereas phenomenologists have made valuable contributions to the analysis of the nature of medicine, the meaning of illness and health as well as clinical practice, there have been comparably few analyses of such issues that combine insights from feminist phenomenology and phenomenology of medicine. This, however, is now gradually changing, a development to which the present volume aims to contribute.

Feminist Phenomenology and Medicine demonstrates the value of bringing together research in the fields of feminist phenomenology and phenomenology of medicine in order to advance more comprehensive analyses of issues such as bodily self-experience, normality and deviance, self-alienation and objectification that are central to both fields. It indicates the relevance of feminist phenomenological perspectives to the field of medicine and health by highlighting difference, vulnerability, and volatility as central dimensions of human experience rather than deviations, and vitalizes the field of feminist phenomenology, as well as the field of phenomenology more generally, by bringing it into conversation with a range of different materials, such as empirical research, case studies, cultural representations, and personal narrative. It also takes into consideration and examines normative cultural practices and structures of meaning that situate different bodies in different ways and with different conditions, and seek to lay bare the constitutive conditions of experience. Finally, by taking seriously the embodiment and situatedness of subjective life and experience and by bringing different forms of embodied existence to description and analysis, *Feminist Phenomenology and Medicine* seeks to develop and sharpen the methodological tools and conceptual framework of phenomenology.

Situated at the intersection of phenomenology of medicine and feminist phenomenology, this volume contributes to furthering phenomenological work in philosophy of medicine and brings out the large scope of the field of medicine including its strong impact on various areas of life that are perhaps not immediately considered medical areas such as sexuality, bodily appearance, and norms of beauty. The essays in the book draw from numerous fields, such as dentistry, midwifery, cosmetic surgery, and psychiatry, as well as other health sciences, and address topics such as cosmetic surgery and complicity, Body Integrity Identity Disorder (BIID), reassignment surgery for intersex children, experiences of heart transplants, and anorexia, to mention again but a few examples.

Phenomenology and Medicine

Phenomenological studies have offered descriptions and analyses of significant relevance for medical practice since its early days, as is evident with the work of Maurice Merleau-Ponty. Recent years have also seen a raise in the number of such studies and we discern mainly two tendencies. First, there is a growing phenomenological literature that analyzes the nature of medicine; the meaning and lived experience of illness, disability, and health; the distinction between immediate experience and scientific exploration; the nature of embodiment; and the interrelation between body, consciousness, and world in experiences of, for example, pain, illness, and disability. This literature sometimes focuses on first-person experience and seeks to lay bare the structures and meanings of such experience. It may also draw on or involve different forms of empirical research or clinical cases with the aim of theoretical elaboration and conceptual development (see for example Merleau-Ponty 1962; Finlay 2003; Bengtsson et al. 2004; Engelsrud 2005; Zeiler and Wickström 2009). This literature can be contrasted with another strand of literature that is phenomenological in the sense that it examines lived experiences of illness and disability from within the social sciences but without a philosophical analysis of these experiences as its primary aim.[1]

This first tendency can be exemplified with phenomenological analyses of embodiment and bodily self-awareness when falling ill and when experiencing pain, illness, and/or bodily alienation

(Buytendijk 1973; Zaner 1981, 1988; Leder 1990; Toombs 2001; Svenaeus 2001, 2009; Carel 2008; Bullington 2009) as well as with analyses of the shareability of pain (Käll 2013). It can also be exemplified
with analyses of how to understand intersubjectivity, communication, and empathic understanding between health care professionals and the sick person and the different perspectives of health care
professionals and patients (Toombs 1993, 2001; Svenaeus 2001). Furthermore, phenomenological work within this strand has contributed with insights of relevance for psychiatry and psychopathology
(Sass and Parnas 2001; Fuchs 2002; Parnas 2003; Ratcliffe 2008, 2011;
Parnas, Sass, Zahavi 2011; Sass, Parnas, Zahavi 2011; Stanghellini
2011), organ donation (Leder 1999; Perpich 2008; Slatman 2009;
Shildrick 2008; Svenaeus 2012), dementia (Matthews 2006, Dekkers
2011, Zeiler 2013b), death (Weiss 2006; Heinämaa 2010), and questioned knowledge production in the development of genetic theory
(Diprose 2005).

Feminist Phenomenology and Medicine contributes to this strand
with, for example, Fredrik Svenaeus' analysis of anorexia as an experience of the body uncanny, Abby Wilkerson's investigation of bodily
self-alienation in depression, Margrit Shildrick's discussion of the
intimations of an otherness within experienced by heart transplant
recipients, and Kristin Zeiler and Lisa Guntram's examination of
bodily self-awareness in relation to young women's stories of coming
to know that they have no womb and no or a small vagina.

Second, there is a less strong but nevertheless persistently growing body of literature that elaborates phenomenological approaches
to ethics and particularly medical ethics. Some such work investigates
the phenomenology of specific moral experiences. They examine
what it feels like to be in a situation that the subject experiences as
ethically sensitive, problematic, or promising, and what being in this
situation means to the subject. In the context of medicine, this can be
exemplified with analyses of experiences of objectification, shame, or
guilt in relation to cases of body dysmorphia and depression (Fuchs
2003). In this volume, Erik Malmqvist's chapter targets such ethically
sensitive situations in a discussion of complicity with unjust social
norms and with a particular focus on cosmetic surgery.

Other studies within the field of phenomenological approaches
to ethics start in an analysis of human being-in-the-world, which also
includes being-with-others and moves from this level of analysis to

an examination of how we ought to live together without examining specific moral experiences. Such phenomenological work can examine how the other is encountered in the forming of the self, including different ways of encountering the other, some of which are seen as better than others (Diprose 2005).[2] It may also distinguish ethics from ontology; emphasize human vulnerability, responsivity, and openness to the other as ethical modes of being; and examine what this means for sensitivity and ethical perception on behalf of health care professionals (Nortvedt 2008). In this volume, Lisa Folkmarson Käll for instance thematizes vulnerability and exposure in addressing the question of the possibility of ethical perception within an objectifying framework and highly controlled clinical research setting of medical science.

Still other studies within the field of phenomenological approaches to ethics critically interrogate dominant modes of being, thinking, feeling, and acting in particular cultural contexts. Within the context of medicine, such research examines how certain norms about bodies can become taken-for-granted and motivate what may be called "normalizing" surgery, that is, surgery that seeks to make bodies conform to prevailing norms (e.g., Shildrick 1999; Weiss 2009; Zeiler and Wickström 2009; Malmqvist and Zeiler 2010; Cadwallader 2010) or how the lived experience of a specific embodiment can affect the structures of imagination and interpretation that people use in moral perception and evaluation of specific cases, such as those of, for instance, "deaf designer babies" (Scully 2003). *Feminist Phenomenology and Medicine* includes discussion of various forms of surgical interventions that in different ways and with different impact contributes to producing "normal" bodies. Gail Weiss, for instance, discusses normalizing interventions in relation to rhetorics of enhancement and notions of naturalness, and Nikki Sullivan raises issues regarding the punitive consequences of resisting and rejecting surgical interventions of normalization in her analysis of how the first hand-transplant recipient was represented in the media.

This last kind of phenomenological ethical work also includes contributions to normative ethics, as when scholars elaborate lines of argumentation for therapeutic cloning (Svenaeus 2007) or engage with phenomenological work in an ethical analysis of the use of new reproductive technologies such as pre-implantation genetic diagnosis (Malmqvist 2008).

Feminist Phenomenology

Feminist phenomenology may be said to have been a vital dimension within phenomenology already in its early formation with the work of Edith Stein and Simone de Beauvoir. In the 1930s, Stein brought the homogeneity and universality of intersubjective relations into question with her phenomenological descriptions of feminine and masculine types of consciousness (1996) and, in her 1949 classic *The Second Sex*, Beauvoir radically situated the embodied subject by bringing the question of woman's being to phenomenological reflection (2010). Beauvoir's commitment to raising the question of sexual difference as a philosophical question through the method of phenomenological inquiry is present throughout her work and has come to form the foundation for further developments of feminist phenomenology.

Much feminist phenomenology has focused on bringing specifically female experiences to careful description, using the conceptual tools and methodological framework of phenomenology to approach areas of experience left uncharted in the phenomenological tradition. Such experiences include, for example, those of pregnancy and giving birth (Bigwood 1991; Lundquist 2008); of menstruation, of having breasts and lactating, of self-alienation (Young 2005; Beauvoir 2010); of eating disorders (Bordo 1993); of embodying the risk of being subjected to sexual violence (Cahill 2001; Käll 2009b); and of bodily self-awareness in which one's body stands forth as a thematic object, in a positive and nonalienating way (Young 2005). These phenomenological descriptions and analyses serve as a critical and corrective complement or expansion of the field of describable experiences. While not explicitly questioning or altering the phenomenological methods and concepts, this approach is of importance for drawing attention to a whole range of experience that philosophers have neglected to consider. Furthermore, feminist phenomenological descriptions of women's experience play a crucial role in dismantling what passes as universal and essential to human experience as reflecting only a limited group and thereby enriching our understanding of the scope and structures of human experience (Oksala 2004, 16–17).

By demonstrating that neglected regions of experience do not all fall into categories of pathology but, rather, belong to the everyday lives of women (and in the case of pregnancy and giving birth, are conditions for the continuation of humanity), feminist phenomenology also throws a critical light on the constitution of normality, both that of the human and that of woman and man. It furthermore brings out the complexities of experiences that deviate and are excluded from the realms of normality in the double sense of falling outside the boundaries not only of what is the accepted, although false, norm for the human but also of what is considered to be a normally *sexed* human being. These circumstances are brought out in this volume in, for instance, Zeiler and Guntram's contribution, in which the authors discuss norms about female embodiment in the light of young women's experiences of atypical sexual development, and in Ellen Feder's analysis of experiences of such double exclusion in her examination of the standards of care of surgical intervention in cases of children born with ambiguous genitalia. In a different way, Cressida Heyes' discussion of cosmetic surgery devotee Lolo Ferrari also demonstrates this double exclusion in the constitution of normalcy.

Using the method of phenomenological description to complement and enrich the field of describable experience furthermore adds an important perspective in discussions on experiential analysis more generally that has been at the core of the development of much feminist theory (Fisher 2000; Alcoff 2000). As much as the conceptual tools and methodological framework of phenomenology have proved resourceful for feminist purposes, however, they have also been put under critical scrutiny by feminist phenomenologists who, instead of dismissing phenomenology altogether, have pointed to its limitations and contributed to its development. Integrating phenomenological and feminist frameworks for analysis more fully, feminist phenomenologists have brought to the fore how proper investigations into the phenomena of, for instance, sexual difference, pregnancy, and birth radically alter phenomenological analysis of the emergence of conscious experience and the birth of the human being (Oksala 2004; Schües 1997). In this regard, already Iris Marion Young (2005) argues that the experience of pregnancy makes manifest a fracturing of the integrity of the embodied subject and questions the unity of the phenomenological subject as a condition of possibility for experience (see Heinämaa 2012).

Indeed, feminist voices have been key in inquiring into the possibilities of accounting for difference and otherness within the framework of phenomenology as a philosophy of the subject or consciousness. Feminist phenomenologists have been careful to stress and investigate different forms of interrelations between self and other as constitutive of subjectivity and experience. *Feminist Phenomenology and Medicine* testifies to the concern with the role of concrete as well as general others in the constitution and understanding of the self. For instance, Jenny Slatman and Gili Yaron's analysis of facial disfigurement highlights, among other things, not only how living with facial disfigurement comes to affect social relations but also how social relations impact and form subjective experience and self-understanding. Also Erik Malmqvist's interrogation of complicity with unjust social norms draws attention to the role of both concrete and general others in self-understanding. Furthermore, the constitutive interrelation between self and other is brought out in a very different way in Sarah LaChance Adams and Paul Burcher's discussion of the experience of "communal pushing" in childbirth.

Of particular interest for feminist phenomenology has been the experience of bodily self-alienation and experience of oneself as other to oneself as normative for women's ways of being in the world (Arp 1995; Beauvoir 2010; Young 2005). Building on Beauvoir's insight that "woman *is* her body as man *is* his, but her body is something other than her" (2010, 41), feminist phenomenologists have continued interrogation of the various ways in which women's bodily self-alienation comes to articulation at intersections of different categories of identity and structures of power and privilege. The issue of bodily self-alienation is, as already mentioned, also a central theme in phenomenological accounts of experiences of illness. It comes to the fore in different ways throughout this volume, and several contributions target the interrelation between illness experience and gender. In this way, Fredrik Svenaeus' analysis of anorexia as an experience of the body uncanny bears out the different gendered dimensions of the illness by situating it in a coercive cultural context involving norms of successful femininity. Abby Wilkerson, too, targets the interrelation between bodily self-alienation and gender in her discussion of the impact of social power dynamics on bodily resonance in depression. The experience of one's own body as other to oneself is present also in Lisa Folkmarson Käll's account of the portrayal in Mike Nichols' film *Wit* of the objectification of a woman's body by medical science and in Margrit Shildrick's chapter on the experience of heart-transplant recipients.

Feminist phenomenology is furthermore characterized by the way it builds, and has built since its early articulations, on strands of phenomenology engaged with different forms of empirical studies and interdisciplinary perspectives. It has played an important role in the work of both deepening and carefully thinking through the relation between empirical work and phenomenological reflection through its emphasis on the constitutive role of embodiment, the situatedness of subjectivity, and the concreteness of lived experience. Such engagement provides feminist phenomenology with a unique position for furthering interdisciplinary scholarship founded in a specific methodology characterized by rigorous self-interrogation of its own grounds and presuppositions. The chapters in this volume bring out the strength and potential of interdisciplinarity both for the furthering of the conceptual tools and framework of phenomenology as well as for the understanding of specific phenomena and experiences. By offering a critical perspective on phenomenology using the tools and methods offered in part by phenomenological philosophy, feminist phenomenology also opens the possibility of taking phenomenology into a broad range of fields of philosophical inquiry such as political philosophy, epistemology, ontology, ethics—and indeed also medical ethics. The latter can be seen already in Simone de Beauvoir's existential-phenomenological analysis in *A Very Easy Death* from 1964 (1985) in which she gives a first-person account of witnessing her mother's dying of cancer and of facing the moral dilemma of whether to tell her about the severity and terminal prognosis of her illness.

While the insistence on the necessary situatedness of subjectivity and its contributions to perceptions of reality is characteristic not only of feminist phenomenology but also of feminist philosophy more generally, the phenomenological method constitutes, in our contention, a productive resource for feminist (and other) attempts at denaturalizing metaphysical and essentialist claims about reality and unveiling the role of subjectivity and intersubjectivity in the constitution of that reality. For feminist phenomenology, this denaturalization concerns to a great extent claims about the nature and essences of bodies and desires, sexual difference, and sexuality, and thereby validates and supports an understanding of gender and sexuality as the effect of power relations, patterns of prejudice and privilege, and social and cultural practices. The phenomenological method implies, in a minimal sense, a self-critical distance on the part of the philosophizing subject, enabling her to investigate the constitutive conditions of her own experiences. This methodological step provides feminist theory with a way of critically approaching its own social, cultural, and historical situation from within. In this volume, Lanei Rodemeyer's critical discussion of how a feminism committed to constructionism should approach scientific claims about hormones is one example of such self-interrogation. A critical position, intrinsic to the reality that is its object of investigation, is essential to the viability of a feminist theory and critical interrogation of social structures and practices that is committed to the idea that reality is, to a greater or lesser degree, socially constituted.

The project of denaturalization is at this point in time perhaps especially urgent in relation to the field of medicine, which exerts an unparalleled power in defining and delimiting human nature and normality. A feminist phenomenological perspective on medicine and medical practice is therefore of utmost importance for dismantling this power and for targeting the force of social, cultural, and historical conditions in the production of reality and what is taken to be natural and normal by the authority of medicine.

Feminist Phenomenology and Medicine in This Volume

Taking its point of departure in the phenomenological understanding of subjectivity as embodied and embedded in the world and in interrelation with others, the chapters in *Feminist Phenomenology and Medicine* offer careful description and analysis of a range of topics within the field of medicine and the health sciences. The volume starts with an account of the importance and necessity of a phenomenological approach in studies on illness, particularly in studies on the experience of illness. In "The Illness Experience: A Feminist Phenomenological Perspective," Linda Fisher argues that a phenomenological analysis captures an experiential immediacy and subjective perspective missing in studies focused primarily on sociocultural constructions of illness and the illness experience, while providing an analytical and methodical framework often lacking in personal or narrative renditions of the illness experience: the capacity to move from the singularity of the standard first-person narrative to an account that seeks to identify and analyze generalities and typical features of the experience as such, while examining how this experience resides within and intersects with the broader lifeworld.

Furthermore, a feminist perspective in the form of a feminist phenomenology can be equally valuable and important in disclosing the ways in which our lived experience is inflected by gender and sexual difference. A feminist phenomenology of illness experience, argues Fisher, will remind phenomenology of the sociocultural and political dimensions and structuring of lived experience, while pursuing the analyses through the lens of gender and sexual difference, not to mention other variables like race, class, and sexuality. With reference to interdisciplinary research focusing on the subjective "view from within" and also drawing on her own illness experience, Fisher argues that a phenomenological approach problematizes any simple distinction between a "view from within" and a "view from without" in accounting for the illness experience.

The next two chapters address a central topic in phenomenology and feminism alike, the relation between self and other, reexamining this relation in two different medical contexts, namely that of organ transplantation and of childbirths in hospitals. In "Visceral Phenomenology: Organ Transplantation, Identity, and Bioethics," Margrit Shildrick offers an alternative understanding of organ transplantation to the standard way in which it is practiced and reported within the biomedical sciences. In contrast to a biomedical emphasis on the notion of "spare part surgery" in which the graft is simply a utility exchangeable between bodies but having no existential status of its own, Shildrick explores experiences of recipients of heart transplants through a feminist-phenomenological analysis that undercuts any split between the psychic and the somatic and that lays the ground for an understanding of organ transfer as a procedure that involves the intimate interaction and connection between two embodied selves. Recognizing the fleshy materiality of the graft as a visceral component of the living self, she shows how questions concerning the significance of the transfer to the recipient can be addressed in new ways. Identity disruption and dysmorphia, for instance, can be taken as predictable and meaningful outcomes of the phenomenological experience rather than as individual failures to deal with the traumatic intervention into the body that transplantation entails at the clinical level. Shildrick contends that the intimations of an otherness within, experienced by organ recipients, must be integrated into a model of embodiment that goes beyond the emphasis on relationality and mutual constitution of self and other, found in phenomenology as well as mainstream feminist bioethics, and that recognizes the viscerality of concorporeal life, providing room for the hybridity of transplant recipients.

The intimate interactions and connections between embodied selves are investigated from a different perspective by Sarah LaChance Adams and Paul Burcher. In "Communal Pushing: Childbirth and Intersubjectivity," Adams and Burcher bring Merleau-Ponty's account of intersubjectivity into dialogue with the phenomenon of "communal pushing," which occurs when the people supporting a woman giving birth also start to push with her. They argue that "communal pushing" illustrates the reversibility between the reflective and pre-reflective body and how embodiment is both shared and particular. Although shared pushing is an example of anonymous intersubjectivity, Adams and Burcher also see it as an example of a connectedness that preserves differentiation of, for instance, gender. While men are equally able to push as women, women of all ages nevertheless seem to push more than men, suggesting a closer connectedness between similarly gendered bodies. According to Adams and Burcher men tend to hold themselves apart not because they cannot push, but because their bodies may not read the meaning of pushing as for them. That is, men learn that birthing is *other* to them. However, men *do* push and thereby transcend a culturally determined meaning for a more immediate body-to-body connection. Finally, Adams and Burcher discuss how some experienced practitioners utilize intercorporeality to facilitate the birth as an alternative to technological or verbal interventions. They influence or encourage group pushing in ways that are deliberately intended to change the laboring woman's pushing.

Keeping the focus on self-other relations, several of the contributions explicitly engage with critical analysis of culturally shared norms. Some of these norms are highly contested in feminist research, and this is the point of departure for Erik Malmqvist's phenomenological analysis of the phenomenon of complicity. In the chapter "Phenomenology, Cosmetic Surgery, and Complicity," Malmqvist suggests that the feminist project of criticizing unjust social norms tends to result in a certain sense of ambivalence when individuals comply with such norms, at once escaping the burden that they create and contributing to making that burden heavier on others. Focusing on cosmetic surgery and standards of feminine appearance, Malmqvist explores the ethics of complicity with unjust social norms through an engagement with Merleau-Ponty's phenomenology, which offers a fresh perspective on the problem at hand by allowing social norms to be understood as working on the embodied, prereflective level of human existence and coexistence. He contends that a person who escapes the suffering that an unjust social norm causes by accommodating to that norm may not be able to avoid responsibility for it, regardless of whether she appropriates the norm or not, as the expressive meaning of her choice is likely to lend the norm legitimacy. Far from blaming the victim, however, Malmqvist's account emphasizes that the perpetuation of unjust norms is fundamentally a shared ethical concern.

The analysis of how norms are reinforced, legitimized, and sometimes questioned, in various medical contexts, is pertinent also in the following four contributions. Focusing, in particular, on the intricate interconnections among what she calls the three Ns—the normal, the natural, and the normative—Gail Weiss argues in her essay "Uncosmetic Surgeries in an Age of Normativity" that, paradoxically, rapid *expansions* in medical technologies often function to reinforce and further entrench the *narrowness* of norms, thereby producing ever more restricted views of what counts as normal and natural. Furthermore, by collapsing the distinction between the real and the ideal, the growing number of "enhancement" surgeries available leads those individuals who refuse such "improvements" or those who actively seek to modify their bodies in nonnormative ways, to be regarded as not only *aesthetically deficient* but also *morally blameworthy*. Through a phenomenological method of description, Weiss aims to address taken-for-granted assumptions that underlie a contemporary "rhetoric of enhancement" and that reflect ideals of corporeal perfection permeating both medical and popular literature regarding cosmetic surgery as well as much analytic bioethical work on this topic. Weiss argues that when we grasp that normativity, normalization, and naturalization are closely intertwined, fundamentally interdependent temporal, spatial, and embodied processes, we can better assess their collective impact in shaping not only ethical but also medical, scientific, legal, economic, and religious conceptions of what it means to be human.

Nikki Sullivan's chapter "'BIID'? Queer (Dis)Orientations and the Phenomenology of 'Home'" also deals with the topic of nonnormative surgeries. Sullivan examines the increasing interest among medical professionals of various persuasions, philosophers, cultural

theorists, legal theorists, and others, in the desire for the amputation of healthy limbs—a desire said to stem from what is now often
referred to as Body Integrity Identity Disorder (BIID). She notes
an almost universal assumption in the existing literature that what
is being referred to as BIID is a (potentially) diagnosable illness that
resides in the psyche or the body of the afflicted individual, and
that this can be cured, or at least treated, by various medical interventions. In contrast to this focus on diagnostic classification and
treatment protocols, Sullivan is concerned with how particular categorizations work and what modes of corporeality and of dwelling
they (dis)enable. When so doing, she seeks to reorient debates about
the desire(s) for amputation, and other forms of "nonnormative"
embodiment, away from the question of integrity and toward a consideration of orientation. Turning to an understanding of orientation
rather than integrity, she brings to light how the source of suffering
for many so-called wannabes is not found in the bodies they want but
do not have but rather in a sense of living a life out of place or not
being at-home-in-the-world.

The concept of nonnormative embodiment can be understood
as implying embodiment that does not harmonize with culturally
shared norms about how bodies should be lived and how they should
look (even though we also need to consider whether this very concept contributes to further marginalization of these examples of
embodiment). In this sense, the contribution by Kristin Zeiler and
Lisa Guntram offers another angle on the issue of nonnormative
embodiment by examining young Swedish women's descriptions of
coming to know that they have no uterus and no vagina or a small
part of the vagina in their teens. In their chapter "Sexed Embodiment in Atypical Pubertal Development: Intersubjectivity, Excorporation, and the Importance of Making Space for Difference," Zeiler
and Guntram examine how different body parts become objects of
attention, are attributed value, or disappear in the women's descriptions of this realization. Via the phenomenological concept of incorporation and its reverse—excorporation—they further examine how
gendered patterns of behavior, including some culturally shared and
bodily expressed expectations and norms about female and male
bodies, can form embodied agency. Shifting focus to young women's
ways of handling the new bodily knowledge and their body-world
relations, after the initial shock has passed, Zeiler and Guntram also
discuss sexed embodiment as a style of being. Such conceptualization

of sexed embodiment, they argue, should preferably be combined with an analysis of asymmetrical relations that make some changes in one's style of being more difficult than others.

Continuing with the focus on sexed embodiment, Ellen Feder offers critical interrogation of normalizing surgical management of children born with ambiguous genitalia in her chapter "Reassigning Ambiguity: Intersex, Biomedicine, and the Question of Harm." The chapter aims at providing better understanding of the consequences of the ongoing focus (particularly in the USA) on relieving parental discomfort, specifically, the nature of the harm that results from the prevailing model of medical management. Feder proposes a framework for understanding the particular harm that normalizing genital surgery in infancy and early childhood may entail in phenomenological terms and notes that the harm she identifies is one not so easily conveyed by the accepted principles of bioethics as it occurs on the level of the so-called body schema. Engaging the narrative of "Jim," a young man who underwent sex reassignment and normalizing surgery as an infant, Feder offers insight into the lasting effects of early normalizing surgeries that remain part of the standard of care, revealing the material and symbolic harms that prevalent forms of evidence in this field inadequately capture. Attending to these harms, she concludes, speaks to the need in medicine for a moral framework that, resting on the relationality of lived embodiment, may provide better guidance for parents and physicians in caring for children with unusual anatomies.

Yet another angle on sexed embodiment is provided by Lanei Rodemeyer in her essay "Feminism, Phenomenology, and Hormones." Through an engagement with Edmund Husserl's now well-established conceptual distinction between *Körper* and *Leib* and a critical reading of psychologist John Money's famous case study of David Reimer, Rodemeyer addresses the question of what a feminism committed to constructionism should do about hormones. What should feminism do if scientific studies do not seem to support important and/or well-established feminist claims (or seem to oppose them)? How can feminist perspectives address scientific studies that show a link between prenatal hormone exposure and postnatal sexual or gender-related behavior? What should feminist perspectives that argue the forcefulness of social construction do about hormones? Rodemeyer suggests that a feminist phenomenology, drawing on Husserlian terminology, can provide a more nuanced description and explanation of embodied experiences. Allowing for various types of experience of the body, she argues, makes it possible for us to acknowledge—and to describe more fully—the experience of the transsexual, when everything in and on the body appears "normal"; or of the (surgically altered) intersex person who "knows" that something happened, other than what has been told to her; or of David Reimer, who knew that the assignment of female didn't belong to him and that further feminizing sexual surgery would be wrong.

In addition to concerns with cultural norms that run through most of the chapters in the volume, some contributions, as mentioned earlier, also focus on the experience of one's own body as other to oneself. This is the core concern in Fredrik Svenaeus' essay "The Body Uncanny: Alienation, Illness, and Anorexia Nervosa." Taking his point of departure in the phenomenological notion of the lived body, Svenaeus discusses different forms of bodily alienation in which one's own body is experienced as uncanny. He draws particular attention to the specific case of anorexia nervosa, which, he argues, clearly introduces the experience of the *body uncanny* while at the same time highlighting ways in which bodily alienation is connected to matters of identity and politics, issues that are either not present, or harder to discern, than in most cases of somatic illness. Svenaeus describes how alienation of the body in anorexia involves objectification in an everyday manner by the gaze of others in a social world. Finding herself in a cultural pattern of norms regarding femininity, health, beauty, and success, the anorexic turns the objectifying gaze of others into an escalating process of self-surveillance in which the image of her own body becomes gradually, increasingly unrealistic and self-punishing. A phenomenological analysis of the uncanniness of anorexic bodily self-experience, argues Svenaeus, has implications for how to treat anorexia beyond a medical model of surveillance and coercion.

Much feminist phenomenological work highlights the difficulties involved in any strict separation between bodily and sociocultural dimensions of human existence when interrogating lived experiences. The value of feminist phenomenological approaches that acknowledge bodily ambiguity in terms of the body always being subject and object, and always material-sociocultural, is given close attention in Jenny Slatman and Gili Yaron's chapter "Toward a Phenomenology of Disfigurement." Turning specifically to facial disfigurements, Slatman and Yaron aim to develop a phenomenological, empirically informed, approach to bodily disfigurement. Their claim is that this approach, which includes the analysis of an individual's embodied self-experience against her or his social-cultural lifeworld, bridges the gap between the realm of the individual and the social. Addressing the double body ontology that is at stake in facial disfigurement, Slatman and Yaron discuss the case of Leah, a facially disfigured woman wearing a facial prosthesis. Leah's story, they argue, not only illustrates the body's double-sided ontology, but also reveals that it is by no means a given, static condition. Slatman and Yaron demonstrate how Leah does not endure her disfigurement passively: coping with her condition means that she develops various ways of "doing" her body anew, which operate both on her body as image and on her body as lived through the condition of appearance. The case of Leah, they contend, illustrates that the impact of disfigurement can only be adequately assessed if we take into account the body's ambiguous ontology.

The three final essays of the volume examine issues of agency and passivity in thought-provoking ways. In the chapter entitled "'She's Research!' Exposure, Epistemophilia, and Ethical Perception through Mike Nichols' *Wit*," Lisa Folkmarson Käll considers the conditions and possibility of ethical perception in relation to the practices of scientific medicine. Through a reading of Mike Nichols' film *Wit*, which is a striking display of the objectification of a human body for scientific purposes, Käll discusses how different forms of exposure lay bare possibilities and limitations of self-objectification and of objectifying frameworks more generally. She argues that the ground for our object-related intentionality and our distancing relation to the world as an object world, as well as to our bodies as objects detached from our minds, is to be found in an original foundational attachment to the world as embodied exposure and openness to experience. Käll identifies this attachment as the site for an ethical relation that is not one of strict separation between autonomous subjects but instead characterized by openness, dependence, and unpredictability. Such an understanding further brings to light the possibility of ethical perception as emerging from the experience of exposure and vulnerability rather than from well-informed deliberation and decision-making. Käll discusses the possibility of moving toward an ethics of exposure on the basis of the display in *Wit* of the failure of ethical perception within the highly controlled clinical research setting of medical science.

The very meaning of passivity is at stake in Cressida Heyes' essay "Anaesthetics of Existence." Heyes turns her attention to the story of cosmetic surgery devotee Lolo Ferrari who claimed to love the oblivion of general anaesthesia and its capacity to suspend her life, allowing her to wake up transformed without any further exercise of agency. Given our culture's emphasis on maintaining sovereignty over one's life and over the territory of one's body, and the importance of these ideas to feminism, Heyes asks whether Ferrari can be seen as anything other than a passive victim? Asking for the feminist meanings of anaesthesia, where the literal meets the metaphorical, she argues that the lived experience of the loss of sensibility may have a political importance in modulating demands for a perpetually self-creating individual. She also examines how the sovereign subject of late liberal capitalism is required to exercise autonomy iteratively, expressing individuality qua capacity to choose in an interminable series of self-determining moments. "Anaesthetic existence" offers a counterpoint to the exhausting and painful experience of willful self-creation, Heyes suggests—and an analysis of the lived experience of anaesthesia as exemplified by Lolo Ferrari's descriptions can capture a pervasive, if often despairing, form of resistance to a masculinist insistence on the centrality of the self-making agent.

The final essay of the volume addresses the experience of depression and the possibilities of agency within the midst of the passivity of depression. In her essay "Wandering in the Unhomelike: Chronic Depression, Inequality, and the Recovery Imperative," Abby Wilkerson brings a phenomenological approach to depression into dialogue with feminist disability studies in order to highlight how the burdens of the recovery imperative that dominate discourse on depression interact with gender and other vectors of oppression. The recovery imperative, she argues, implies a particularly heavy burden for members of oppressed groups, who face depressogenic social transactions regularly. According to Wilkerson, oppressed people are not only more vulnerable to depression; if they do become depressed, the ongoing nature of such transactions imposes obstacles to recovery. While arguing that a phenomenological framework offers significant advantages for illuminating possibilities for agency, she also notes that concepts of pathology and normalcy are central in the medicalization and life experience of depression. These concepts require further scrutiny than has yet emerged in phenomenology. Closer attention to social contexts can advance ongoing efforts to critique the medicalization of affect and the normalizing functions of these processes—while providing a more detailed account of the majority of cases of depression. Wilkerson's chapter elaborates a framework that offers ways to recognize and legitimate the suffering of depression, points toward paths for relieving it without reifying conservative notions of pathology, and generates critique toward social change.

By bringing together sophisticated phenomenological insights with concrete human conditions, the essays in this volume demonstrate the depth and richness feminist phenomenological perspectives can offer in relation to medicine. Through careful analysis of experience and its conditions, they uncover taken-for-granted and in this sense "hidden" assumptions, beliefs, and norms that we live by, that we strengthen by repeated action, and that we can sometimes question and radically alter. It is our hope that the collection will contribute to continued interrogation of what feminist phenomenological work in relation to and within the field of medicine might entail and provoke further questions concerning the conditions of normative frameworks and structures of experience.

Acknowledgments

This volume was initiated within the collaborative framework of the research network Humanities Forum: Gender and Health, financed by Riksbankens Jubileumsfond and Linköping University, and the Body/Embodiment Research group in the GenNa Program at the Center for Gender Research, Uppsala University. The contributions within the volume were presented and discussed at the conference Feminist Phenomenology and Medicine in May 2011. We would like to thank all the speakers and participants at the conference for contributing to making it such a successful event. We are also most grateful to Riksbankens Jubileumsfond, the Swedish Council for Working Life and Social Research, the Swedish Research Council, Linköping University, and Uppsala University for the financial support that made this three-day conference possible. Finally, we owe gratitude to Andrew Kenyon and Diane Ganeles at State University of New York Press.

Notes

1. Such studies can be influenced by a phenomenological emphasis on subjective experience and meaning-making and contribute to

the understanding of such meaning-making but are commonly removed from the conceptual framework and method of phenomenological philosophy.

2. "Better," here, does most often *not* mean a search for criteria for a morally just action but, as put by Sarah Ahmed (2000, 139–140), that some ways better "may allow the other to exist beyond the grasp of the present" and enable the protection of "the otherness of the other."

References

Ahmed, Sarah. 2006. *Queer Phenomenology: Orientations, Objects, Others.* Durham, NC: Duke University Press.

Ahmed, Sarah. 2007. "A Phenomenology of Whiteness." *Feminist Theory* 8: 149–168.

Alcoff, Linda Martín. 1999. "Towards a Phenomenology of Racial Embodiment." *Radical Philosophy* 95: 15–24.

Alcoff, Linda Martín. 2000. "Phenomenology, Post-Structuralism and Feminist Theory on the Concept of Experience." In *Feminist Phenomenology*, edited by Linda Fisher and Lester Embree, 39–56. Dordrecht: Kluwer.

Al-Saji, Alia. 2010. "Bodies and Sensings: On the Uses of Husserlian Phenomenology for Feminist Theory." *Continental Philosophy Review* 43: 13–37.

Arp, Kristana. 1995. "Beauvoir's Concept of Bodily Alienation." In *Feminist Interpretations of Simone de Beauvoir*, edited by Margaret A. Simons, 161–177. University Park: The Pennsylvania State University Press.

Beauvoir, Simone de. 1985. *A Very Easy Death.* New York: Pantheon Books/Random House.

Beauvoir, Simone de. 2010. *The Second Sex*, translated by Constance Borde and Sheila Malovany-Chevalier. New York: Alfred A. Knopf.

Bengtsson, Jan, Kristin Heggen, and Gunn Engelsrud (eds). 2004. "Livsvärldsfenomenologi och vårdforskning" [Life-world Phenomenology and Health Research]. Special issue of *Norsk Tidsskrift for Sykepleieforskning* [Norwegian Journal of Nursing Research] 6 (3): 3–6.

Bigwood, Carol. 1991. "Renaturalizing the Body (with the Help of Merleau-Ponty)." *Hypatia* 6 (3): 54–73.

Bullington, Jennifer. 2009. "Embodiment and Chronic Pain: Implications for Rehabilitation Practice." *Health Care Analysis* 17 (2): 100–119.

Butler, Judith. 1988. "Performative Acts and Gender Constitution: An Essay in Phenomenology and Feminist Theory." *Theatre Journal* 40 (4): 519–531.

Butler, Judith. 1989. "Sexual Ideology and Phenomenological Description: A Feminist Critique of Merleau-Ponty's *Phenomenology of Perception*." In *The Thinking Muse: Feminism and Modern French Philosophy*, edited by Jeffner Allen and Iris Marion Young, 85–100. Bloomington: Indiana University Press.

Buytendijk, F. J. J. 1973. *Pain*, translated by Eda O'Shiel. Westport, CT: Greenwood Press.

Cadwallader, Jessica Robyn. 2010. "Archiving Gifts." *Australian Feminist Studies* 25: 121–132.

Carel, Havi. 2008. *Illness*. Stocksfield: Acumen.

Dekkers, Wim. 2011. "Dwelling, House and Home: Towards a Home-Led Perspective on Dementia Care." *Medicine, Health Care and Philosophy* 14 (3): 291–300.

Diprose, Rosalyn. 2002. *Corporeal Generosity*. Albany: State University of New York Press.

Diprose, Rosalyn. 2005. "A 'Genethics' That Makes Sense: Take Two." In *Ethics of the Body: Postconventional Challenges*, edited by Margrit Shildrick and Roxanne Mykitiuk, 237–258. Cambridge, MA: MIT Press.

Engelsrud, Gunn. 2005. "The Lived Body as Experience and Perspective: Methodological Challenges." *Qualitative Research* 5 (3): 267–284.

Finlay, Linda. 2003. "The Intertwining of Body, Self and World: A Phenomenological Study of Living with Recently Diagnosed Multiple Sclerosis." *Journal of Phenomenological Psychology* 34 (2): 157–178.

Fisher, Linda. 2000. "Phenomenology and Feminism: Perspectives on Their Relation." In *Feminist Phenomenology*, edited by Linda Fisher and Lester Embree, 17–38. Dordrecht: Kluwer.

Fuchs, Thomas, 2002. "The Challenge of Neuroscience: Psychiatry and Phenomenology Today." *Psychopathology* 35 (6): 319–226.

Fuchs, Thomas. 2003. "The Phenomenology of Shame, Guilt and the Body in Body Dysmorphic Disorder and Depression." *Journal of Phenomenological Psychology* 33 (2): 223–243.

Heinämaa, Sara. 2003. *Towards a Phenomenology of Sexual Difference.* Lanham: Rowman and Littlefield.

Heinämaa, Sara. 2010. "Phenomenologies of Mortality and Generativity." In *Birth, Death, and Femininity: Philosophies of Embodiment,* edited by Robin May Schott, 73–156. Bloomington: Indiana University Press.

Heinämaa, Sara. 2012. "Beauvoir and Husserl: An Unorthodox Approach to *The Second Sex.*" In *Beauvoir and Western Thought from Plato to Butler,* edited by Shannon M. Mussett and William S. Wilkerson. Albany: State University of New York Press.

Heinämaa, Sara, and Lanei Rodemeyer. 2010. "Introduction." *Continental Philosophy Review* 43: 1–11.

Käll, Lisa Folkmarson. 2009a. "A Being of Two Leaves: On the Founding Significance of the Lived Body." In *Body Claims,* edited by Janne Bromseth, Lisa Folkmarson Käll, and Katarina Mattsson, 110–133. Uppsala: Uppsala University.

Käll, Lisa Folkmarson. 2009b. "'. . . looking at myself as in a movie . . .' Reflections on Normative and Pathological Self-Objectification." In *Normality/Normativity,* edited by Lisa Folkmarson Käll, 225–250. Uppsala: Uppsala University.

Käll, Lisa Folkmarson. 2010. "Fashioned in Nakedness, Sculptured and Caused to Be Born: Bodies in Light of the Sartrean Gaze." *Continental Philosophy Review* 43 (1): 61–81.

Käll, Lisa Folkmarson. 2013. "Intercorporeality and the Shareability of Pain." In *Dimensions of Pain: Humanities and Social Science Perspectives,* edited by Lisa Folkmarson Käll, 27–40. London and New York: Routledge.

Leder, Drew. 1990. *The Absent Body.* Chicago: University of Chicago Press.

Leder, Drew. 1999. "Whose Body? What Body? The Metaphysics of Organ Transplantation." In *Persons and Their Bodies: Rights, Responsibilities, Relationships,* edited by Mark J. Cherry, 233–264. Dordrecht: Kluwer.

Lundquist, Caroline. 2008. "Being Torn: Toward a Phenomenology of Unwanted Pregnancy." *Hypatia* 23 (3): 136–155.

Malmqvist, Erik. 2008. *Good Parents, Better Babies: An Argument about Reproductive Technologies, Enhancement and Ethics.* Dissertation. Linköping: Linköping University.

Malmqvist, Erik, and Kristin Zeiler. 2010. "Cultural Norms, the

Phenomenology of Incorporation and the Experience of Having a Child Born with Ambiguous Sex." *Social Theory and Practice* 36 (1): 157–164.

Matthews, Eric. 2006. Dementia and the Identity of the Person. In *Dementia: Mind, Meaning and the Person*, edited by Julian C. Hughes, Stephen J. Louw and Steven R. Sabat, 163–178. Oxford and New York: Oxford University Press.

Nortvedt, Per. 2008. "Sensibility and Clinical Understanding." *Medicine, Health Care and Philosophy* 11: 209–219.

Oksala, Johanna. 2004. "What Is Feminist Phenomenology? Thinking Birth Philosophically." *Radical Philosophy* 126: 16–22.

Oksala, Johanna. 2006. "A Phenomenology of Gender." *Continental Philosophy Review* 39: 229–244.

Parnas, Josef. 2003. "Self and Schizophrenia: A Phenomenological Perspective." In *The Self in Neuroscience and Psychiatry*, edited Tilo Kircher and Anthony David, 217–241. Cambridge: Cambridge University Press.

Parnas, Josef, Louis Sass, and Dan Zahavi. 2011. "Phenomenology and Psychopathology." *Philosophy, Psychiatry & Psychology* 18 (1): 37–39.

Pellegrino, Thomasma. 2004. "Philosophy of Medicine and Medical Ethics: A Phenomenological Perspective." In *Handbook of Bioethics*, edited by George Khushf, 183–202. Dordrecht, Boston, London: Kluwer.

Perpich, Diane. 2010. "Vulnerability and the Ethics of Facial Tissue Transplantation." *Journal of Bioethical Inquiry* 7 (2): 173–185.

Ratcliffe, Matthew. 2008. *Feelings of Being: Phenomenology, Psychiatry and the Sense of Reality*. Oxford: Oxford University Press.

Ratcliffe, Matthew. 2011. "Phenomenology Is Not a Servant of Science." *Philosophy, Psychiatry & Psychology* 18(1): 33–36.

Sass, Louis, and Josef Parnas. 2001. "Phenomenology of Self-Disturbances in Schizophrenia: Some Research Findings and Directions." *Philosophy, Psychiatry & Psychology* 8 (4): 347–356.

Sass, Louis, Josef Parnas, and Dan Zahavi. 2011. "Phenomenological Psychopathology and Schizophrenia: Contemporary Approaches and Misunderstandings." *Philosophy, Psychiatry & Psychology* 18 (1): 1–23.

Schües, Christina. 1997. "The Birth of Difference." *Human Studies* 20 (2): 243–252.

Scully, Jackie Leach. 2003. "Drawing lines, crossing lines: ethics and the challenge of disabled embodiment." *Feminist Theology* 11 (3): 265–280.

Shildrick, Margrit. 1999. "The Body Which Is Not One: Dealing with Difference." *Body & Society* 5: 77–92.

Shildrick, Margrit. 2008. "The Critical Turn in Feminist Bioethics: The Case of Heart Transplantation." *International Journal of Feminist Approaches to Bioethics* 1 (1): 28–47.

Slatman, Jenny. 2009. "A Strange Hand: On Self-Recognition and Recognition of Another." *Phenomenology and the Cognitive Sciences* 8 (3): 321–342.

Stanghellini, Giovanni. 2011. "Clinical Phenomenology: A Method for Care?" *Philosophy, Psychiatry & Psychology* 18 (1): 25–29.

Svenaeus, Fredrik. 2001. *The Hermeneutics of Medicine and the Phenomenology of Health: Steps towards a Philosophy of Medical Practice.* Dordrecht: Kluwer.

Svenaeus, Fredrik. 2007. "A Heideggerian Defence of Therapeutic Cloning." *Theoretical Medicine and Bioethics* 28 (1): 31–62.

Svenaeus, Fredrik. 2009. "The Phenomenology of Falling Ill: An Explication, Critique and Improvement of Sartre's Theory of Embodiment and Alienation." *Human Studies* 32 (1): 53–66.

Svenaeus, Fredrik. 2012. "The Phenomenology of Organ Transplantation: How Does the Malfunction and Change of Organs Have Effects on Personal Identity?" In *The Body as Gift, Resource and Commodity: Exchanging Organ, Tissues and Cells in the 21st Century*, edited by Martin Gunnarson and Fredrik Svenaeus, 58–79. Stockholm: Södertörn University College.

Toombs, S. Kay. 1993. *The Meaning of Illness: A Phenomenological Account of the Different Perspectives of Physician and Patient.* Dordrecht: Kluwer.

Toombs, S. Kay (ed.). 2001. *Handbook of Phenomenology and Medicine.* Dordrecht: Kluwer.

Weiss, Gail. 1999. *Body Images: Embodiment as Intercorporeality.* London: Routledge.

Weiss, Gail. 2006. "Death and the Other: Rethinking Authenticity." In *The Voice of Breast Cancer in Medicine and Bioethics*, edited by Mary C. Rawlinson and Shannon Lundeen, 103–116. Dordrecht: Springer.

Weiss, Gail. 2009. "Intertwined Identities: Challenges to Bodily Autonomy." In *The Body Within: Art, Medicine, and Visualization*, edited by Renée Van de Vall and Robert Zwijnenberg, 173–186. Leiden, the Netherlands: Brill Academic.

Young, Iris Marion. 2005. *On Female Body Experience: "Throwing Like a Girl" and Other Essays*. Oxford: Oxford University Press.

Zaner, Richard. 1981. *The Context of Self: A Phenomenological Inquiry Using Medicine as a Clue*. Athens: Ohio University Press.

Zaner, Richard. 1994. "Phenomenology and the Clinical Event." *Phenomenology of the Cultural Disciplines' Contributions to Phenomenology*, edited by Mano Daniel and Lester Embree, 39–66. Dordrecht: Kluwer.

Zeiler, Kristin. 2013a. "A Phenomenology of Excorporation, Bodily Alienation and Resistance: Rethinking Sexed and Racialised Embodiment." *Hypatia: A Journal of Feminist Philosophy* 28 (1): 69–84.

Zeiler, K. 2013b. "A Philosophical Defense of the Idea that We Can Hold Each Other in Personhood: Intercorporeal Personhood in Dementia Care." *Medicine, Health Care and Philosophy*. Early Online view.

Zeiler, Kristin, and Anette Wickström. 2009. "Why Do 'We' Perform Surgery on Newborn Intersexed Children? The Phenomenology of the Parental Experience of Having a Child with Intersex Anatomies." *Feminist Theory* 10 (3): 355–374.

2

THE ILLNESS EXPERIENCE

A Feminist Phenomenological Perspective

LINDA FISHER

R esearch and writing on the illness experience has been growing at a rapid rate over the last several decades. While the traditional orientation to illness reflected an emphasis on the objective
biomedical elements, researchers began distinguishing between the
biomedical condition as a disease-state and the subjective experience of illness.[1] In signaling the experiential and ontological dimensions of illness, studies of the illness experience have thus focused
on the experience and meanings of illness from a lived, subjective
perspective.

Much, if not most, of this research, especially earlier studies, has
come from the social sciences, where crucial analyses include the
impact of illness on interpersonal relations and sociality, as well as
issues related to sociopolitical and institutional structures. Other studies examine issues of subjectivity and identity in illness and how individuals express and represent their experience of illness in personal
accounts or "illness narratives." While not disputing the merit of these
studies, and indeed acknowledging their significant contribution, I
wish to argue for the importance and necessity of a phenomenological approach to the illness experience.

As the descriptive analysis of the nature, structures, and meanings
of lived experience, phenomenology is particularly well suited to an

investigation of the illness experience. Phenomenological analysis can access and capture an experiential immediacy and subjective perspective missing in studies focused primarily on sociocultural constructions and discourses of illness and the illness experience, while providing an analytical and systematic framework often lacking in personal or narrative renditions of the illness experience: the capacity to move from the singularity of the standard first-person narrative to an account that seeks to identify, describe, and analyze generalities and typical features of the experience as such, while examining how this experience resides within and intersects with the broader lifeworld. As such, a phenomenological approach affords particular tools and strategies for the task of grasping and understanding the nature and the experience of illness and of being ill.

Correspondingly, a feminist perspective in the form of a feminist phenomenology can be equally valuable and important in disclosing the ways in which our lived experience is inflected by gender and sexual difference. To the extent that lived experience, including many illness experiences, are highly conditioned by gender, among other variables—are manifestly always already gendered on the existential and empirical level—then addressing the illness experience from a feminist and gendered perspective is clearly indicated. At the same time, the feminist perspective underscores the sense in which the lifeworld is also an eminently social and political lifeworld, and it is the intrinsic attunement and vested engagement to issues connected to this lifeworld that feminism also brings to phenomenology as feminist phenomenology. This attunement and commitment to the lived sociopolitical and existential context as feminist phenomenology informs and provides the horizon for what follows.[2]

Having thus indicated what phenomenology can bring to discussions of the illness experience and what feminism brings to phenomenology, I want to circle back to the wider discourse on the illness experience. I am a strong advocate of both a return to the "doing" of phenomenology, in addition to the (often overemphasized) historical scholarship, as well as incorporating relevant empirical research into phenomenological analyses: in both senses this is ground-level phenomenology. A phenomenology of illness experience makes the importance of such orientations especially apparent. As such, I take a phenomenology of illness experience to necessarily entail incorporating source material from medical and social science research, along with personal accounts and illness narratives. And a feminist phenomenology of illness experience reminds phenomenology of the sociocultural and political dimensions and structuring of lived experience, while pursuing the analyses through the lens of gender and sexual difference, along with other modalities like race, class, sexuality, and disability/ability. This is not to suggest that feminism is alone in emphasizing the significance of these dimensions and their various intersections; but it has played an unmistakable and pivotal role in situating them in the center of contemporary discourse. Once again, it is these existential and sociopolitical commitments that feminism can reinforce and unfold within feminist phenomenology.

I begin by discussing illness and health and the illness experience, with some reference to the social science research. In looking at the emphasis in accounts of illness experience on the subjective perspective, I interweave observations about "the view from within" and "the view from without." I then proceed to a discussion of phenomenology and illness experience, starting with an analysis of how "the view from within" and "the view from without" are problematized in a phenomenological approach and then moving to some reflections about the framing of illness experience in phenomenological and feminist phenomenological perspectives.

Illness and the Illness Experience

Illness v. Health

In the everyday sense, illness is seen broadly as a situation of disrupted or compromised good health. This does not necessarily mean any state of less than total well-being—since at any given time no one is in such an idealized state—but nevertheless a state in which there has been some marked interruption or disruption of well-being due to a specific factor or set of conditions, be they physiological, psychological, cognitive, or some combination of these.[3] As such, illness tends to be defined in juxtaposition not just to health but to the sense of "good health" already implied by "health," if not to an imagined ideal health. In the *OED* definition of "illness," along with synonyms or alternate terms such as disease, ailment, and sickness, and a somewhat circular definition of illness as "the condition of being ill," the definition also states, indeed, leads off with the following: "bad or unhealthy condition of the body." In fact, this is the third entry, the first two being obsolete meanings:

1. Bad moral quality, condition, or character; wickedness, depravity; evil conduct; badness;
2. Unpleasantness, disagreeableness; troublesomeness; hurtfulness, noxiousness; badness.[4]

Thus we see the framing of illness as not just the compromising but the negation of health, along with an unequivocal moral valorization, made even more explicit in the obsolete meanings, where it is extended to encompass moral character and conduct and a host of highly undesirable traits.[5]

Negative attitudes about illness are understandable, of course, and I do not wish to argue that illness is a good thing; although, as some have pointed out, there are aspects of illness and the illness experience that can be seen in a more positive way, such as the possibility of gaining new or enhanced perspectives on one's life and experiences, on values and priorities. Moreover, a distinction can be made between "bad" and "negative," especially as regards the social intersubjective world. Here is where the difference between the "view from within" and the "view from without" first comes into play. A situation that is not good—that is, conventionally considered bad and unwanted—can be construed very differently depending on the epistemic location, whether the experiential horizon of the person living in or outside the immediacy of the experience. While the person living this experience of illness will doubtless consider it less than good, undesirable, even bad, the outsider perspective can be more judgmental, seeing it in prevailingly negative terms, the negativity rippling outward from the initial syndrome or biomedical event to the general situation and possibly even including the afflicted individual herself or himself. Perhaps some of these readings of illness are officially obsolete, but many of the negative and discriminatory attributions still persist nonetheless, including implicit or explicit associations of illness with some kind of character flaw or moral failing. Early attitudes toward HIV/AIDS are a salient example of this, but there are many instances—the smoker who develops respiratory problems, the overweight person with heart disease—where the ill person is seen as not only responsible but morally blameworthy for their illness, the illness seen as their fault, even as deserved.[6] However, even in the absence of such attributions of responsibility and blame, there is still frequently an overriding moral negativity and anxiety about illness, a negativity and anxiety, once again, that can extend to the ill person herself, even if unwittingly.

Whether such negative social framings of illness are latent or on the surface, whether mild or strong, they serve to constitute illness and the ill person as Other. Illness is the deviation from health, the Other to health, and as with numerous other cultural and historical examples of constituted deviance, difference, and otherness, it serves the normative function of designating what counts as normality and the desirable status quo. In this manner, health is defined in opposition to illness, as the absence of or resistance to this ever-threatening Other, the negative foregrounding and delineating the positive.

We began by defining illness in juxtaposition to health, as the negation of health or as nonhealth, to come full circle to the framing of health in opposition to illness, as a relative absence of illness; but this is an absence manifested not negatively, as a diremption, but (ironically) as a positive wholeness: the state of being healthy. I am not suggesting here that health and illness can be generally strictly defined in a binary or either/or manner; the boundaries between them are not so precisely demarcated and their own definitions not so delimited. Rather, they coexist and intersect in a complex and interconnected relation within an embodied and situated experiential continuum. However, I do wish to underscore the extent to which conventional and popular conceptions of health and illness are often framed in positive/negative terms, and that this has profound consequences for the lived illness experience. As such, these mutual characterizations of illness and health can be seen as intertwined and dialectical, with considerable social and cultural significations embedded within these characterizations.

Illness/Disease

If we move from these generalized cultural construals of illness to more specialized and scholarly analyses, interpretations of illness are obviously less malignant and more formalized. While many, even within medicine, might have used the terms "disease" and "illness" interchangeably (mirroring the dictionary rendering as synonyms), over the last several decades it has become increasingly common to differentiate between disease and illness both within medicine and medical humanities and social science scholarship. Discussions and debates in these fields about the distinctions between health, illness, and disease are lively and ongoing, and I will not rehearse them here. However, a key distinction, now widely accepted and implemented, is that between disease and illness as objective and subjective states respectively. While the traditional emphasis in medicine was on the objective biomedical components of the disease/illness state, critiques of the one-sided approach of biomedicine, and an increased aware-ness of the importance of subjective elements of illness/disease led to distinguishing between the disease-state and the subjective expe-rience: disease is the biomedical condition, and illness is the lived experience of that condition in all its varied aspects. As such, we *have* a disease, but we *are* ill, signaling the experiential, ontological, and situational dimensions of illness.

At the same time, just as with health and illness, disease and ill-ness do not simply coexist as the two sides of a given biomedical phenomenon. As Patricia Benner states, "Illness and disease do not exist in a one-to-one relationship. One can be cured of one's disease and still experience illness or, alternatively, disease can be silent with no illness experience" (Benner 2001, 353). For example, David Jen-nings points out that "one can be seriously diseased without being ill, [as] with silent hypertension" (Jennings 1986, 866). Another variable are cases of "health within illness" (Lindsey 1996) where even with pronounced disease-states the individual may feel, and be, otherwise healthy, thus resisting the traditional "sick role" while complicating the division between health and disease. People living with motor neuron disease (aka amyotrophic lateral sclerosis), for instance, often report that they can feel quite well, and aside from the disease they are dealing with, they consider themselves to be generally healthy. To be sure, while the body has certainly experienced various clear effects of the disease, most notably loss of muscle mass and strength and motor function, and there are significant ramifications of this, yet there can be an absence of the symptoms and manifestations ordinar-ily associated with being "sick," and in fact this individual can other-wise be quite healthy.[7] Indeed, this is why some people with MND consider it more a disability than an illness per se.[8] At the same time, such cases do not preclude an illness experience as such. Rather, the scope of such an experiential horizon encompasses disease, "illness," and many disability experiences. At the same time the illness experience extends beyond the experienced biomedical condition and even beyond the localized first-person subjective experience of that condition, as I discuss further below.

Toward the Illness Experience

There is a daunting amount of material pertaining to the illness experience, ranging from medical and humanities/social science research to a myriad of personal accounts and illness narratives, autobiographies and illness memoirs, both academic and nonacademic, not to mention countless internet resources such as personal websites, online newspaper columns and features, blogs, and patient forums; these latter and other nonacademic accounts often serving as important source material for the research. Discussing the rise of autobiographical literature chronicling experiences of illness and disability, Kristin Lindgren observes that

> Its current proliferation and popularity can be attributed to several factors, including the rise of the literary memoir, the growing interest in previously marginalized voices, and the culturally sanctioned questioning of medical authority. Narratives of illness and disability are also, perhaps above all, products of a cultural moment in which talk of bodies and selves saturates both academic and popular discourse. (Lindgren 2004, 146)[9]

By the same token, clearly illness experience discourse and research has been active and growing for some time. In her comprehensive survey of illness experience research, Janine Pierret tracks the emergence of this research from the 1960s and 1970s when social scientists were working from Talcott Parsons' concepts of illness and the sick role, to studies of illness behavior in the 1980s that also factored in social and demographic variables, along with aspects such as stress and coping. Alongside these developments were case studies dating from the early 1960s of "how people lived with and made sense of conditions such as tuberculosis, polio, visible disabilities and dying" (Pierret 2003, 6).

Another important development in illness experience discourse and research are the aforementioned illness narratives.[10] Comprising both actual illness narratives and studies and analyses of the nature of narrative and of illness narratives specifically, illness narratives explore the capacity of narrative to both illuminate and address a situation of illness. Along with being a means of expressing and communicating an experience of illness, the illness narrative also discloses and brings to the fore salient features and meanings of illness experience, which has significance for both academic investigations and clinical practice. In addition, to the extent that illness is often characterized as life interruption or "biographical disruption" (Bury 1982), compromising not just body or mind but also the sense of self and identity, illness narratives are also seen as an important coping and rebuilding strategy, the act of expression and storytelling serving the function of helping to make sense of the experience, to reorder one's existence, and to repair and reconstruct one's identity and sense of self.

What these various materials and approaches have in common is a shift in focus to the subjective experiential perspective: looking at individuals' meanings and representations of their illness, the lived experience and subjectivity of the ill person, the immediacy and force of the first-person voice and perspective in illness accounts, and the implications for intersubjective relations and interactions with the broader social structure within illness experience. Prevalent themes include an altered and/or intensified awareness of the body; a changed relation to the body, often instilling a sense of distance between or separation of body and mind or self and body; the body experienced as alienated from or as other to the self; within the self, a sense of disrupted, destabilized, or embattled identity, a dramatically altered self (old self vs. new self) or loss of self, or tensions between private self and public social identity; and experiences of shame or stigma, exclusion and social isolation, or alternately enhanced and deepened relationships but generally transformed relations with others and with the social world.

Exploring such themes thus entails an intermingled process of examining the subjective experience of the individual in illness— that is, situating the investigation in the subjective field—while both attending to and incorporating the voices of illness in order to accurately represent and elucidate the themes of body, self, and world in illness experience and to ground the investigation in the first-person and subjective experiential perspective. Such a scientific and discursive (re-)orienting serves not only the obvious purpose of illuminating such subjective experience and dimensions but also has clear implications for biomedical research and practice: in highlighting and thematizing the subjective experience of the patient in illness, the "other side" of the biomedical situation is given its place and, hopefully, due consideration. Not that this displaces or even necessarily disturbs an emphasis on the objective biomedical condition in some contexts; but it makes it one part of the overall situation rather than the only part and sole focus. This balancing, or at least supplementing, has important applications, for example, in clinical practice, in the clinical experience, and in interactions between patients and medical professionals. Indeed, in terms of the overall situation of this experiential horizon, we see that the biomedical condition and the subjective experience are also not a binary but, from the perspective of lived embodiment, are two aspects of an intertwined and mutually conditioning phenomenon, which for the purposes of analysis can be distinguished in terms of biomedical disease and illness experience: the objective condition of the subject and the subjective situation occasioned by the condition.

All these benefits and consequences of recognizing and listening to subjective experience in discussions of illness, not to mention the inherent epistemic worth, and even morality and activism, of giving voice to those living a given experience, make the significance of attending to the view from within self-evident. But while the epistemic and phenomenological benefits furnished by the view-from-within perspective may be obvious, considering the effects of some view-from-without accounts and perspectives provides additional support. I turn now to some examples in order to demonstrate that such perspectives, particularly if dominant, can lead to misplaced and potentially even harmful conceptions of an illness experience.

The View from Without: Some Examples from ALS

Motor neuron disease, also known as amyotrophic lateral sclerosis, or ALS (known additionally as Lou Gehrig's Disease), is a progressive degenerative neuromuscular disease. It occurs when the upper and lower motor neurons in the brain and spinal cord are compromised, for some reason, and degenerate. As motor nerve cells begin to die, voluntary muscles are affected, weakening and atrophying, resulting eventually in the loss of muscle control and function in muscles needed to move, speak, eat, and breathe. Worldwide the incidence of ALS is one to three people per 100,000. The cause is unknown, there is no effective treatment let alone a cure. The prognosis is not good: 80 percent of people with ALS die within two to five years of diagnosis, some die even sooner, while approximately 10 percent can survive ten years or longer.

Despite the difficulties of this condition, and the sobering prognosis, however, studies have found that many people living with ALS report a comparatively positive quality of life. Losing muscle functionality, while certainly limiting and frustrating, can be managed and adapted to in the absence of an imminent life-threatening event. There are certainly some individuals who have greater difficulty coming to terms with their condition, manifesting more morose and fatalistic attitudes—my informal and unscientific survey of blogs and ALS forums suggests that these attitudes seem to be somewhat more prevalent among men with ALS than women, but this could also be due to the fact that a greater percentage of men acquire ALS than do women. However, there have not been significant studies of gendered attitudes and behavior with ALS, and I think this would be an important analysis to pursue. At the same time, many ALS memoirs and narratives do in fact reflect a more positive outlook, with themes of hope, coping, and adaptation, and a sense of getting on with life despite significant challenges. This is borne out also by scholarly studies. Nevertheless, such a situation is often exceedingly difficult for many outsiders to fathom, when the prospect of life with a wheelchair is commonly seen as unbearable, not to mention all the other aspects and syndromes, present and future, entailed by ALS. In popular and media accounts the ALS experience is invariably framed as a tragi-heroic narrative—a framing common to representations of illness and disability generally—but even in the case of a largely upbeat heroic account, the narrative still has the element of tragedy, frequently accompanied by a dash of poignancy—the touching hopefulness of the patient in what we know to be a hopeless situation. There are also dramatic and iconic paradoxes: starting with Lou Gehrig, the star athlete, announcing his retirement from baseball at the height of his career due to a disease that will take his name, and extending to Stephen Hawking, the brilliant scientist who cannot move or speak, that brain trapped in *that* body, with all the ironic necessity of being a theoretical physicist.

Such framings are well illustrated by an episode Albert Robillard recounts in his book *Meaning of a Disability: The Lived Experience of Paralysis* (Robillard 1999). Robillard is a faculty member in the Department of Sociology at the University of Hawaii at Manoa and is living with ALS. When his university's press office wanted to do a story on him, he told the reporter that he did not want something on the order of "look at what happened to Britt and his poor family." Nevertheless, the story was firmly situated in the tragi-heroic narrative. Since 1989, the story stated, "he has had virtually no muscle control, causing him to slump in his wheelchair. He cannot move his hands, arms or fingers." Continuing, Robillard writes, "There followed a litany of what I cannot do, eat, drink, and speak. Then the story shifted to how I am dependent on my translators for my productivity and my ability to assist in my own care. Then it told, from the *viewpoint of colleagues*, how I once was 'young, aggressive, bright, pushy, hardworking and smart' but now have become a heroic figure, struggling to live life to its fullest" (Robillard 1999, 118; my emphasis). Not only is this the usual outsider perspective, focusing on everything he is not or cannot do, but it also reduces his entire lived being to helplessness and dependence and an object of pity.

Even much of the medical and social science research on the ALS experience takes its point of departure not from a neutral investigation of the experience of ALS but from a presumption of prevailing negativity. Studies with titles such as "Severity of Depressive Symptoms and Quality of Life in Patients with Amyotrophic Lateral Sclerosis" (Kübler et al. 2005) and "Correlates of Suffering in Amyotrophic Lateral Sclerosis" (Ganzini et al. 1999), not to mention a somewhat morbid fascination with assisted suicide, foster a particular impression. Many such studies begin with a hypothesis postulating significant levels of depression and poor quality of life in people with ALS. What many studies find instead is that reported and measured quality of life is frequently not only satisfactory but surprisingly high.[11] Moreover, there is not clear evidence for appreciably higher levels of depression—while depression can occur, some researchers offer other explanations, arguing for example that incidence of depression among people with ALS is not significantly different from the general population, or alternatively that proclivity to depression might be due to certain psychological tendencies in the individual that predate the onset of ALS.

As such, as one study concludes, "There is no empirical basis for the fatalistically postulated correlation of ALS with depression" (Lulé et al. 2008, 401). This study, titled "Depression and Quality of Life

in Patients with Amyotrophic Lateral Sclerosis," begins with a more
open and positive disposition toward the issue of the ALS experience, stating at the outset that conversations with patients and their
relatives and associated medical professionals reveal that these other
people often possess "no accurate knowledge of the actual emotional
situation of patients with severe impairment of motor function in
general, or, more specifically, of patients with amyotrophic lateral
sclerosis" (Lulé et al. 2008, 397). They go on to note that despite this
lack of certain knowledge, decisions about life-terminating measures
are often made or at least highly influenced by physicians and relatives, adding that evidence suggests that, in the Netherlands today,
one in five ALS patients dies either by euthanasia or by assisted suicide. And this situation is a running motif and backdrop to their study,
which concludes, "The authors hope that these empirical data on
the emotional state of severely impaired patients will serve as firmer
scientific ground for future discussions of physician–assisted suicide
(PAS), and that they will pave the way for further studies that share
the goal of putting the emphasis on the patient's perspective" (Lulé
et al. 2008, 402).

So not only can placing the emphasis on the patient's perspective
in studies examining the lived experience of illness furnish important knowledge about that subjective experience, along with allowing
these often muted patients' voices to be heard, but it can counteract
detrimental and potentially serious consequences of ignoring that
perspective.

Illness Experience and Phenomenology

Beyond the View from Within and the View from Without

I noted previously that the biomedical condition and the subjective experience are two aspects of an interconnected and mutually
conditioning situation in the experiential horizon. While lived and
experienced by a subject, it is clearly co-constituted as the relation of
corporeal situation and subjective experiencing of the situation; this is
true of any lived bodily situation for the body-subject, whether under
consideration is a situation characterized by illness, or the sexed and
gendered bodily situation, or the phenomenological baseline, as it

were, of any lived embodiment intertwined with lived and living subjectivity.

The examples in the preceding section point to a crucial feature of the illness experience, indeed, of the constitution of any such interpersonal experience. I also noted earlier that the illness experience extends beyond both the biomedical condition and the subjective experience of that condition. Like these other bodily situations, the illness experience is intersubjectively constituted as the interaction and interrelation between self and other in the shared social world. This coexistence and copresencing in that world forms the basis of that interaction, an interaction that takes a multitude of forms—perception, acknowledgment, negotiation, reciprocity, encroachment, delimitation, even menace. The nature of intersubjective co-constitution extends to the constitution of the ill individual's experience of living this condition, interactively and hermeneutically constituted in terms of the experience from within and from without; meaning here the experience as internally lived, interpreted, and framed, interwoven and codetermined by the experience as externally perceived, interpreted, framed, and, frequently, circumscribed.

Moreover, insofar as this intersubjective codetermining process unfolds and is embedded in the wider social world, it is not just a matter of subject/subject or self/other but involves a complex sociopolitical context characterized in turn by prevailing systems and structures informed by and reinforcing normative frameworks and belief systems and asymmetrical power relations and hierarchies. Far from being immune to these systems and processes, the medical world and experience is thoroughly conditioned by them. As such, the illness experience is correspondingly conditioned by these systems and cannot be read outside of or in isolation from this context.

I would contend that given the often inequitable relational dynamics that obtain in a medical situation, whether it be the clinical setting or the broader social one, along with the frequently lesser or weaker, more vulnerable subjective and social positioning on the part of the ill person, this can result in an asymmetrical relation with myriad implications. With respect to an intersubjective constitution of the illness experience, one possible implication is a greater influence and authority given to the view from without, resulting in the latter exercising a disproportionate effect on the interpretation and framing of the illness experience. As a result, the illness experience, purportedly an account of the subjective experience and the individual's account of the interpretation and experience of illness, can be too strongly characterized by an outsider perspective, on the one hand, or, on the other hand, heavily colored by the reception, construal, and treatment of the individual in the wider social context. Either way, or together, it would appear that the subjective illness experience is considerably, if not largely, defined and conditioned by the wider interpersonal social horizon. As such, a significant component, and challenge, of my experience of living with ALS is not just my relation to my bodily experience and the travails my body is currently undergoing, but also the broader sociocultural context and how that framing of me frames in turn my illness experience.

Toward a Phenomenology of Illness Experience

Insofar as many studies and illness narratives employ phenomenological vocabulary and approaches, phenomenology is already frequently situated in this discourse. Language of "the lived experience of . . ." and attention to phenomenological themes and concepts, as well as the implementing of phenomenological methodology such as versions of bracketing, attest to the value of phenomenology to illness research and accounts of illness experience.

There are potential limitations to the approaches to illness research I discussed earlier: medical and social science research using case studies, measurement instruments, and interviews can remain at a level of tabulating and reporting results, albeit with analysis of the data, but not necessarily taking the step to the wider conceptual and existential implications of their findings. Illness narratives and memoirs run the risk of being solipsistic rather than subjective, or potentially too constructed and performative, raising concerns for some about reliability and methodological validity. But these are the challenges facing any account situated in the subjective or first-person perspective: how can the reliability of the account be established throughout potentially distorting intervening factors? How do we move from an individual, possibly idiosyncratic, account to one that is more representative of the experience as such?

These, of course, are precisely the kinds of questions that phenomenology starting from Husserl endeavors to answer. This obviously requires a much longer discussion than space permits. But on the whole we can say that phenomenology, in attempting to answer such questions, looks to identify patterns and common threads, thematic and structural continuities, among the often highly variegated experiential accounts and representations, without losing the immediacy and the rich diversity and specificity of individualized experiences; as Merleau-Ponty notes, elaborating a structure that captures and expresses both generality and particularity (Merleau-Ponty 1962). Moreover, the aim of phenomenology is not just to observe and describe experience but to analyze and philosophize on the basis of the observed and described experience, deriving insights and knowledge about the nature of lived experience and the shared intersubjective world in all their complexity. By the same token, while Husserl considered reflection to generally be sufficient, subsequently phenomenologists began increasingly to incorporate empirical material and social scientific research into their analyses, and once again, when it comes to phenomenological investigations of illness and illness experience, such a multifaceted approach is requisite.

At the same time I am arguing for the necessity of a philosophical, and in particular, phenomenological approach to and treatment of illness and the illness experience. To date there has been very little philosophical attention given to these themes and issues, but increasingly philosophers and phenomenologists are turning their attention to them and the field of medicine generally, and they can and are making important contributions to the discussion and research.[12]

In speaking about the challenges inherent in the endeavor to tease out common strands and patterns from the variegated experiential accounts, and the further methodological challenges in assessing which features are more structural, that is, endemic to the experience as such, and which are perhaps more of the status of variations on that structural experience, I believe that analyses of illness and illness experience illustrate these challenges in a particularly striking way. Within the disability community the notion of disability is often framed more globally and collectively, for example, "disabled people," for reasons of identification and solidarity, not to mention for political and activist purposes, all the while it is recognized that this is of course somewhat misleading, since there is such a variety of disabilities and circumstances in which disability is lived and negotiated that it makes it difficult to generalize about disability as such, particularly in terms of experiences of disability. This is no less true with the case of illness experience. Different illnesses can entail different kinds of experiences; different sociocultural contexts inform the experience and interpretation of illness; and specificities of gender, class, ethnicity, and sexuality are further variables in the effort to delineate features of the illness experience as such.

For all these reasons phenomenology provides an invaluable conceptual and strategic approach and framework for investigations of the illness experience. At the same time, such illness experience investigations highlight the unique challenges facing a project that seeks to philosophize from a first-person perspective on the basis of lived experience. Phenomenology has much to lend to illness and illness-experience research, and correspondingly such areas and themes prod phenomenology out of what is often a textual slumber, to reinvigorate the "doing" of phenomenology as a vital, living descriptive and critical analysis.

Acknowledgments

The research for this chapter was sponsored by Central European University Foundation, Budapest (CEUBPF).

Notes

1. To distinguish between the biomedical condition and the subjective experience does not necessarily imply a binary or dichotomy, although some researchers frame the distinction more strongly. As I discuss later, these are two interconnected aspects of one experiential horizon.
2. For further discussions of feminist phenomenology, see Fisher 2010, Fisher 2000, and Fisher 1999.
3. While clearly any illness entails an illness experience as such, I am using "illness" and "illness experience" here in keeping with the usual meaning in these discussions: a chronic illness, that is, a significant health event, in particular a serious, and/or prolonged, and/or life-threatening illness.
4. *OED Online*, second edition, 1989; online version March 2011. http://www.oed.com:80/Entry/91493.
5. In *Illness as Metaphor* Susan Sontag discusses the ways in which diseases are given a meaning, invariably moralistic. Pointing to epidemic diseases as a "common figure for social disorder," she

traces early meanings of pestilence and its derivations, the latter heavily imbued with moralistic attributions: "From pestilence (bubonic plague) came 'pestilent,' whose figurative meaning, according to the *Oxford English Dictionary*, is 'injurious to religion, morals, or public peace—1513'; and 'pestilential,' meaning 'morally baneful or pernicious—1531.' Feelings about evil are projected onto a disease. And the disease (so enriched with meanings) is projected onto the world" (Sontag 1979, 58).

6. Susan Sontag also notes the long history of punitive notions of disease, along with the attendant sense of culpability: "Ostensibly, the illness is the culprit. But it is also the cancer patient who is made culpable. Widely believed psychological theories of disease assign to the ill the ultimate responsibility both for falling ill and for getting well" (Sontag 1979, 57).

7. I consider myself to be an example of this. Living with ALS/MND, I am sometimes asked, particularly by someone I just met, when I "got sick." I usually answer that I don't consider myself to be sick as such, rather I am living with a particular disease. The usual reaction to this is one of apparent disbelief: not accustomed to making such distinctions or more nuanced conceptualizations of illness and disease, and confronted with a visual display of what most people see as strong evidence of "sickness," many people demur, no doubt convinced that I am simply in denial.

8. To take an iconic example, Stephen Hawking has referred to his situation as someone living with MND/ALS as his "disability." At one time his website had a page where he discussed his experience of living with MND/ALS, which used to be entitled "Disability Advice" but was later called "Living with ALS." See See http://www.hawking.org.uk/living-with-als.html.

9. I would add to this a certain contemporary impulse, partly motivated by individual psychology, and fostered and fed by a confessional and celebrified culture, to "tell my story"; an impulse all the more powerful when that story involves a particularly dramatic or life-changing event or a compelling personal journey. The impulse to tell one's story has, of course, always existed, as the large body of work in this genre attests. I am referring rather to a more contemporary phenomenon wherein an impulse becomes more like an imperative, fueled, no doubt, not only by an enabling culture but also by the ubiquitous contemporary desire for fame.

10. The literature on illness narratives is vast and I cannot do it justice here. Some key references, however, are: Bury 2001; Frank 1995, 1993, and 1991; Gunaratnam and Oliviere 2009; Hydén 1997; Kleinman 1988; and Nelson 2001 and 1997.
11. See also Young and McNicoll 1998.
12. Representative work in phenomenology and illness includes Carel 2012 and 2008; Svenaeus 2000a and 2000b; and Toombs 1990 and 1988.

References

Benner, Patricia. 2001. "The Phenomenon of Care." In *Handbook of Phenomenology and Medicine*, edited by S. Kay Toombs, 351–369. Dordrecht: Kluwer.
Bishop, Jeffrey P. 2012. "Subjective Experience and Medical Practice." *Journal of Medicine and Philosophy* 37: 91–95.
Bury, Michael. 1982. "Chronic Illness as Biographical Disruption." *Sociology of Health and Illness* 4: 167–182.
Bury, Michael. 2001. "Illness Narratives: Fact or Fiction?" *Sociology of Health & Illness* 23 (3): 263–285.
Carel, Havi. 2008 *Illness: The Cry of the Flesh.* Stocksfield, UK: Acumen.
Carel, Havi. 2012. "Phenomenology as a Resource for Patients." *Journal of Medicine and Philosophy* 37: 96–113.
Fisher, Linda. 1999. "Sexual Difference, Phenomenology, and Alterity." *Philosophy Today* 43 (Supplement): 68–75.
Fisher, Linda. 2000. "Phenomenology and Feminism: Perspectives on Their Relation." In *Feminist Phenomenology*, edited by Linda Fisher and Lester Embree, 17–38. Dordrecht: Kluwer.
Fisher, Linda. 2010. "Feminist Phenomenological Voices." *Continental Philosophy Review* 43 (1): 83–95.
Frank, Arthur W. 1993. "The Rhetoric of Self-Change: Illness Experience as Narrative." *The Sociological Quarterly* 34 (1): 39–52.
Frank, Arthur W. 1995. *The Wounded Storyteller: Body, Illness, and Ethics.* Chicago: University of Chicago Press.
Frank, Arthur W. 1991. *At the Will of the Body: Reflections on Illness.* Boston: Houghton Mifflin.
Ganzini, Linda, Wendy S. Johnston, and William F. Hoffman. 1999.

"Correlates of Suffering in Amyotrophic Lateral Sclerosis." *Neurology* 52 (7): 1434–1440.

Gunaratnam, Yasmin, and David Oliviere (eds.). 2009. *Narrative and Stories in Health Care: Illness, Dying and Bereavement.* Oxford: Oxford University Press.

Hydén, Lars-Christer. 1997. "Illness and Narrative." *Sociology of Health & Illness* 19 (1): 48–69.

Jennings, D. 1986. "The Confusion between Disease and Illness in Clinical Medicine." *Canadian Medical Association Journal*: 865–870.

Kleinman, Arthur. 1988. *The Illness Narratives: Suffering, Healing and the Human Condition.* New York: Basic Books.

Kübler, Andrea, Susanne Winter, Albert C. Ludolph, Martin Hautzinger, and Niels Birbaumer. 2005. "Severity of Depressive Symptoms and Quality of Life in Patients with Amyotrophic Lateral Sclerosis." *Neurorehabilitation and Neural Repair* 19 (3): 182–193.

Lindgren, Kristin. 2004. "Bodies in Trouble: Identity, Embodiment, and Disability." In *Gendering Disability*, edited by Bonnie G. Smith and Beth Hutchison, 145–165. New Brunswick: Rutgers University Press.

Lindsey, Elizabeth. 1996. "Health within Illness: Experiences of Chronically Ill/Disabled People." *Journal of Advanced Nursing* 24: 465–472.

Lulé, Dorothée, Sonja Häcker, Albert Ludolph, Niels Birbaumer, and Andrea Kübler. 2008. "Depression and Quality of Life in Patients with Amyotrophic Lateral Sclerosis." *Dtsch Arztebl Int* 105 (23): 397–403.

Merleau-Ponty, Maurice. 1962. *Phenomenology of Perception*, translated by Colin Smith. London: Routledge and Kegan Paul. Originally published as *Phénoménologie de la perception*. Paris: Éditions Gallimard, 1945.

Nelson, Hilde Lindemann, ed. 1997. *Stories and Their Limits: Narrative Approaches to Bioethics.* New York: Routledge.

Nelson, Hilde Lindemann. 2001. *Damaged Identities, Narrative Repair.* Ithaca: Cornell University Press.

Pierret, Janine. 2003. "The Illness Experience: State of Knowledge and Perspectives for Research." *Sociology of Health & Illness* 25: 4–22.

Robillard, Albert B. 1999. *Meaning of a Disability: The Lived Experience of Paralysis.* Philadelphia: Temple University Press.

Sontag, Susan. 1979. *Illness as Metaphor*. New York: Vintage Books.

Svenaeus, Fredrik. 2000a. "The Body Uncanny: Further Steps Towards a Phenomenology of Illness." *Medicine, Health Care and Philosophy* 3: 125–137.

Svenaeus, Fredrik. 2000b. "Das Unheimliche: Towards a Phenomenology of Illness." *Medicine, Health Care and Philosophy* 3: 3–16.

Toombs, S. Kay. 1988. "Illness and the Paradigm of Lived Body." *Theoretical Medicine* 9: 201–226.

Toombs, S. Kay. 1990. "The Temporality of Illness: Four Levels of Experience." *Theoretical Medicine* 11: 227–241.

Young, Jenny M., and Paule McNicoll. 1998. "Against All Odds: Positive Life Experiences of People with Advanced Amyotrophic Lateral Sclerosis." *Health & Social Work* 23 (1): 35–43.

3

VISCERAL PHENOMENOLOGY

Organ Transplantation, Identity, and Bioethics

MARGRIT SHILDRICK

Organ transplantation in the twenty-first century has become so
well established as a biomedical practice—and a predominantly
successful one—that it scarcely raises any special interest unless the
procedure is entering into new territory such as that opened up by
face transplants. With few exceptions, the standard way in which the
field is reported both within the biomedical sciences and in lay media
heavily emphasizes the notion of spare part surgery in which the graft
is simply a utility, exchangeable between bodies but having no existential status of its own. At the same time the procedure is deemed
to have few or no implications for the phenomenological sense of
the being-in-the-body of the recipient but is judged as a success or
failure solely on the evidence of immunological acceptance and subsequent functionality. Nonetheless many ostensibly fully successful
operations, in which the signs of ongoing clinical recovery are strong,
result for the transplant recipients in significant degrees of psychic
disturbance to their sense of self, which range from feelings of unease
and uncertainty through to complete breakdown. In short the radical modification of the bodies of recipients, even when it is scarcely
discernible at a visual level, can have profound implications for the
supposed continuity of the embodied self.

In this chapter, I take heart transplantation as my specific focus in order to problematize and explore the issues through a phenomenological perspective in two interrelated ways. First, the approach undercuts any putative split between the psychic and the somatic, and second, it lays the ground for an understanding of organ transfer as a procedure that involves the intimate interaction and connection between at least two embodied selves. In recognizing the fleshy materiality of the graft as a visceral component of the living self, questions concerning the significance of the transfer to the recipient can be addressed in new ways. The substantive research that underpins my more speculative mode here is based in an international multidisciplinary project—the Process of Incorporating a Transplanted Heart (PITH)— that explicitly sets out to use a phenomenological perspective to gain insight into the nonmedical aspects of transplantation.[1] Instead of reading off the biomedical markers of recipients to ascertain the levels to which they are supposedly restored to health, the project with which I am involved seeks to engage with heart recipients in terms of their lived experience, asking them how they *feel* about their new forms of embodiment. The results to date have been startling in the degree of self-uncertainty and distress that is exhibited both through verbal interchanges and through bodily comportment. The question "Who am I?" takes on new meaning that can only be understood—as phenomenological theory would already indicate—through the body. What has emerged from the research indicates very high levels of identity disruption and dysmorphia across the sexes, but rather than seeing such reported experiences as evidence of an individual failure to deal with the traumatic intervention into the body that transplantation entails at the clinical level, a phenomenological perspective would take those disturbances as predictable and meaningful outcomes of the embodied experience. In deploying the theoretical resources of feminist philosophy and phenomenology, the PITH team is engaged in an analysis that demands a profound rethinking of the practices of organ transplantation.

Before describing in more detail the specific dimensions of the problematic around heart transplantation, I want to briefly outline a broader view of phenomenology—derived from the work of Maurice Merleau-Ponty—that fundamentally challenges the Cartesian split between mind and body that authorizes biomedical interventions into the body. In the conventional model, an originary core self is immune from assaults on the corporeal substance to the extent that, as Descartes famously put it, "Although the whole mind seems to be united to the whole body, nevertheless, were a foot or an arm or any other bodily part amputated, I know that nothing would be taken away from the mind" (1980, 97). In consequence, procedures that disassemble, cleave, suture, or transform the body, particularly when it is reduced to its component parts, are deemed to have limited impact on the transcendent self, whose interest in the corpus is predominantly that of a property relationship. It is not that such interventions are without significance—the personal body is after all putatively inalienable[2]—but the materiality of their effects in the biomedical sphere exist alongside a belief that it is within the power of health care to restore not just health but the well-being of a subject temporarily obscured or disarrayed by corporeal breakdown. Once the body itself has healed, then the core self is enabled to reemerge unscathed. For Merleau-Ponty, in contrast, the embodied self is reducible to neither mind nor body alone; a human being is not "a consciousness *in* a body," but rather establishes what he calls being-in-the-world through the potentialities of bodily activity. As he puts it: "We have no idea of a mind that would not be *doubled* with a body, that would not be established on this *ground*" (Merleau-Ponty 1968, 259). Moreover, what we understand as "I"—our sense of self-identity—comes into being through our corporeal engagement with the world: "there is no inner man, man is in the world, and only in the world does he know himself" (Merleau-Ponty 1962, xii). The significance of this for biomedicine is profound and suggests at the very least that a phenomenological approach that focused on the lived body might be a more adequate model from which to understand the actual experiences of the recipients of health care in all its manifestations.

The contestation of the separation of mind and body is, however, just one of a series of moves made by Merleau-Ponty that interrogate the binary structure of the modernist logos. A further highly evocative point arising from his work, and one that has been particularly developed in feminist thinking (Grosz 1994; Weiss 1999; Diprose 2002), concerns the intercorporeal possibilities suggested by the phenomenological notion of reversibility. For Merleau-Ponty (1968), reversibility signals a series of correspondences in which sight and touch always intend "being seen" and "being touched," a mutuality of perception and affect that troubles the distinction between self and other. The theme of an ambiguous intersubjectivity is apparent from the earlier work (Merleau-Ponty 1962), but it is in his posthumous text *The Visible and the Invisible* (1968) that Merleau-Ponty lays the ground for a crossing of the boundaries not only between an embodied subject and embodied object but between exterior and interior. While the thematic of intercorporeality—although never mentioned as such—is strongly implied in the chiasmatic relation between bodies, the further step of *con*corporeality, the coming together of bodies, is there to be developed.

In engaging with Merleau-Ponty, feminist scholars see such ideas as speaking to a pre-existing feminist stress on connection and relationality, which ground a limited ethics at least, although I posit a more appropriate postconventional ethics later in the chapter. For now, what matters is the notion that bodies cannot be seen in terms of the absolute separation and distinction demanded of the sovereign subject of modernity. For phenomenologists, feminist or otherwise (Toombs 1993; Diprose 2002; Rothfield 2005), bodies are always in communication and co-construction, even where distance is maintained as in Merleau-Ponty's reimagining of the chiasmatic relation between the seer and the seen in *The Visible and the Invisible*. More specifically, I suggest that the late work might provide significant new insights into the operations of what, in the context of organ transplantation, is essentially the construction of a hybrid body.

Aside from the question of the mutuality of embodiment, a further important insight taken from Merleau-Ponty concerns his concept of flesh ontology. What he appears to imply in this notion is that in excess of the human-to-human interconnection that channels the co-construction of embodiment, we are all immersed within, profoundly touched, and constituted by the elemental medium of the "flesh of the world," the undecidable environment in which the encounter between self and other takes place. Indeed the use of the terms "self" and "other" cannot be taken to refer to the binary distinction of the modernist logos, for that is precisely what is thrown open to question. Rather we experience distance through proximity, a folding over of flesh that creates the possibility of difference within a unified but undifferentiated medium. As Sue Cataldi (1993, 28) puts it, "things simultaneously envelop or *copresently* implicate each other." More importantly for the present project, the concept of flesh enables us to "think through embodiment beneath subject-object dualism by developing a radically unified ontology" (Cataldi 1993, 58). What Merleau-Ponty is attempting to do is to express a fundamental unity of existence without being centered on a knowing and sovereign subject. In insisting that we are all part of the same flesh where "the world of each opens upon that of the other," he seeks to instantiate "other landscapes besides my own" (Merleau-Ponty 1968, 141) that are nonetheless interwoven with mine through the reversibility of seer and seen, subject and object. As Merleau-Ponty uses it, the central notion of reversibility developed in his later work does not imply any merging of subjectivities but rather a coming together in difference, a point of both convergence and divergence. This becomes important in my account of heart transplant recipients, who I argue are both self and other, constituted as hybrid but never comfortably merged into a new unified whole.[3]

Taking the particular strand of phenomenology developed by Merleau-Ponty as its starting point, then, the PITH research project seeks to establish how heart-transplant recipients perceive their hearts both pre- and post-transplant, whether they experience disruptions to bodily integrity or personal identity, and how they imagine and speak about the relation to their donors. For critical theorists over many disciplines and for philosophers, it might seem obvious that such issues need to be addressed if more ethically adequate biomedical procedures are to be put in place, but strangely there is an entrenched reluctance within the professions allied to transplantation to countenance the relevance of those questions. With regard to the goals of organ transfer, the discourse of biomedicine remains firmly within the realm of heroic interventions that result in the promise of prolonged life, with enhanced functionality, and the expectation that the recipient will be restored to her original self. The replacement of the diseased heart with a healthier model is accomplished without pause for thought as to the sociocultural or psychic significance of intercorporeality, in large part because the operative mode of discourse reproduces the modernist mind-body split in which the meaning of embodiment is entirely occluded. As Drew Leder (1992, 23) remarks: "At the core of modern medical practice is the Cartesian revelation: the living body can be treated as essentially no different from a machine." The lay terminology of "spare part surgery" succinctly sums up what is perceived to be at stake, and the machine model of the body is widely cited by recipients themselves, but that does little to allay an underlying and widespread sociocultural anxiety as to the real meaning of suturing body parts together. As Margaret Lock (2002b, 1410) puts it:

It is abundantly clear that donated organs very often represent much more than mere biological body parts; the life with which they are animated is experienced by recipients as personified, an agency that manifests itself in some surprising ways, and profoundly influences subjectivity.

Worse still, the authorized narrative of clinic gives no credence to recipient doubts and fears other than as manifestations of psychological disturbance. For most patients attending clinic sessions, the only appropriate—the only allowable—response to the question "how are you?" is to respond with reference to measures of diet, energy levels, respiration, pulse rate, and so on, all the expected biomedical markers of recovery. What is scarcely mentioned in such settings is any sense of the lived body and its affects.

The question of what other considerations should be attended to has been raised repeatedly by philosophers (Varela 2001; Nancy 2002), social anthropologists (Lock 2002b; Sharp 2006), critical cultural theorists (Waldby 2002), and sociologists (Haddow 2005; Fox and Swazey 1992) but very rarely from within biomedicine and then usually only by those in "supporting" therapeutic roles (Forsberg et al. 2000; Sadala and Stolf 2008). Issues include not only those concerning disruptions to the embodied self, but wider concerns about the commodification of organs (Joralemon 1995; Scheper-Hughes 2003), the nature of consent (Koenig and Hogle 1995), the socioeconomic costs in the context of scarce resources (Mitchell et al. 1993; Dewar 1998,) and the experience of donor families (Haddow 2005). All of these are important issues, but my focus here remains on the relatively underresearched area of the experience of recipients. In a move away from the more usual phenomenological dimensions of the lived body, which might concern the scope of activity in the world and the continuing interactions within a social network, it is the very viscerality of transplantation that needs to be addressed. As the analysis of the PITH data confirms, heart recipients experience a range of affects and emotions including distress, loss, guilt, joy, and gratitude, which while subjective in the usual sense of the word are also embodied. They are not simply mental states but experiential modes of being that engage precisely with transformations within. It is not so much the exteriority of experience that concerns me, then, as the frequently unexpressed and often inexpressible meaning of a body effectively rendered hybrid. Arthur Frank (2001, 355) begins to catch some aspects of the problematic when he remarks, "suffer-ing is the unspeakable," but it is more than that, not simply a failure of words or even conceptualization but a disordering of embodi-ment that throws into question the very possibility of a singular "I" as Frank himself recognizes: "the medical model, so potent against what can be located, identified, and acted upon, is equally impotent against suffering that resists location, identification, and action."

What is called for is a visceral phenomenology that understands changes to the interiority of the body as having as much import to being-in-the-world as our external interactions. As Drew Leder puts it: "Beneath the surface flesh, visible and tangible, lies a hidden vital-ity that courses within me. 'Blood' is the metaphor for this viscerality" (1999, 204). My intertwining with the other is a relation of flesh *and blood*, and must therefore take account of the interior organs and tis-sues. The flesh of the world does not stop at the skin, and from that perspective, organ transplantation could never be simply spare part surgery, a matter of technical proficiency stripped of any implications for the embodied self. Leder explicitly sites the maternal/fetal bond as an example of Merleau-Ponty's chiasmatic identity-in-difference—"the two bodies are enfolded together, sharing one pulsing blood-stream" (1999, 206)—and for feminist scholars, pregnancy has become a powerful trope for, to use Irigaray's term (1985), the body that is not one (Young 1984; Diprose 1994). I have previously written about the shared embodiment of conjoined twins in such a phenomenologi-cal mode (Shildrick 2001), and it seems that to extend the notion to encompass transplantation is a further inevitable step.

A visceral phenomenology, nonetheless, faces real difficulties of acceptance particularly when the transfer of internal organs is com-pared to the newly emergent procedures of hand and face transplants. To take one example, a recent brief article in *The Lancet*—a journal not renowned for its exploration of abstract ideas beyond the medical model—made a strong, albeit unnamed, phenomenological claim that "the identity of an individual extends beyond him or herself" (Caro-sella and Pradeu 2006, 183), before reassuring the reader that because *organ* transplants are internal and nonvisible, "the self-identity of the organ recipient was not in question" (Carosella and Pradeu 2006, 183). In contrast, the authors assert, hand or face transplants are more ethi-cally complex, because they imply "accepting the constant presence of another person, and even a modified expression of the recipient's personality [. . .] a deep identity split occurs" (Carosella and Pradeu

2006, 183). One cannot doubt that the visibility of the graft does entail distinct problems, but what is remarkable is that Carosella and Pradeu's account could just as easily have been describing the experiences of many of the PITH respondents. For them the interiority of the graft—as with pregnant women—did not circumvent the question of an otherness within.

That the substantive issues of organ transplantation could be usefully rethought through a philosophical phenomenological perspective is becoming increasingly clear, but before further exploring the theorization of hybrid bodies, I want to note that the *methodology* of the PITH project is equally indebted to an understanding of phenomenology. Although the broad basis of gathering data operates through the familiar vehicle of semi-structured interviews, the preferred qualitative choice for researchers working with fairly limited data sets, those interviews are conducted with phenomenological principles in mind.[4] Each encounter between the potential or actual heart-transplant recipient and researcher is not only audiotaped but also video-recorded to capture the bodies of *both* the participants[5] and something of the environment in which the interview takes place. Recipients are given the choice of where to meet with the interviewer, and with relatively few exceptions, their everyday domestic setting is the preferred option, the usual alternative being a comfortable "sitting" room within the hospital that is deliberately distanced from the clinic itself. In the majority of interviews, then, the recording captures speech, posture and dress, bodily gestures, environmental artifacts, and the embodied interaction between interviewer and interviewee. All of these in a phenomenological sense are aspects of communication, much of which takes place in the prelinguistic mode. Human beings habitually engage in a complex body language of gestures, facial expression, movement, and tone of voice that precedes and supports speech itself, a formal structure that could not have developed, Merleau-Ponty asserts, without this prior form of communicative activity. Language in its prelinguistic form "creates itself in its expressive acts, which sweeps me on from the signs toward meaning" (Merleau-Ponty 1973, 10). In the context of contemporary health care, Christian Heath is one of the few empirical researchers who both uses and offers a justification of visual methodologies (Heath 2002; Heath, Hindmarsh, and Luff 2010). As he notes: "Through gesture, bodily comportment and talk, [respondents] render visible what would otherwise remain hidden and unavailable for inspection" (Heath 2002, 615). Moreover, in the context of the "flesh

of the world"—although Heath does not offer an explicitly phenomenological analysis—we should expect that the environmental aspects
of the interviews would not be without their own contribution to
meaning.

The recording of the respondents' body language, then, gives an
extra dimension to the analysis of what they actually have to say, but
what is striking is the extent to which such expressiveness goes beyond
or even contradicts the spoken word. The respondents' narratives,
whether verbal or otherwise, engage with all the ambiguity surrounding what Merleau-Ponty calls being-in-the-world, and what I refer to
as becoming-in-the-world, a never-ending process of construction that
belies any reference to a core self. Given that our grammatical structures presuppose a stable speaking subject transparent to herself, the
difficulty that post-transplant recipients may experience in articulat-
ing in words alone the undecidable nature of the disruptions to a
sense of self fully justifies the use of video-recording. As Heath puts
it: "The inner and the subjective are overlaid on the outer surface of
the body and rendered visible and objective" (2002, 603). Although
I cannot share Heath's somewhat uncritical assumption of a truth to
be told, or, more problematic yet, of an explicit intentionality on the
part of the respondent, his approach is surely enriched by the engagement with body language. One strongly recurring feature of participant videos was the incidence of clear incongruities between spoken
words and embodied expressions and gestures, which was observed
in nineteen of the twenty-five records. These could be classified as
either *upgrades* where recipients displayed guarded body comportment or distressed expressions while voicing positive feelings ("I'm
a 100 percent satisfied" spoken in an assertive voice while holding
oneself in a comforting hug); or *downgrades* in which body language
was assessed as nondistressed and open, despite the markedly negative content of verbal communication (the laughing participant who
spoke of the "expiry date" of the transplanted organ). Artifacts also
played a significant part in complicating the narrative structure, as
for example in the case of a woman, three years post-transplant, who
showed her inner tensions, even despair, not only by speaking in a
slow pained monotone but by constantly banging a water bottle on
her own lap, albeit the message she was attempting to convey to the
interviewer was one of survival and hope. Indeed she had chosen to
be interviewed under a prominent wall sign spelling out the word
"Hope." Another recipient, who was highly successful in deflecting

the interviewer's questions away from any in-depth appraisal of how he felt about himself post-transplant, used the medium of taking apart a heart-sized and -shaped Inuit puzzle sculpture to visually signal his fear that his own "broken heart" could not be put together again.

What is perhaps surprising in the biomedical literature surrounding transplantation is that despite the general acceptance of a mechanistic Cartesian model of the body that would appear devoid of nonnormative dimensions, a number of papers recognize that post-transplant recipients do in fact have strategies to negotiate anxieties that remain largely unspoken. In a discussion of defense mechanisms in heart-transplant recipients that concentrates on attitudes toward the donor, Bunzel, Wollenek, and Grundböck (1992), for example, claim that almost 73 percent are in either complete or partial denial with respect to their relationship with the donor; while a paper by the psychiatric team, Inspector, Kutz, and David, on the role of magical thinking reveals that just under half of their sample of heart recipients "despite sophisticated knowledge of anatomy and physiology [. . .] had an overt or covert notion of potentially acquiring some of the donor's personality characteristics along with the heart" (2004, xx). While such work uncovers the disparity between a rationalist and "fantasy" approach[6] that may nevertheless both be present in an individual recipient, studies that rely on a range of formal instruments and semi-structured interviews alone cannot fully encompass the lived experience of the respondent. The assumptions of the researchers, moreover, that the post-transplant recipients were alone in their resort to defense mechanisms is surely undermined by Margareta Sanner's observation that "[a]voidance, suppression and denial were the most common defence mechanisms, *all of which seemed to be supported by the medical context*" (2003, 391; my emphasis). The authorized narrative of the clinic is far from neutral, and, as I have analyzed elsewhere, may work not only to silence anxieties but to promote seemingly contradictory epistemological frameworks (Shildrick 2008; Shildrick et al. 2009).

The PITH team makes no claims as to its own neutrality, and clearly the interpretation of the video and audio recordings cannot escape a certain partiality, but to expect otherwise—that there could be a wholly objective truth of the matter to uncover—goes entirely against the spirit of the phenomenological perspective that has informed the project from the beginning. The attempts to minimize researcher bias comply with standard advice in some respects—such as having repeated team and individual viewings of the videos in order to pull out themes that have then been encoded using NVivo8—but with a strong feminist component to the team, we have attempted too to be critically self-reflective, rather than unbiased, in our engagement with what has often been highly disturbing material. We have no desire to replicate the subject-object, mind-body divides, undone by phenomenology but usually demanded of biomedical and social science research. Viewing the depth of dysphoria and distress evidenced in the videos has not been an easy task if we are to acknowledge, rather than cover over, our own embodiment in such an enterprise. With a team equally divided between clinicians and feminist academics in the social sciences and humanities, we have not always agreed on the best way to gain credibility in both spheres for the findings of the project, but none of us has attempted to deny the depth of our own emotional and affective engagement with what we have discovered.[7] Referring to that sense of being emotionally drained, one member of the team, Jen Poole, comments: "Sitting through the tapes, we have watched participants speak of identity disruption, distress, depression, dreams of the donor, and a loss so palpable that we have had trouble shifting from our seats at the end of these days" (Poole et al. 2009, 36). Moreover, in line with recent postconventional and feminist thought, the team has been less concerned to attempt to impartially engage with the descriptive question of the "how?" of the data set—and here we depart from a more classical Husserlian phenomenology—than to ask the question "why?"

At the heart of the matter—and it is instructive how ubiquitous such metaphors are in Western languages—lies a concern with the integrity of embodiment, an integrity that for most, if not all, organ recipients will have been severely tested by the onset of life-threatening illness and disease. Although few of us may actually experience ourselves in terms of a Cartesian duality whereby a controlling self simply exercises the machinery of the body, there is a taken-for-granted sense in which the body is assumed to be not so much at our disposal as simply a responsive, but largely unthought, material medium through which our agency is expressed. That sense constitutes what Leder (1990) calls the absent body, a state that cannot prevail in the face of illness, breakdown, or even such ordinary corporeal transformations as pregnancy. Perhaps the normative Cartesian body—the other of the lived body of phenomenology—is something of an illusion, but what is undeniable is that although the individual mind/body split may have a limited hold in the social imaginary, we do still maintain a belief in the separation and distinction between one body and another. It is predominantly in situations of material disruption that the vulnerability, unpredictability, and interconnectedness of corporeality explicitly claim our attention. The body itself may become an alien other, disengaged from the self and threatening to the integrity of the embodied subject. As Leder puts it: "The body is no longer alien as forgotten, but precisely as re-membered, a sharp searing presence threatening the self" (1990, 91). For many phenomenologically inclined sociologists of health and illness (such as Kleinman 1988), the goal of health care is the recovery of the unified self and the restoration of forgetfulness, as though the normative body were not already vulnerable, unstable and open to its others. Patient narratives often provide support for the idea of getting back to one's old self, where the integrity of embodiment is once again taken for granted. Alongside what he calls the restitution model, Arthur Frank (1997), however, identifies two further alternatives: first, the chaos narrative in which the patient expects no respite from the alienation of illness, and second, the quest narrative in which the experience of bodily breakdown is seen as a transformatory one that enables the sick person to become someone new. In bioethical terms, it is the latter that best expresses an optimistic scenario for organ recipients. Despite an insistent authorized narrative of transplantation that mirrors restitution, the recorded experiences of heart recipients speak to a complex and disturbing alienation in the embodied self that might be most effectively addressed by the bioethical goal of facilitating an acceptance of transformation.

The difficulty, as I understand it, lies in the notion—indeed the reality—of hybridity, for despite an everyday acknowledgment of our external communication and connection with others, the psychosocial imaginary maintains the illusion that each embodied subject is self-complete and occupies a clearly demarcated territory sealed by the boundary of the skin.[8] The body that is less than bordered, distinct, and wholly itself is the matter of deep anxiety, literally the stuff of nightmares or horror movies where alien elements may breach the boundaries of the body to effect a mode of concorporeality that subverts the embodied subject from within. In the context of transplantation, relatively few of the PITH respondents reported feeling a sense of renewed wholeness but rather were acutely aware that their sutured bodies spoke to a different mode of being-in-the-world.

As Catherine Waldby points out, the "organ recipient is involved in the most direct and literal form of intercorporeality" (2002, 249), and I would go further and name that experience as concorporeality. The post-operative patient knows that something fundamental has changed and in order to live well must find ways to accommodate the reality of a corporeal transformation that instantiates the hybrid body, whether that devolves on the incorporation of human or mechanical organs. Although heart recipients are encouraged to see the transplanted organ as their own, the difficulty of sustaining that ownership is evident in the uncomfortable and inconsistent shifts between "my heart" and "his/her heart" that most respondents verbalize. That difficulty, moreover, is heightened insofar as the recipient body now hosts alien DNA that will never lose the specificity of its otherness and that will continue to provoke an unremitting immunological response that would reject the transplant organ. In consequence all recipients are obliged to take a cocktail of immunosuppressant and counteractive drugs for the remainder of their lives, without, however, being given adequate information as to precisely the hybrid nature of their embodiment. In effect—and despite any expectations of recovering oneself—the other is both incorporated within and irreducibly alien to that self. The embodied self is, then, inevitably transformed, the body that is no longer one. As Luce Irigaray puts it, the body is "always at least double [. . .] it is plural, more diversified, more multiple in its differences, more complex, more subtle than is commonly imagined—in an imaginary rather too narrowly focused on sameness" (1985, 28). One of the most sustained reflections on the broadly phenomenological significance of having a heart transplant comes from the philosopher Jean-Luc Nancy, who underwent the procedure in the early 1990s. In *L'Intrus* (The intruder), Nancy makes explicit what other recipients leave implicit—that his account cannot "disentangle the organic, the symbolic, and the imaginary" (2002, 3). Unlike many others, however, Nancy is indifferent to the identity of his donor and refuses to sentimentalize the experience of otherness within. Where I have been arguing that phenomenology might see the hybridity of the transplanted body as a point of felt connection that escapes the binary of self and other, Nancy focuses instead what is unassimilable.

In a gesture more akin to Derrida than Merleau-Ponty, *L'Intrus* opens with a deliberation on the in-coming of the stranger, whom we briefly suppose to be a metaphor for the grafted heart, until

it quickly becomes apparent that for Nancy, his *own* failing heart
is the originary stranger. As corporeal breakdown has forced itself
on his attention, the absent presence of the healthy body has been
superseded by the "dysappearance"—to use another of Leder's terms
(1990)—of his heart as an element now threatening the previously
assumed integrity of his embodiment. Nancy's failing heart becomes,
he says, "an elsewhere 'in' me" (2002, 6), such that the self/other relation is experienced as an internal condition. After transplantation, as
his immune system attempts to reject the substitute organ, Nancy
refuses the metaphor of either ownership or connection, reflecting
instead on a self-alienation in which the meaning of *l'intrus* comes to
figure equally the original heart, the graft, the multiple viruses and
bacteria that inhabit any body, the effects of the immune system and
the drugs that suppress it, the onset of a cancerous tumor, and above
all death itself. There is no possible restoration of the self but only
the recognition of hybridity as the condition of all forms of embodiment. As Nancy concludes: "The *intrus* is none other than me, my
self" (2002, 13), a transformed self exposed as multiple, excessive, and
always in a state of becoming. Where other recipients attribute their
feelings of alienation to the troubling incorporation of the donor
heart, Nancy uses the experience of transplantation to reflect that
embodied selfhood is never unified but rather inherently fissured. As
a phenomenological insight into what it means to be embodied, the
account speaks clearly to disintegration, but does it mean that such a
mode of thinking must give up on the intimation of connection that
Merleau-Ponty seemed to foreshadow?

One answer might be to posit a critical feminist use of phenomenology that would endorse the trope of the disorganization of personal embodiment but see that precisely as the condition of possibility
for connection with others. If the self-contained and impermeable
subject of modernity is an illusion, operative only in the sociocultural imaginary, then an inherent openness to otherness is the starting
point. In the face of the contingency and vulnerability of embodiment where becoming-in-the-world is always mediated by others
(Shildrick 2002), self and other are always concorporeal, intertwined
but not encompassed by sameness, and what postconventional feminist theory has always stressed has been the fluidity between bodies
that does not stop at the skin (Irigaray 1985; Grosz 1994; Weiss 1999).
It mobilizes, as Irigaray puts it, "Nearness so pronounced that it makes

all discrimination of identity, and thus all forms of property, impossible. [. . .] This puts into question all prevailing economies" (1985, 31). Although Irigaray refers here to what she sees as elements of an unrealized notion of the feminine, her words are suggestive of the encounter between self and other in the context of transplantation, where questions of self-identity and the ownership of body parts become equally meaningless. And like the feminine, they require another mode of thinking. Unlike Merleau-Ponty—to whom she gives serious if critical consideration (see Irigaray 1993)—Irigaray is fully engaged with a visceral phenomenology that does not depend on perception alone. Her project is always a deeply ethical one, which should remind us of the urgent need to mobilize a bioethics of transplantation that does not rely of issues of rational consent, property in the body, contract, or the proper determination of donor death.

A possible way forward is suggested, I think, by the work of Rosalyn Diprose (2002), who has developed an ethics of what she calls "corporeal generosity." In a productive reworking of the notion of the gift—which is a central and generally unproblematized trope in explaining what is taken to be simply an exchange relationship between donor and recipient—Diprose takes up the Derridean elaboration of the gift without return (Derrida 1992). Where her approach is particularly relevant to transplant ethics is in the understanding of corporeal generosity as figuring what literally happens between bodies and yet is intrinsically excessive to the notion of the bounded body.[9] The gift, as Diprose sees it, "exceeds [. . .] contractual relations between individuals," and she goes on to name affect as "the basis of the production and transformation of the corporeal self through others" (2002, 75). Her model challenges the viability of the legitimated biomedical narrative of an unchanged self. As the PITH project has shown, for recipients, the donor heart is always more than an object of exchange; it is the locus of a heightened experience of the lived body reliant on the coming together, but never merging, of the giver and receiver. Corporeal generosity itself, in Diprose's terms, comes into play precisely in the event of difference, which must be both preserved and responded to. As she puts it: "intercorporeal generosity maintains alterity and ambiguity in the possibilities it opens [. . .] generosity is only possible if neither sameness nor unity is assumed as either the basis or the goal of an encounter with another" (Diprose 2002, 90–91). In the mode of transplantation, what this suggests is that the heart recipient's intuitive grasping of an otherness within should not be denied—the organ is *not* mine to assimilate; the irreducibility of difference must be responded to rather than covered over. Corporeal generosity sets out an openness to the other that is not reliant on exchange, on denial, or on the expectation of integration. With the account offered by Nancy's *L'Intrus* in mind, it is instructive too that Diprose is not proposing a rerun of early second-wave feminist touchy-feely notions of mutuality; she recognizes that the gift may be disturbing and disruptive. The opening to the other is at least always ambiguous and uncertain.

What I want to take from Diprose is the possibility of an ethics that includes the "affective material offering of our body to the other" (2002, 191), and to that I would add the acceptance by the donee of such an offering. As I understand it, mainstream feminist bioethics has long had a commitment to relationality, but that has not readily challenged the propriety—the completion and closure—of individual bodies. The model, I am proposing here, goes further, then, than the standard feminist recognition of the embodied mutuality of becoming to potentially address a mode of concorporeality that might include the hybridity of the heart-transplant recipient. If nothing else, a phenomenological enquiry into the acquisition of a donor organ should make us aware that to have a sense of self at all is to accept oneself as both in a process of coconstruction and as open to more radical transformations. The putative incorporation of the heart of another is not a once and for all event but a lifelong disturbance to the self that continues to pose the question "Who am I?" The task, then, is to find ways to accommodate the hybrid self without a complete loss of personal identity. And lest we imagine that it is only the heart that invokes such issues, I would point to the words of the recipient of a liver graft:

> I take tentative steps, consider everything as only a tentative understanding, a lost cartographer with no maps. [. . .] We are left to invent a new way of being human where bodily parts go into each other's bodies, redesigning the landscape of boundaries in the habit of what we so definitely used to call distinct bodies. (Varela 2001, 161)

It is difficult to see how organ recipients and, indeed, the transplant professionals themselves, can flourish unless the intimations of otherness within experienced by respondents, such as those in the PITH cohort, are openly accepted and integrated into a model of embodiment that stresses not just the mutual construction and dependency of self and other—as phenomenology has always done —but the viscerality of truly intercorporeal life.

Acknowledgments

I am grateful to Gail Weiss for her detailed commentary on this chapter at the Feminist Phenomenology and Medicine Conference.

Notes

1. PITH project REB File # 07-0822-BE. The team—Heather Ross, Susan Abbey, Jennifer Poole, Patricia McKeever, and Margrit Shildrick—consists of the medical director of the transplant clinic where the empirical elements of the research are based, the unit's psychiatrist, a mental health researcher, medical sociologist, and a philosophically trained critical cultural theorist, as well as two nurse-trained research assistants who are familiar with transplant procedures. Data analysis of the post-organ transplant cohort is complete, and the team is now investigating recipient and intending recipient responses to the incorporation of a mechanical heart, that is, a left ventricular assist device, commonly known as an LVAD.

2. The inalienability is undermined both by the notion that one may consent to certain assaults on the body—though curiously not to others—and by entering into a contract in which body parts, such as organs, tissue, ova, blood, and so on, are subject to commodification in an exchange economy.

3. I do not want to imply that some "natural" bodies are beyond the ascription of hybridity (Waldby and Mitchell 2006; Hird 2007) but to make the point that although the term is very rarely used in either clinical or lay literature, the recipient of a donor organ—or for that matter a mechanical LVAD (left ventricular assist device)—is undeniably constituted as hybrid. In phenomenological terms there is nothing exceptional about that: we are all embodied, or come into being, through our intrinsic intercorporeality with an array of others.

4. It should be made clear that the PITH project uses phenomenology as a theoretical orientation derived from the philosophy of Merleau-Ponty rather than as a methodology *per se.* Many empirical researchers in the social sciences—and particularly those subscribing to grounded theory—claim to use a phenomenological methodology in the aim of "describing a general or typical essential structure, based on descriptions of experiences of others" (Norlyk and Harder 2010, 427), but they are more often drawing on the work of Husserl, which underpins notions such as reduction, bracketing, and the discovery of core essences derived from the text alone. The PITH focus is on the inseparability of embodied responses, affect, and verbal expression regarding transplantation.

5. The majority of the videos show just two participants, but it is not unusual for recipients to choose to be interviewed in the presence of a family member or for others—along with a variety of pets—to be in and out of the background of the defined location.

6. The PITH team is not concerned with the truth value of respondent accounts but with the phenomenological experience that produces such accounts. When the records of the first cohort of heart-transplant participants were unblinded, it became apparent that there was very little correspondence between what was imagined of a donor and who that donor actually was.

7. Fox and Swazey attributed their decision to cease research in the field of transplantation to "participant-observer burnout," but they made clear not only their own distress at observing the disturbance to other people's lives but also their disquiet with biomedicine's "zealous determination to maintain life at any cost; and a relentless, hubris-ridden refusal to accept limits" (1992, 199). The PITH team has similar concerns.

8. One thinks immediately of Donna Haraway's challenging assertion: "even the most reliable western individuated bodies [. . .] neither stop nor start at the skin" (1989, 18). Indeed Haraway's notion of the cyborg has much in common with the hybrid bodies I describe, particularly in the interface between the human and technological. The crucial difference is that in her conception the cyborg is lived as *posthuman*, whereas transplant recipients are caught up in a psychosocial imaginary that can recognize only the human.

9. Myra Hird (2007) has usefully worked through the implications of corporeal generosity in terms of the movement of cellular material from the maternal to fetal body.

References

Bunzel, B, G. Wollenek, A. Grundböck. 1992. "Living with a Donor Heart: Feelings and Attitudes of Patients toward the Donor and the Donor Organ." *Journal of Heart and Lung Transplant* 11 (6): 1151–1155.

Carosella, Edgardo, and Thomas Pradeu. 2006. "Transplantation and Identity: A Dangerous Split?" *The Lancet* 368: 183–184.

Cataldi, Sue L. 1993. *Emotion, Depth, and the Flesh: A Study of Sensitive Space*. Albany: State University of New York Press.

Derrida, Jacques. 1992. *Given Time: I. Counterfeit Money*, trans. Peggy Kamuf. Chicago: University of Chicago Press.

Descartes, René. 1980. *Discourse on Method and Meditations on First Philosophy*, trans. Donald A. Cress. Indianapolis: Hackett.

Dew, Mary A., and Andrea F. DiMartini. 2005. "Psychological Disorders and Distress after Adult Cardiothoracic Transplantation." *Journal of Cardiovascular Nursing* 20 (5)(Supplement): 51–66.

Dewar, Diane. 1998. "Allocating Organ Transplant Services: What Can Be Learned from the United States Experience?" *Review of Social Economy* 56: 157–174.

Diprose, Rosalyn. 1994. *The Bodies of Women: Ethics, Embodiment and Sexual Difference*. London: Routledge.

Diprose, Rosalyn. 2002. *Corporeal Generosity: On Giving with Nietzsche, Merleau-Ponty, and Levinas*. Albany: State University of New York Press.

Forsberg, Anna, Lars Bäckman, and Anders Möller. 2000. "Experiencing Liver Transplantation: A Phenomenological Approach." *Journal of Advanced Nursing* 32 (2): 327–334.

Fox, Renée, and Judith Swazey. 1992. *Spare Parts: Organ Replacement in Human Society*. Oxford: Oxford University Press.

Frank, Arthur. 1997. *The Wounded Storyteller: Body, Illness, and Ethics*. Chicago: University of Chicago Press.

Frank, Arthur. 2001. "Can We Research Suffering?" *Qualitative Health Research* 11 (3): 353–362.

Grosz, Elizabeth. 1994. *Volatile Bodies: Towards a Corporeal Feminism*. Bloomington: Indiana University Press.

Haddow, Gill. 2005. "The Phenomenology of Death, Embodiment and Organ Transplantation." *Sociology of Health and Illness* 27 (1): 92–113.

Haraway, Donna. 1991. "A Cyborg Manifesto: Science, Technology, and Socialist-Feminism in the Late Twentieth Century." In *Simians, Cyborgs, and Women: The Reinvention of Nature.* London: Free Association Books.

Heath, Christian. 2002. "Demonstrative Suffering: The Gestural (Re)embodiment of Symptoms." *Journal of Communication* 52: 597–616.

Heath, Christian, Jon Hindmarsh, and Paul Luff. 2010. *Video in Qualitative Research.* London: Sage.

Hird, Myra. 2007. "The Corporeal Generosity of Maternity." *Body & Society* 13 (1): 1–20.

Inspector, Y., I. Kutz, and D. David. 2004. "Another Person's Heart: Magical and Rational Thinking in the Psychological Adaptation to Heart Transplantation." *Israeli Journal of Psychiatry and Related Sciences* 41 (3): 161–73.

Irigaray, Luce. 1985. *This Sex Which Is Not One*, trans. Catherine Porter. Ithaca: Cornell University Press.

Irigaray, Luce. 1993. *An Ethics of Sexual Difference*, trans. Carolyn Burke and Gillian Gill. Ithaca: Cornell University Press.

Joralemon, Donald. 1995. "Organ Wars: The Battle for Body Parts." *Medical Anthropology Quarterly* 9: 335–356.

Kleinman, Arthur. 1988. *The Illness Narratives: Suffering, Healing and the Human Condition.* New York: Basic Books.

Koenig, Barbara, and Linda Hogle. 1995. "Organ Transplantation (Re) examined?" *Medical Anthropology Quarterly* 9 (3): 393–397.

Leder, Drew. 1990. *The Absent Body.* Chicago: University of Chicago Press.

Leder, Drew. 1992. "A Tale of Two Bodies: The Cartesian Corpse and the Lived Body." In *The Body in Medical Thought and Practice*, edited by Drew Leder, 17–35. Dordrecht: Kluwer.

Leder, Drew. 1999. "Flesh and Blood: A Proposed Supplement to Merleau-Ponty." In *The Body: Classic and Contemporary Readings*, edited by Don Welton, 200–210. Oxford: Blackwell.

Lock, Margaret. 2002a. *Twice Dead: Organ Transplants and the Reinvention of Death.* Berkeley: University of California Press.

Lock, Margaret. 2002b. "Human Body Parts as Therapeutic Tools: Contradictory Discourses and Transformed Subjectivities." *Qualitative Health Research* 12: 1406–1418.

Merleau-Ponty, Maurice. 1962. *The Phenomenology of Perception.* London: Routledge and Kegan Paul.

Merleau-Ponty, Maurice. 1968. *The Visible and the Invisible.* Evanston, IL: Northwestern University Press.

Merleau-Ponty, Maurice. 1973. *The Prose of the World,* trans. John O'Neill. Evanston, IL: Northwestern University Press.

Mitchell, S.V., R. A. Smallwood, P. W. Angus, and H. M. Lapsley. 1993. "Can We Afford to Transplant?" *Medical Journal of Australia* 158 (3): 190–194.

Morstyn, Ron. 2009. "Merleau-Ponty and Me: Some Phenomenological Reflections upon My Recent Bone Marrow Transplant." *Australasian Psychiatry* 17 (3): 237–239.

Nancy, Jean-Luc. 2002. *L'Intrus,* trans. Susan Hanson. Ann Arbor: Michigan State University Press.

Norlyk, Annelise, and Ingegerd Harder. 2010. "What Makes a Phenomenological Study Phenomenological? An Analysis of Peer-Reviewed Empirical Nursing Studies." *Qualitative Health Research* 20: 420–431.

Poole, Jennifer, Margrit Shildrick, Patricia McKeever, Susan Abbey, and Heather Ross. 2009. "'You might not feel like yourself': Heart Transplants, Identity and Ethics." In *Critical Interventions in the Ethics of Healthcare: Challenging the Principle of Autonomy in Bioethics,* edited by S. Murray and D. Holmes, 33–45. Farnham: Ashgate.

Rothfield, Philippa. 2005. "Attending to Difference: Phenomenology and Bioethics." In *Ethics of the Body: Postconventional Challenges,* ed. Margrit Shildrick and Roxanne Mykitiuk, 22–49. Cambridge, MA: MIT Press.

Sadala, Maria Lúcia Araújo, and Noedir Antônio Groppo Stolf. 2008. "Heart Transplantation Experiences: A Phenomenological Approach." *Journal of Clinical Nursing* 17 (7b): 217–225.

Sanner, Margareta. 2003. "Transplant Recipients' Conceptions of Three Key Phenomena in Transplantation: The Organ Donation, the Organ Donor, and the Organ Transplant." *Clinical Transplantation* 17 (4): 391–400.

Scheper-Hughes, Nancy. 2003. "Rotten Trade: Millennial Capitalism, Human Values and Global Justice in Organs Trafficking." *Journal of Human Rights* 2 (2): 197–226.

Sharp, Leslie. 1995. "Organ Transplantation as a Transformative Experience: Anthropological Insights into the Restructuring of the Self." *Medical Anthropology Quarterly, New Series* 9 (3): 357–389.

Sharp, Leslie. 2006. *Strange Harvest: Organ Transplants, Denatured Bodies, and the Transformed Self.* Berkeley: University of California Press.

Shildrick, Margrit. 2001. "Some Speculations on Matters of Touch." *Journal of Medicine and Philosophy* 26 (4): 387–404.

Shildrick, Margrit. 2002. *Embodying the Monster: Encounters with the Vulnerable Self.* London: Sage.

Shildrick, Margrit. 2008. "The Critical Turn in Feminist Bioethics: The Case of Heart Transplantation." *International Journal of Feminist Approaches to Bioethics* 1 (1): 28–47.

Shildrick, Margrit, Patricia McKeever, Susan Abbey, Jennifer Poole, and Heather Ross. 2009. "Troubling Dimensions of Heart Transplantation." *Medical Humanities (BMJ Supplement)* 35 (1): 35–38.

Toombs, Susan Kay. 1993. *The Meaning of Illness: A Phenomenological Account of the Different Perspectives of Physician and Patient.* Dordrecht: Kluwer.

Varela, Francisco. 2001. "Intimate Distances: Fragments for a Phenomenology of Organ Transplantation." *Journal of Consciousness Studies* 8 (5–7): 259–271.

Waldby, Catherine. 2002. "Biomedicine, Tissue Transfer and Intercorporeality." *Feminist Theory* 3 (3): 239–254.

Waldby, Catherine, and Robert Mitchell. 2006. *Tissue Economies: Blood, Organs, and Cell Lines in Late Capitalism.* Durham, NC: Duke University Press.

Weiss, Gail. 1999. *Body Images: Embodiment as Intercorporeality.* London: Routledge.

Young, Iris Marion. 1984. "Pregnant Embodiment: Subjectivity and Alienation." *Journal of Medicine and Philosophy* 9: 45–62.

4

COMMUNAL PUSHING

Childbirth and Intersubjectivity

SARAH LACHANCE ADAMS AND PAUL BURCHER

I remember an example of "shared pushing" that influenced the outcome of a birth according to the mother involved. The woman wanted a VBAC for her second birth.[1] Her first birth had occurred in Mexico and had been an unplanned emergency caesarean and her baby did not survive. She was strongly motivated to have a vaginal birth with her second baby, but her second stage of labor was quite prolonged. I called the physician on call with me after she had been pushing two hours. She was still distant from delivery and I was concerned about the resilience of the baby and the mother. The physician arrived and received report and discussed delivery options with the patient. He offered her a caesarean delivery, which she vigorously declined. As he watched her pushing efforts, he became more and more involved. At first he only directed her pushing with words and then he began to watch for the beginnings of the push, keep eye contact, hold his breath, and mimic her body posture. They pushed together for another hour.

At her post-partum visit, we discussed her birth experience. She had a vaginal birth after a twelve-hour labor and a three-and-a-half-hour second stage. The baby was admitted to NICU with metabolic acidosis and had a very difficult course there. The mom explained to me that she was very pleased with her birth and that the doctor who "pushed with" her was key to her success. She identified her husband as not helpful during this part of labor as he simply stood by her side and held her hand. The team pushing really encouraged her. To my surprise, she identified me as another person who had "shared pushing" with her. For me, it was done unconsciously.

—Cindy Hunter, personal communication

In so far as I am born into the world, and have a body and a natural
world, I can find in that world other patterns of behavior with which my
own interweave [. . .].
        —Maurice Merleau-Ponty, *Phenomenology of Perception*

The communal push is when those supporting a woman in childbirth also find themselves pushing with the muscles of the pelvic
floor, often with held breath and red faces. It seems to happen most
frequently when the laboring woman is *struggling* to push the baby
out; women having an easy time of pushing do not seem to elicit this
response in their support group.

Communal pushing is not universal among laboring women,
even when there is close support, but it happens frequently enough
that labor nurses, midwives, and obstetricians are aware of the phenomenon. It is clear from the unanimity of the response that it does
not seem to be a remembered bodily reaction occurring only in
those who have been in the same position as the laboring mother.
A midwife known to the second author of this essay remarked that
in her experience young girls are often the best "support pushers"
even though they have never pushed a baby out or even seen another
birth. Communal pushing is often not consciously chosen or willed.
Typically, one does not decide or "get the idea" to push with the
laboring women, it usually begins without any direct acknowledgment. Communal pushing is not entirely gendered either; although
men are more likely to stand apart from the pushing, both fathers
and male partners often find themselves pushing. In a room where
the laboring woman has become the total focus of the family attention, frequently only the professional care providers stand outside the
communal push. Yet labor nurses report that they find themselves
pushing when it is their daughter or close friend who is now in labor.

The complexity of the communal push gives it a strength and
richness that tests any theory of embodied intersubjectivity to
explain. The bodily support is unconsciously offered to the laboring
woman—and by unconsciously we mean that the body is responding
directly to another body without any reflection or cognitive choice.
As Merleau-Ponty (1968, 130) states, reflection already relies on the
prereflective body. Yet these prereflective acts parallel the reflectively
chosen support being offered. The woman is the center of the group's
attention, thought, and conversation, but Merleau-Ponty would argue

that this support and the bodily support are parallel—the body is not following the mind—they are acting in unison:

> When we say that the life of the body, or the flesh, and the life of the psyche are involved in a relationship of reciprocal *expression*, or that the bodily event always has a psychic *meaning*, these formulations need to be explained. Valid as they are for excluding thought, they do not mean that the body is a transparent integument of the Spirit. The return to existence, as to the setting in which communication between body and mind can be understood, is not a return to Consciousness or spirit [. . .]. (Merleau-Ponty 1958, 185)

The "reciprocal expression" of the communal push is that the body is acting without there necessarily being a conscious choice to support another body, *but* the history and situation that compel the shared push is actually shared by both the body and reflective consciousness. That is, the body does not need the assent of reflection. In a sense, it understands it is acting to support someone who the reflective self wishes to support.

Perhaps it would even be better to go further and argue that the bodies lead, although within confines that the conscious self would concur with if asked. The laboring woman's body—meaning not an objective body but a lived body in behavior—is immediately known to the other family members and friends as a body that carries the significance it has taken on through time in their relationship, and that it needs the support of others. In this sense the laboring woman's body has a different meaning for the family members present than it does for the health professionals in the room, and so their bodies typically respond differently to this different meaning. But the point here is that the body's response frequently precedes reflection: people push without realizing it and are sometimes embarrassed to find themselves pushing. There is an intimacy to pushing with another that can sometimes seem inappropriate when brought to light—particularly because it happens in the quasi-public sphere of a hospital room with professional onlookers also present. Those who share in the pushing can find themselves being drawn closer than the boundaries they may have consciously chosen given reflective thought on the situation. The other reason we suspect people sometimes express

embarrassment over finding themselves pushing is the seeming futility of it. Within the realm of "objective reality" what possible good
could be accomplished by getting red in the face and bearing down
with a woman giving birth? After all, only she can actually push out
the baby.

Using the classical feminist distinction between the sexing of a
body that is biological and the gendering that is largely (or completely, depending upon the author) culturally constructed, the communal push provides some answers about how our anonymous bodies
are different and yet also mutually intersecting. There is a clear gender
divide in that women of all ages push more than men, but it is not
an absolute division. It would perhaps be correct to say that the connectedness between similarly gendered bodies is greater. Men can and
do push with the same muscles and pelvic floor that women have—
much of the anatomy of pushing is shared and the medical term "Val-
salva" makes no gender distinction between a women bearing down
with her abdominal muscles to push out a baby and a man bearing
down to facilitate a bowel movement. The joke on labor units is that
everyone—male and female—gets hemorrhoids from helping the
women push. Our sense is that the sexual difference is not the reason
men push less than women, and that the gender roles play a larger
part. Men tend to hold themselves apart not because they cannot
push, but because their bodies may not read the meaning of pushing
as for them. That is, men are born without an ability to birth a baby,
but to a greater degree they learn that birthing is *other* to them. But
what is probably most important to this analysis is the relativity of it:
men *do* push. In doing this they are transcending a culturally determined meaning for a more immediate body-to-body connection in
someone for whom they care.

Merleau-Ponty's Contribution

The chapter in *Phenomenology of Perception* in which Merleau-Ponty
first explains his philosophy of intersubjectivity is set apart from much
of what precedes it by the relative lack of examples and psychological
experiments to illustrate the argument he is making. Most notably
missing are strongly visceral examples of bodily interconnectedness—
instead examples of vision and language are used that are less *fleshy*
than his powerful philosophical descriptions of interweaving, especially in *The Visible and the Invisible*. Yet, we are struck by the power

of Merleau-Ponty's work to explain some of the most profound and gritty examples of bodily interconnectedness. By giving a stronger example of embodied interweaving than found in Merleau-Ponty's work—communal pushing—our hope is to retrieve Merleau-Ponty from the misunderstandings of some of his commentators. Notably, we respond to some feminist critics who fail to see the potential in Merleau-Ponty's work for understanding both gender difference and commonality. Although Merleau-Ponty may be lacking adequate examples illustrating both unity and particularity, he correctly understands that the intersubjective body is both distinct and prereflectively united to others.

In the *Phenomenology of Perception*, Merleau-Ponty emphasizes our sense of coherence with the world. Prior to reflection, one does not stand out as situated over and against the world and others. We are immersed in a reality whose qualities and meanings appear as both shared and self-evident. "My consciousness [. . .] is hardly distinguishable from what is offered to it [. . .]" (Merleau-Ponty 1958, 278). The sensory is open to me "through a gift of nature, with no effort made on my part" (Merleau-Ponty 1958, 251). There is no immediate distinction between myself and my perceptions. There is no *I* or *world* over and against one another, rather these two poles are found in and through each other. Our primary engagement is always already present and carries on in the background even when we think of ourselves abstractly. Our underlying engagement with the world typically remains *anonymous*.

For Merleau-Ponty, one's sense of continuity with the world extends also to other people. In the natural attitude, others are not inaccessible; we share a public, sensible world as fellow sentient beings. I do recognize that others have a distinct view upon the world, and their differing perceptions add depth and new dimensions to my own. This communication with others is fundamental to understanding the world as possessing a truth. We do not begin as a singular point of view to which others are added; infants require a human *community* not only to survive, but for perceptual confirmation. Our gestures *establish* a common meaning (Merleau-Ponty 1958, 215–216); an infant's primary caregivers endow the world with its significance. For a human being, others contribute to the constitution of my world before I am even aware of it.

Merleau-Ponty argues that babies and young children are fully immersed in the public world and that the earlier we look into their development, the more pervasive is their sense of anonymity (1958, 413). In "The Child's Relations with Others" he describes the child as not reflectively aware of himself as holding a unique perspective. As we mature, he believes, we come to realize our differentiation from others, but anonymous intersubjectivity continually underlies all of our interactions. Merleau-Ponty (1958, 417) states that: "although I am outrun on all sides by my own acts, submerged in generality, the fact remains that I am the one by whom they are experienced." Each body has its own boundaries, but these same boundaries are also the point of contact between oneself and the sensible world. We simultaneously inhabit a sensuous unity and suffer a division. Even the pregnant mother maintains her own bodily integrity in this manner. She does not taste her amniotic fluid as the fetus breathes it in. Our bodies establish points of contact that also keep us from merging.

Feminist Readings of Merleau-Ponty

Scholars agree that Merleau-Ponty does not have any explicit theory of sexual difference, and he has been critiqued for this neglect. For example, Judith Butler (1989, 95), Jeffner Allen (1982–1983, 245), Shannon Sullivan (1997, 2001), and Beata Stawarska (2006, 103–104) raise a number of important concerns. First among them is that Merleau-Ponty has no explicit theory of sexual difference. While this may be true, Merleau-Ponty does not consider all bodies to be the same. Critics mistake his theory of anonymity for universality. Sex and gender will *necessarily* be a factor in embodied experience because Merleau-Ponty argues that the body is always situated within a biological, social, and historical context, even in its anonymous mode. The second major concern of Merleau-Ponty's feminist detractors is that he denies alterity. However, reading Merleau-Ponty on his own terms, we think it is clear that his critics underestimate the importance of alterity to his philosophy.

In fact, Merleau-Ponty's work has tremendous feminist potential. Throughout *The Structure of Behavior* and *Phenomenology of Perception* he demonstrates great interest in bodily differences. His insightful remarks on pregnancy in his lectures on child psychology and pedagogy are good evidence for a specific interest in female embodiment. And, many feminists have found that Merleau-Ponty contributes useful resources for thinking about sexual difference, especially some helpful theoretical groundwork for thinking about women's embodied experience.[2] Furthermore, Merleau-Ponty's work describes an *ambiguous* intersubjectivity that also makes sense of alterity. The prereflective sense of unity with others does not deny that there is also an écart between self and other. Furthermore, the prereflective experience of continuity does not deny the possibility of alienation. The world still escapes our grasp at times, even as we inhabit it. Although there are disparities of interpretation in the secondary literature on Merleau-Ponty, on the issue of alterity there is primarily a difference in *emphasis*. Some scholars concentrate on Merleau-Ponty as overcoming dichotomy, describing a profound connection between self and other, others focus on the *distinctness* between self and other. Yet Merleau-Ponty finds *both* of these aspects essential. We believe that the communal push provides a vivid example of how this plays out, while offering a valuable illustration of sexual difference and interconnection.

Merleau-Ponty and the Communal

Although shared pushing is an example of prereflective embodied sharing, in keeping with Merleau-Ponty's philosophy of embodied intersubjectivity, it is not an example that argues for a universal connectedness that lacks differentiation. Although the communal push originates in that "common" core shared by all bodies, there are differences between bodily responses to a laboring woman's pushing. If we are really all the same at the pre-personal level, then we could not account for the differences that do exist. Indeed, Merleau-Ponty understands that we do not simply read other bodies as a projection of our own body's intentionality; we do not just see others only as we see ourselves. Although we share embodiment with others, we never share in a way that implies total reversibility; we always remain within our own bodies—there is no possibility of role reversal. Merleau-Ponty writes:

> I enter into a pact with the other, having resolved to live in an interworld in which I accord as much place to others as to myself. But this interworld is still a project of mine, and

it would be hypocritical to pretend that I seek the welfare of another as if it were mine, since this very attachment to another's interest still has its source in me. (1958, 415)

This raises different questions for how communal pushing is to be understood. Is there some breakdown in the boundary between our body and the other's body when we push with them, which can be equally understood as trying to push *for* them, which is impossible in a direct sense? If so, the helpful pusher would seem to be forgetting his or her place in the "interworld."

Nevertheless, the communal push represents support without a complete loss of bodily identity. That is, the body understands it is creating a shared space in which the pushing woman feels that others are focusing with her on the task that is still ultimately hers alone. The fact that the hardest pusher is always the woman herself would lend support to communal pushing being more a *sharing* than a true *transference* or role reversal. But the sharing that occurs includes a "forgetting" of place—a *partial* loss of individuality. Indeed, when people are made aware of the fact that they are pushing with the woman in labor, they generally stop pushing, at least for a time. They resume their expected place in the setting, until the powerful urge to help compels them to join the laboring woman again.

The effect of space and proximity is also an interesting one. A midwife coworker of the second author of this essay, who believes in facilitating communal pushing, told him that she often crowds a non-pushing male partner into the circle of pushers without sharing her motives for doing so. Usually, she reports putting him within a circle of pushers will make him a pusher. Whether this is proximity to the laboring women or an additive effect of being surrounded by other pushers is not clear, but it is clear that the farther one is from the pushing the more likely one is to adopt an attitude of spectator rather than participant. The closing of distance certainly parallels the blending that we believe is occurring at a deeper level—we are trying to give our strength when we push with another. Intimate physical proximity coincides with the merging of bodily intentions, the twinning of muscle groups that increases the laboring woman's expulsive efforts.

The temporality of shared pushing is also telling. In instances of spontaneous communal pushing, the laboring woman sets the pace and timing of pushing—the others follow her and she leads. However, sometimes experienced midwives and obstetricians will intentionally push with a woman to override her pushing rhythms and "reset" her timing, particularly if she has become frantic and ineffectual in her pushing. Then the midwife will, with conscious intent, choose to push in a way that gives herself the lead, and the laboring woman now follows. The other supporters will follow the midwife, and the distinction between unconscious pushing and conscious support has now become blurred as some will just unconsciously follow along unaware of the change, and others will understand what has occurred and will consciously follow the midwife's lead to help with the resynchronization of pushing to a slower, more efficacious pacing. This shows that although shared pushing arises unconsciously, it is often recognized by the people doing it, and once this happens they must make a choice about whether to continue it or not. Furthermore, it can be consciously manipulated by experienced practitioners in ways that are deliberately intended to change the way a woman pushes without having to verbally explain it to her—an approach that is dramatically less effective especially toward the end of labor.

But perhaps the most important question raised by communal pushing is whether or not the communal push aids the woman in labor. That is, is it *really* a communal push—is the apparent bodily intertwining genuine? We assert the laboring woman is genuinely supported to the extent that she perceives herself to be. One woman shared that she had a much easier birth at home than in the hospital, because she felt her family had been inhibited from pushing with her at the hospital but had pushed together with her at home, and that she found the pushing easier because of their support. For Merleau-Ponty (1958, 30), perceptual reality is the ground of all other realities; science and empiricism are secondary truths that begin in perceptual truth. Yet even without Merleau-Ponty's reversal of objective and perceptual reality, it would be ridiculous to argue that a woman who feels support from others around her is not actually being supported. Numerous studies have documented better labor outcomes measured by several variables in women who have better social supports during labor, although none have focused specifically on supportive pushing. It is an unfortunate aside that in the hospital setting shared pushing is often made note of by health professionals in a way that makes light of it and tends to extinguish the behavior. Given its benefits, this is another area where hospitals may be dehumanizing at the deepest possible level—severing connections between caring, loving individuals.

Merleau-Ponty asserts that there is a parallel between the close intertwining of personal consciousness and the anonymous body and the connection between other bodies in the world. Both show reciprocal relatedness but nonidentity. Without the strong example of shared pushing this analogy is seemingly tenuous because the connectedness between bodies would appear far more distant than the connection our reflective consciousness has with our bodies. But to the extent that shared pushing can be seen as an example of bodily connectedness anticipated and explained by Merleau-Ponty's work, we can argue that the connection between bodies more closely fits the model of one's reflective consciousness and one's own body. If this seems to be an overstatement, a reflection on the opacity of our own body to our reflective consciousness may be helpful. Merleau-Ponty (1958, 296) describes the relation as follows:

> There is, therefore, another subject beneath me, for whom a world exists before I am here, and who marks out my place in it. This captive or natural spirit is my body, not the momentary body which is the instrument of my personal choices and which fastens upon this or that world, but the system of anonymous 'functions' which draw every particular focus into a general project.

There is an otherness to our own bodies just as there is an otherness between bodies. Similarly we argue, just as consciousness can actually lose itself in the body, two or more bodies can collaborate in a shared purpose.

Merleau-Ponty's critics are correct about his relative neglect of sexual difference but are wrong to then believe that his work cannot account for this difference, or that this produces an androcentric theory crippled by its inability to recognize sexual and gender differences. Perhaps his failure to convincingly illustrate the complexity of his own theory is partially to blame for controversies among feminists. His examples of shared perception do not suggest the deep level of corporeal intertwining that his philosophy describes. We find that communal pushing better exemplifies the complexity of human intersubjectivity, the way in which interweaving is both ubiquitous and unique, each individual responding differently to the bodily need of another. We are suggesting that this sharing does include the potential for bodies to care for one another in ways that actually *move* us at the prereflective level.

Notes

1. Vaginal birth after cesarean—delivering a baby vaginally after a previous baby was delivered via cesarean section.
2. See, for example, Beauvoir 1952, Young 1990, Bigwood 1991, Grosz 1994, Simms 2006, Wynn 2002, and Heinämaa 2003.

References

Ainsworth, Mary, Mary C. Blehar, Everett Waters, and Sally Wall. 1978. *Patterns of Attachment: A Psychological Study of the Strange Situation*. Hillsdale: Lawrence Erlbaum Associates.

Allen, Jeffner. 1982–1983. "Through the Wild Region: An Essay in Phenomenological Feminism." *Review of Existential Psychology & Psychiatry: Merleau-Ponty and Psychology* 18: 241–256.

Beauvoir, Simone de. 2010. *The Second Sex*. New York: Alfred A. Knopf.

Bigwood, Carol. 1991. "Renaturalizing the Body (with the Help of Merleau-Ponty)." *Hypatia* 6 (3): 54–73.

Butler, Judith. 1989. "Sexual Ideology and Phenomenological Description: A Feminist Critique of Merleau-Ponty's *Phenomenology of Perception*." In *The Thinking Muse: Feminism and Modern French Philosophy*, edited by Jeffner Allen and Iris Marion Young, 85–100. Bloomington: Indiana University Press.

Grosz, Elizabeth. 1994. *Volatile Bodies: Toward a Corporeal Feminism*. Bloomington: Indiana University Press.

Grosz, Elizabeth. 1999. "Merleau-Ponty and Irigaray in the Flesh." In *Merleau-Ponty, Interiority and Exteriority, Psychic Life and the World*, edited by Dorothea Olkowski and James Morley, 145–166. Albany: State University of New York Press.

Heinämaa, Sara. 2003. *Toward a Phenomenology of Sexual Difference: Husserl, Merleau-Ponty, Beauvoir*. Lanham, MD: Rowman & Littlefield.

Hunter, Cindy. 2011. Personal communication.

James, Beverly. 1994. *Handbook for the Treatment of Attachment-Trauma Problems in Children*. New York: Lexington Books.

Karen, Robert. 1994. *Becoming Attached*. Oxford: Oxford University Press, 1994.

Merleau-Ponty, Maurice. 2010. *Child Psychology and Pedagogy: The Sorbonne Lectures 1949–1952*, translated by Talia Welsh. Evanston: Northwestern University Press.

Merleau-Ponty, Maurice. 1958. *Phenomenology of Perception*, translated by Colin Smith. London: Routledge.

Merleau-Ponty, Maurice. 1964. "The Child's Relations with Others," translated by William Cobb. In *The Primacy of Perception*, edited by James M. Edie, 96–155. Evanston: Northwestern University Press.

Merleau-Ponty, Maurice. 1968. *The Visible and the Invisible*, translated by Alphonso Lingis. Evanston: Northwestern University Press.

Merleau-Ponty, Maurice. 2002. *The Structure of Behavior*, translated by Allen Fisher. Pittsburgh: Duquesne University Press.

Simms, Eva-Maria. 2006. "Milk and Flesh: A Phenomenological Reflection on Infancy and Coexistence." *Journal of Phenomenological Psychology* 32 (1): 22–40.

Stawarska, Beata. 2006. "From the Body Proper to Flesh: Merleau-Ponty on Intersubjectivity." In *Feminist Interpretations of Maurice Merleau-Ponty*, edited by Dorothea Olkowski and Gail Weiss, 91–106. University Park: Pennsylvania State University Press.

Sullivan, Shannon. 1997. "Domination and Dialogue in Merleau-Ponty's *Phenomenology of Perception*." *Hypatia* 12 (1): 1–19.

Sullivan, Shannon. 2001. *Living Across and Through Skins*. Bloomington: Indiana University Press.

Wynn, Francine. 2002. "The Early Relationship of Mother and Pre-Infant: Merleau-Ponty and Pregnancy." *Nursing Philosophy* 3: 4–14.

Young, Iris. 1990. *Throwing Like a Girl and Other Essays in Feminist Philosophy and Social Theory*. Bloomington: Indiana University Press.

5

PHENOMENOLOGY, COSMETIC SURGERY, AND COMPLICITY

ERIK MALMQVIST

Consider the following case. Anne is a successful lawyer in her fif-ties, happily married and proud mother of two daughters. How-ever, despite these outer marks of success she has grown increasingly unhappy with her life over the last several years. The reason is her face. It looks so wrinkled and tired, as if it belonged to a much older person or had been worn out by late nights and excessive drink-ing, not at all representative of the healthy and energetic person she is. Recently, a couple of colleagues have dropped casual but deeply hurtful remarks about her apparent age. Her husband is too consider-ate for such remarks, of course, but Anne nonetheless senses that he is reluctant to look at and touch her face in the ways he used to. She is also finding inquisitive glances from strangers increasingly difficult to disregard. These experiences have made her acutely and painfully self-conscious. Her facial appearance keeps occupying her thoughts, and she feels strangely inhibited in social situations that she used to find pleasurable, somehow isolated from strangers and acquaintances alike.

Anne has contemplated a face-lift for some time, but her feminist sympathies have always made her brush aside the idea. However, now the situation has become unbearable. She contacts a well-reputed cos-metic surgery clinic and is scheduled for consultation and, eventually, surgery. The operation goes well. While the recovery is long and pain-ful, Anne feels quite satisfied with the end result. Her face now looks younger, healthier, and more energetic—much more representative of who she really is. Her husband, who has cautiously supported her decision all along, is quite enthusiastic about her new look, and she is delighted to receive flattering comments from friends and colleagues.

Several months after the surgery, Anne has coffee with an old friend—also a feminist—who she has not seen for a long time. She is taken aback by her friend's reaction to her new appearance. The friend is not only surprised by Anne's changed face but also highly critical of her choice to undergo cosmetic surgery. They engage in a heated discussion:

> Friend: I can't believe you had a face-lift! You used to call yourself a feminist!
> Anne: Well, I still do, I think.
> Friend: And yet you caved in to the pressure.
> Anne: You're getting it all wrong! It's not like anybody forced me to have the surgery. And I didn't do it to please my husband or anybody else. It was my own choice, and I did it for myself.
> Friend: But you chose to follow sexist standards of beauty that keep women down and that feminists should fight.
> Anne: I completely agree that standards of female beauty are sexist and bad. But you seem to forget that failing to meet them causes real suffering to real women. We have a right to escape that suffering if we can.
> Friend: Even by making things worse for other women? You're *complicit* with the very standards you reject.
> Anne: It's absurd to hold *me* responsible for society's standards of beauty. Surely, they exist regardless of whether I have surgery or not.

Feminists tend to feel ambivalent about cases of this kind. Some feminist scholars endorse one or more of the criticisms that Anne's friend levels against her choice (Little 1997; Bordo 1998), while oth-ers are more sympathetic toward the points that Anne herself raises in defense (Parker 1993; Davis 1995). Most, however, recognize some truth in both positions. I think that this reflects a tension between two different feminist commitments. On the one hand, feminists seek to criticize oppressive social norms and the individual actions that are shaped by and sustain them. On the other hand, they sympathize with the plight of the women victimized by these norms. Hence the ambivalence. Should feminists celebrate women who seek surgery to escape the burden of dubious standards of female appearance or criticize them for making the burden heavier on others?

I approach this thorny issue by exploring a particular objection that Anne's friend raises, namely, that Anne's choice of cosmetic surgery makes her *complicit* with dubious norms of female beauty. Feminists sometimes frame women's involvement in cosmetic surgery and other beautifying practices in precisely such terms (Little 1997; Bordo 1998). The issue is not only of interest to feminists, however. Analogous concerns about complicity with racist beauty standards arise when Asian Americans request surgery to make their eyes or noses look more European (Kaw 1993), for instance, or when Jews seek to surgically efface their so-called Jewish noses (Elliott 2003). Yet the ethics of complicity with questionable social norms remains largely unexplored, with a few notable exceptions (Little 1997; 1998).[1] What is the basis and nature of such complicity? When and why are people responsible for morally dubious norms when they follow them? Do responsibilities differ from one agent to another and, if so, why?

Note that these questions are not about moral wrongness. In particular, my aim is not to determine whether Anne or others like her should choose cosmetic surgery or not. Rather, I want to explore the concern that accommodating unjust social norms by surgical or other means, whether ultimately right or wrong, involves taking up a morally problematic position vis-à-vis these norms. Even if ethics is about determining how we should act all things considered—a question on which I remain neutral in this chapter—judgments about complicity is but one of several ingredients in such a global assessment; one may well both be complicit *and* do the right thing.

Moral philosophers have begun addressing the broader problem of complicity, of conceptualizing individual responsibility for collective harm. However, I argue that the general frameworks proposed so far are of little use for understanding the specific case of complicity with social norms. I then turn to Maurice Merleau-Ponty's phenomenology in order to outline a better framework for such complicity. Phenomenology is unlikely to resolve the ethical ambivalence surrounding the issue, but it may help us understand it a little better.

The Problem of Complicity

I begin by anticipating an objection to my inquiry. Investigating women's complicity with dubious standards of beauty when they seek cosmetic surgery may seem too much like blaming the victim. It may be argued that critical analyses of cosmetic surgery should instead focus on the individuals or industry that offer it or the sexist social order that makes women want it. I certainly agree that social structures and cosmetic surgeons merit critical scrutiny. However, three tendencies in feminist thinking converge to make the question of women's own responsibility difficult to escape altogether.

First, feminists regard norms of feminine beauty—the norms that women who request cosmetic surgery seek to meet—as morally suspect. The details of their assessments differ, but they agree that these norms oppress women in some way or other. Second, feminists increasingly emphasize that women who fix their appearance (surgically or otherwise) in accordance with such norms are not forced or duped into doing so. Explanations of female beautification in terms of coercion or false consciousness appear to have gone out of fashion (Tong and Lindemann 2006). For instance, Kathy Davis' influential study of cosmetic surgery in the Netherlands makes a strong case for regarding women who choose surgery not as "cultural dopes" but as "active and knowledgeable agents who negotiate their lives in a context where their awareness is partial and the options limited" (Davis 1995, 170). Third, feminists often stress the importance of everyday individual agency to the workings of gender norms. Individuals constantly reproduce and reinforce such norms when they comply with them.[2] Together these tendencies bring individual responsibility into focus. If people actively and knowingly follow oppressive norms and if they thereby help reproducing these norms, it seems that they are in some sense morally responsible for the oppression of others. But, again, how should such responsibility be conceptualized?

The problem is not, in a general form, unique to this context. It arises whenever individuals are implicated in harms or wrongs that come about only through collective agency. How should one make sense of, for instance, the responsibility of an individual car owner for global warming, that of a taxpayer for the unjust wars of her government, or that of a single member of a six-person-strong firing squad for the death of an executed victim? Moral philosophers have tried to answer such questions in terms of either causality (Gardner 2007) or intentions (Kutz 2000). Is either of these strategies capable of making sense of individual responsibility for dubious social norms?

The causal strategy is deeply rooted in commonsense morality. We hesitate to hold people accountable for harms that would have occurred regardless of what they did—that is, when their actions did not make a causal difference to the harmful outcome. The problem is that many collectively brought about harms are causally overdetermined or occur only through a multitude of marginal contributions. The individual marksman makes no difference to the victim's death if five others fire deadly bullets simultaneously. The emission from one car is so small that an individual driver makes no difference to a natural disaster caused by global warming. And since the same is true of each marksman and each driver, nobody seems responsible on causal grounds (Kutz 2000). Individual responsibility for questionable social norms seems equally inexplicable on such grounds. It makes little difference to the existence or pervasiveness of society's standards of feminine beauty whether or not Anne has a face-lift.

In an important book, Christopher Kutz (2000) conceptualizes individual implication in collective harms in terms of intentions rather than causality. He suggests that individuals are accountable for such harms when they intentionally participate in the collective endeavors that cause them. We act as a group when each of us conceives of his or her action as furthering the group's end and there is sufficient overlap between our respective conceptions. Each one is then accountable for the actions of every other group member and for the consequences of our joint project, regardless of whether he or she contributes causally to these actions and consequences. This explains, for instance, why all bomber pilots participating in an area bombing campaign are accountable for the resulting mayhem even if no single pilot makes a difference (a case that Kutz discusses with much insight).

The problem with making sense of complicity with dubious social norms in such terms is that people do not seem engaged in any joint project when they follow these norms. When people fix their appearance in accordance with dominant standards of beauty, for instance, they do so in response to individual predicaments, not as self-identified members of a group. There is no plausible way of conceptualizing Anne's choice of cosmetic surgery as an intentional contribution to a collective end. Yet the confluence of her choice and the choices of countless others uphold standards of appearance that cause women real suffering. The analogous problem arises with respect to complicity with other large and diffuse harms, such as environmental damage (Williams 2002). There is no plausible sense in which individual car owners or air travelers are joined in intentional pursuit of a shared end. Yet what they do together accelerates global warming, causing floods and droughts that shatter the lives of millions.

Aware of the difficulty of extending his model to such "unstructured collective harms," Kutz (2000) introduces the notion of "quasi-participation." While environmental harms are not the results of concerted collective action, he notes, they are brought about by a shared way of life supported by certain values and institutions with their ultimate origin in individual motivation. The driver who chooses his car over cleaner means of transportation takes part in this way of life, endorses these values, and depends on these institutions. This provides some ground for regarding him as accountable for the harmful collective effects of that way of life even in the absence of a fully fledged participatory intention.

The problem with this variety of the intentional approach is that it spreads responsibility too broadly and too indiscriminately. The person who rides her bike to work may not be less committed to individualistic and consumerist values and the institutions that support them than the driver of a fuel guzzling SUV; her choice of vehicle may reflect her economic means, not her values. Yet the two are intuitively not equally implicated in the large-scale harms that an individualistic and consumerist lifestyle causes. Similarly, the fact that dubious social norms are supported by shared institutions and values may help explain why these norms are everyone's concern (a point I shall return to) but not why people's responsibilities for them appear to differ. It does not explain, for instance, why a woman who fixes her appearance surgically seems complicit with oppressive beauty standards in a different way and to a different degree than, on the one hand, a woman who wears makeup and, on the other hand, a cosmetic surgeon who makes a living pandering to these standards.

This rather cursory review suggests that making sense of individual responsibility for dubious social norms might require going beyond models based on causal contribution and intentional participation. In fairness, Kutz's rich book contains material (albeit underdeveloped) for alternative conceptions. He suggests that "[a]gents are accountable not only by virtue of what they have done or caused" but also "in virtue of who they are" and because of what their actions symbolize (Kutz 2000, 190). I attempt to develop an account of complicity with social norms that follows the direction that these remarks indicate. My account relies on themes from Merleau-Ponty's (2002) seminal work, *Phenomenology of Perception*, which I explicate here. The reason why that work looks promising for addressing the problem at hand is that it conceptualizes human agency and social relations in terms of neither causality nor intentions or other mental states.

Merleau-Ponty and the Lived Body

The central theme of *Phenomenology of Perception* is embodiment as the sine qua non of human experience in all its variety. For Merleau-Ponty, we exist as perceiving and acting subjects capable of thought, language, sociality, and emotion only by virtue of inhabiting a body that prereflectively opens up a world of meaning to us.

This view implies a radical break not only with Cartesian mind-body dualism but also with other dominant philosophical and scientific conceptions of the body. My body, Merleau-Ponty argues, is not a mere piece of matter placed alongside other pieces of matter in the objective world of causal relations described by the natural sciences. It is *my* body, as I live it in first-person experience. Correspondingly, the relation that it establishes to the things around me is primarily a relation of meaning, not of cause and effect. In action and perception my body seamlessly aligns its different parts, projecting me into a world structured as a system of possibilities. This world is also irreducibly a *shared* world, always already rendered meaningful by others and infused with cultural and historical significance.

Importantly, the notion that I am my body implies as radical a rethinking of subjectivity as of the body. Against various idealist and transcendental philosophies, Merleau-Ponty stresses the primordial *practical* and *prereflective* layer of human existence. Subjectivity, he suggests, should not be understood as a pure and transparent thinking consciousness separated from and constituting its world. And the world is not primarily an object of thought or a representation. Our capacity for grasping things in thematic reflection presupposes a more immediate prethematic bodily familiarity with the world. As Merleau-Ponty puts it: "Consciousness is not in the first place a matter of 'I think that' but of 'I can'" (2002, 159).

Norms, Incorporation, and Expression

It is useful to think of social norms as working to a large extent on the prereflective yet meaningful bodily layer of human existence and coexistence that Merleau-Ponty explores. More precisely, the influence of such norms can be analyzed in terms of *incorporation* (Malmqvist and Zeiler 2010).

Incorporation is the process by which our bodily grasp on the world is extended and transformed through the appropriation of external objects and technologies. Merleau-Ponty's (2002) well-known illustration is the blind man's stick, which is no longer encountered as a thing among others but is absorbed into the corporeal resources that allow the man to engage the world in perception and action. As such, it expands the space in which he confidently moves about and gives the objects around him a more determinate location and structure. As a correlate of this experiential extension and refinement, the stick itself recedes from attention. In Drew Leder's (1990) useful terminology, incorporated objects are absorbed into the "focal disappearance" that characterizes body parts when they open up a space for action or perception—the absence of the eye from the visual field, for instance, or the disappearance of my hands from explicit attention as I struggle to type a sentence. As extensions of the acting and perceiving body, they become part of that *from* which one attends *to* something else and can as such not simultaneously be attended *to* (Leder 1990).

Acquiring skills and habits involves the same sort of corporeal transformation (Leder 1990; Talero 2006; Crossley 2001). Indeed, habituation can be understood as the temporal element of incorporation—as the sedimentation process whereby activity conceals itself as a bodily past, opening up new experiential possibilities (Malmqvist and Zeiler 2010). Learning how to dance, for instance, initially requires paying close attention to and painstakingly imitating each step my partner or instructor makes. But practice makes such thematization increasingly redundant, allowing me first to shift focus to more complex movements, then to project my attention toward my partner or even further away. I simultaneously acquire the capacity to coordinate my feet, hips, and arms in new ways and a new sense of coordination with my surroundings. I can move to the rhythm without stepping on my partner's feet or bumping into other people, and the dance floor itself takes on an increasingly hospitable feel.

As Merleau-Ponty (2002) points out, these changes are effected neither by explicit thought nor by mechanical responses to stimuli but through practical bodily appropriation.

Many cultural patterns of understanding and behavior, for instance standards of female beauty, can plausibly be thought of as incorporated habits. These patterns are appropriated practically, and continued practice consolidates them within our prereflective bodily being. They are thus taken up into our taken-for-granted view of the world, shaping movements and feelings as well as our perception and judgments of others and ourselves. Conceptualizing the influence of social norms in this way brings out how such norms often elude explicit thought and voluntary control (Malmqvist and Zeiler 2010). Because they form part of the bodily resources *from* which we attend to the things and people around us they rarely present themselves as something to be attended *to*.

While the relationship between social norms and individual experience and action can be elucidated in terms of incorporation, more needs to be said about the intersubjective nature of such norms. The notion of expression is useful here. Merleau-Ponty's (2002) claim that embodied existence is expressive reflects his ambition to move beyond both the subject-object dichotomy and the related radical separation between self and other.

Expression—whether linguistic, artistic, gestural, or other—is not the outer manifestation of some prior inner significance but constitutes significance itself. Speech, for instance, "does not translate ready-made thought, but accomplishes it" (Merleau-Ponty 2002, 207). It follows that the meaning of what others express is not hidden from me within them and, conversely, that I lack privileged access to the meaning of my own expressions. "Faced with an angry or threatening gesture," Merleau-Ponty writes, "I do not see anger or a threatening attitude as a psychic fact hidden behind the gesture, I read anger in it" (2002, 214). The other's anger is immediately present to me, grasped not by any operation of thought but by a form of bodily apprehension.

In short, expression takes place "in a shared space between self and other" (Käll 2009, 78). At the same time, however, the phenomenon of expression transcends both perspectives in different ways (Käll 2009). While the other's anger is immediately accessible to me in her gesture, its first-person quality escapes me; the anger remains *hers* and is thus not fully reducible to its observable manifestation. Conversely, the angry gesture has an independent meaning for me not fixated by the other's feelings or intentions. Finally, the expression transcends us *both* insofar as it is carried forth by its wider social, cultural, and historical resonance. As expression, the body is thus fundamentally ambiguous, not quite possible to pin down from any one perspective.

Insofar as social norms belong to the habitually incorporated, they are also corporeally expressed. An important dimension can thus be added to the previous analysis. Not only do individuals *appropriate* pervasive social norms through prereflective bodily praxis. The same praxis *communicates* these norms to others, constituting them as inter-subjective expressive phenomena.[3] This brings out a further way in which their influence outruns individual attention and control. The meaning of what I express is not mine alone to determine, whether consciously or unconsciously, but may always be carried in unexpected directions by others.

Nothing said so far implies that the influence of deeply entrenched social norms is wholly irresistible or unintelligible. While such norms elude thematization through incorporation, they may conversely emerge as potential objects of reflection and control through *excorporation* (Malmqvist and Zeiler 2010). Incorporated instruments and habits sometimes cease to smoothly and silently extend our bodies into a lived space. This happens, for instance, in Martin Heidegger's (1996) famous example of the hammer.[4] When working properly, the hammer is a transparent medium through which the carpenter unreflectively accesses a complex network of meaning surrounding the construction of a house. But when it breaks, the hammer no longer extends the carpenter's body in such a taken-for-granted way. Instead it stands forth as an obstacle blocking his access to the meaning structure surrounding his activity, making that structure itself explicit as something beyond his reach.

Similarly, my habitually appropriated dance moves may become embarrassingly conspicuous to me through the critical gaze of a spectator, thus failing to silently allow my body to inhabit the dance floor and giving the dance floor itself an intimidating look. Widely shared cultural patterns of behavior may emerge from their usual bodily concealment in the same way. If I travel to a foreign country, my ordinary forms of greeting or politeness may suddenly be brought to my own awareness because they stand out as odd to my hosts, no longer permitting me to fit effortlessly into social life.

A crucial thing to note about such excorporation is its reflective and critical potential. When our habits fail to extend our bodies in their usual ways, they lose their transparency and stand out as something to which we may adopt a certain distance. This provides an opportunity to reflect on, criticize, and resist them. But note also that such opportunities are not created through introspection. Incorporated habits are often too intimate to be grasped by voluntary acts of consciousness. And while individual habits (such as corny dance moves) are often conspicuous enough to be excorporated via the other's gaze, widely shared forms of bodily behavior (such as standards of physical appearance) tend to go unnoticed because they so smoothly conform to what everyone else does and expects. Excorporation then typically happens unexpectedly—much like in the hammer example—taking the form of an unintended breakdown of our shared habits that makes it possible to grasp how these habits shape our experience.

Toward a Phenomenology of Complicity

With this theoretical background in place, let us return to the problem of complicity posed earlier. In an insightful essay on complicity and cosmetic surgery, Margaret Olivia Little (1997, 160) writes: "To be complicitous is to bear some improper relation to the evil of some practice or set of attitudes. Just what relation is it?" I have already suggested that the salient relation between agents and dubious social norms is neither causal nor mediated by intentional participation in collective activities. Little (1997) indicates further possibilities: agents may be complicit with dubious norms by endorsing them and by benefiting from them. There seem to be concerns about complicity that cannot be made sense of in these terms either. Take the case of Anne again. She does not reflectively endorse the beauty standards that make surgery attractive to her; indeed, she rejects them. Nor does she seem to benefit from these standards in the sense Little has in mind: her choice is better described as "alleviating a harm" than as "gaining a benefit" (1997, 160). But Little offers yet another, more promising, suggestion: agents may be complicit with questionable norms by virtue of the meaning of their actions for others. I draw on the notion of norms as incorporated and expressive developed in the previous section to sketch an account of complicity that unpacks and complements that suggestion.

The first thing to note about habitually incorporated norms is that they are much more *intimate* than the causal and intentional models discussed earlier admit. They are not simply some state of affairs that our individual actions make a difference to or that results from the joint projects in which we intentionally participate. As part of our taken-for-granted bodily resources for making sense of the world, they shape our perceptions, thoughts, feelings, and behavior in pervasive ways across a wide range of circumstances. They are, in an important sense, part of who we are. And we are sometimes responsible not only for doing certain things but also for being in certain ways (Kutz 2000; Goldie 2004).

Of course, people are not responsible for *all* aspects of their identities. It seems appropriate to hold somebody responsible for being a cruel person but not for being a forgetful person. The reason, I think, is that cruelty reliably disposes its bearer to respond to people and situations in morally suspect ways.[5] A cruel person does not see somebody's desperation as a reason to offer assistance, but to the contrary, as a reason to withhold it. She does not feel troubled by other people's suffering or humiliation; instead she feels amused. And so on. Forgetfulness is a different sort of trait. A forgetful person may fail to remember to do something that she morally should do—such as visiting a sick and lonely relative—but there is nothing intrinsic or reliable about the connection between the trait and the culpable omission. She may just as likely forget to do something that she should *not* do. Standards of feminine beauty are more like cruelty in this respect (although they differ from cruelty in other respects). Internalizing these standards makes people reliably disposed to different morally suspect responses in a wide range of situations. It makes people feel disgust or contempt at the sight of a woman's nonconforming appearance, perceiving it as a reason to pass judgment on her character. It makes women feel shame or embarrassment at their own perceived defects, seeing them as something to be hidden or effaced, perhaps through expensive and risky surgery. Like cruelty but unlike forgetfulness, the disposition to respond in these ways is a trait for which one is responsible.

So one way to be complicit with a questionable social norm is to have made that norm one's own, part of who one is. Call this *complicity on grounds of identity*. One way to interpret Anne's friend's criticism, then, is as a complaint that Anne has, however reluctantly, appropriated society's oppressive beauty standards as the standards by which she judges herself. But this is not the whole story of complicity. It still needs to be explained why people who follow norms without having appropriated them as their own may also be complicit with them. Anne may well respond to her friend that she did not fix her appearance in accordance with society's standards of beauty because she judges herself by these standards but exclusively in order to avoid being so judged by others. If this is true, she is not complicit in the sense that I have outlined, but her friend may insist that she is complicit nonetheless.

Here it is important to recall the expressive nature of many social norms. The meaning of what people do when they follow these norms does not simply flow from their individual psychologies. Rather, it is constituted in an irreducibly intersubjective setting where it is shaped in different ways by other people's interpretations and larger social, cultural, and historical currents. This implies that an innocent motive does not fully exempt one from responsibility when one acts in compliance with a dubious norm. "Our responsibilities outstrip our intentions and desires," as Little (1997, 162) aptly notes. One's action may end up reinforcing and legitimizing the norm whether or not one intends or wants it to. So even if Anne truthfully claims not to have made society's beauty standards her own, she may still be implicated in them by virtue of what her choice of surgery means in the eyes of others. Call this *complicity on grounds of expressivity*.

A crucial but perhaps surprising feature of this form of complicity is that it extends not only to agents themselves. If a person's action reinforces or legitimizes a dubious norm partly because of other people's interpretations, these other people carry some responsibility for that reinforcement or legitimization as well. Part of the reason why questions about complicity with unjust norms are disturbing, I think, is that such complicity is irreducibly a widely shared phenomenon. Most of us are implicated in some way or other.

More remains to be said about degrees and nuances of complicity. My account so far implies that everyone who has internalized a questionable norm is responsible for it on grounds of identity and that everyone who takes part in the social interplay where its meaning is constituted is responsible on grounds of expressivity. I think that this is right, in a weak sense of the term "responsible"; the deeply

collective nature of the problem cannot be stressed too much. However, I also think that people's responsibilities for dubious norms differ a lot depending on their position vis-à-vis those norms and on
how they relate and respond to them. We should be able to explain,
for instance, what makes Anne different from a woman who complies
with beauty norms by wearing makeup or from a cosmetic surgeon
who makes money by tapping into women's anxiousness to live up
to these norms.

Justice is probably part of the story. Roughly speaking, the worse
off somebody is because of an unjust system of norms, the less implicated in that system are we likely to think she is when she participates
in it in order to improve her situation. On the one end of the spectrum here is somebody who—like Anne and arguably like the typical cosmetic surgery patient (Davis 1995)—seeks surgery as the only
way out of what is perceived as an unbearable situation. On the other
extreme is someone who is already privileged by the system in which
she participates—think of an already well-off surgeon who exploits
women's anxieties about their bodies to become even wealthier.

Justice aside, complicity on grounds of identity admits of nuances
and degrees. A questionable social norm can be more or less "one's
own," just like a character trait can be more or less one's own. More
specifically, it can be a more or less "robust" (Goldie 2004) part of
a person's outlook, shaping her perceptual, emotional, and behav-
ioral responses to things and people with more or less predictability
and across a narrower or wider range of circumstances. How implicated she is varies accordingly. A person who orients her everyday
life around dominant beauty standards—who meticulously monitors
and adjusts her appearance in every way in order to meet them, feels
terrible whenever she falls short of what they demand, never fails to
measure others against them, and so on—seems more deeply implicated in these standards than a person for whom they play a minor
role on special occasions.

Further, a dubious norm can be one's own in different ways
depending on if and how one reflectively relates to it. As incorporated, social norms tend to shape our experience in ways that elude
reflective consciousness. But while one cannot grasp or control each
single way such a norm manifests itself, one may be generally aware
of, and take different stances toward, its place in one's worldview. The
contours of complicity differ accordingly. Altering the case of Anne

in various ways helps to bring out some important nuances here. In the original case, if society's beauty standards are at all Anne's own—we have seen that they need not be—they are so in a rather weak sense; she recognizes and regrets their hold on her. Now suppose instead that Anne was not aware of being influenced by these standards but followed them completely unreflectively. Or suppose that she was aware of their influence on her but was indifferent toward rather than critical of them. Or suppose again that she reflectively endorsed them, welcoming them both as part of her own motivational structure and as socially shared ideals. In each alternative case the standards would be hers in a different sense than in the original one; what is more, they would be hers in a *stronger* sense, especially in the last case, thus implicating her more deeply.

The expressive meaning of people's actions when they follow dubious social norms also admits of large variation, implicating them in different ways and to different degrees. One reason why seeking surgery seems to be a more problematic way of accommodating beauty standards than dressing up or wearing makeup is the greater willingness to bear risks and inconveniences that one indicates. The message is that living up to these standards must be worth all the trouble. Further, what people communicate through their actions depends on their social position and status. The involvement of medical professionals in beautification practices is especially problematic in this regard. The norms that drive these practices are very easily perceived as sanctioned by one of society's most respected institutions (Little 1998). Similarly, one potential concern about celebrities who choose to fix their looks surgically is that their influence helps elevate the norms motivating their choice.[6]

Also, the expressive significance of a single action may vary considerably depending on one's other actions and commitments. As Little (1997) points out, a woman's choice of cosmetic surgery is much less likely to express support for society's standards of appearance if she actively fights these standards elsewhere. So even though complicity on grounds of expressivity is determined by other people's interpretations of one's actions, it is not completely inescapable or arbitrary because these interpretations are not themselves completely beyond one's influence.

An important upshot of all this is that there is some scope for individually negotiating the danger of becoming complicit with dubious social norms. However, and even more importantly, in view of the near-ubiquitous nature of such complicity, the most promising responses are likely to be collective rather than individual. One is implicated in the reinforcement and legitimization of social norms partly through other people; conversely, as my earlier remarks on excorporation suggest, the gaze of another may provide a rare opportunity to reflectively grasp a norm and resist participating in its reproduction. Complicity is more easily avoided where there is a certain sort of shared circumspection about the unspoken social meanings of our actions, a preparedness not to take what oneself and others do at face value. In that sort of environment one is less likely to unreflectively appropriate unjust norms and one's actions are less prone to endorsing them in other people's eyes. Cultivating such circumspection on a societal level is surely a slow and arduous process, but it has been and continues to be an important part of the feminist project as I understand it.[7]

Conclusion

I end by returning to the feminist ambivalence that I noted at the outset. Feminists should want to side with the people who suffer the most from unjust social norms while maintaining a critical view on how these people themselves help to shape these norms. My remarks on complicity might seem to tend too much toward the critical side, but they are reconcilable with a sympathetic stance. I have suggested that a person who escapes the suffering that an unjust social norm causes by accommodating that norm—for instance by surgically fixing her looks—may not be able to avoid responsibility for it. She may but need not have appropriated that norm as part of her own embodied, evaluative outlook; in either case, the expressive meaning of her choice is likely to lend the norm legitimacy. But the responsibility in question is fundamentally a shared one, and it will often weigh more heavily on others than the agent herself. Correspondingly, avoiding or reducing complicity is a shared task. Thus explicated, concerns about complicity are by no means reducible to a desire to blame the victim. Also, it is important to remember that such concerns are just one part of a complex moral picture. Keeping one's hands clean is hardly an absolute duty, and it may be relatively unimportant in a context where deep suffering is at stake.

Notes

1. More general questions about complicity are certainly not new to feminist thought. For instance, Christina Thürmer-Rohr (1991) argues that women are deeply implicated in the essentially patriarchal historical trajectory that has brought humanity to the brink of nuclear apocalypse. I set aside such very broad questions about complicity to be able to focus on the much narrower problem of complicity with specific social norms.

2. This is one element of Judith Butler's (1990) theory of performativity, for instance.

3. In Sara Ahmed's (2006) terms: incorporation-expression creates and reproduces collective "lines" that "orientate" our bodies in certain ways and toward certain things.

4. Heidegger himself does not mention the body in this passage, but others have linked his example to an analysis of embodiment (Leder 1990; Ahmed 2006; Malmqvist and Zeiler 2010).

5. I am inspired here by Peter Goldie's (2004) suggestion that we are only responsible for personality traits that are "reason-responsive," that is, traits that reliably dispose people to act on morally good or bad reasons. However, I think that the responsiveness that makes traits objects of moral evaluation includes not only sensitivity to reasons for action but also emotional and perceptual aspects not directly action related.

6. I do not want to overemphasize this point. Some celebrities' uses of cosmetic surgery have arguably been spectacular (indeed strange) enough to have an excorporating rather than legitimizing effect on ordinary beauty standards.

7. However, the hold of unjust norms cannot be reduced through long-term, deliberate efforts alone. Because of the bodily taken-for-grantedness of many such norms, critique and change often presuppose their sudden and unexpected excorporation (Malmqvist and Zeiler 2010).

References

Ahmed, Sara. 2006. *Queer Phenomenology: Orientations, Objects, Others.* Durham, NC: Duke University Press.

Bordo, Susan. 1998. "*Braveheart, Babe,* and the Contemporary Body." In *Enhancing Human Traits: Ethical and Social Implications,* edited by

Erik Parens, 189–221. Washington, DC: Georgetown University Press.

Butler, Judith. 1990. *Gender Trouble: Feminism and the Subversion of Identity*. New York: Routledge.

Crossley, Nick. 2001. "The Phenomenological Habitus and Its Construction." *Theory and Society* 30 (1): 81–120.

Davis, Kathy. 1995. *Reshaping the Female Body: The Dilemma of Cosmetic Surgery*. New York: Routledge.

Elliott, Carl. 2003. *Better Than Well: American Medicine Meets the American Dream*. New York: Norton.

Gardner, John. 2007. "Complicity and Causality." *Criminal Law and Philosophy* 1 (2): 127–141.

Goldie, Peter. 2004. *On Personality*. London: Routledge.

Heidegger, Martin. 1996. *Being and Time*, translated by Joan Stambaugh. Albany: State University of New York Press.

Käll, Lisa Folkmarson. 2009. "Expression between Self and Other." *Idealistic Studies* 39 (1–3): 71–86.

Kaw, Eugenia. 1993. "Medicalization of Racial Features: Asian American Women and Cosmetic Surgery." *Medical Anthropology Quarterly* 7 (1): 74–89.

Kutz, Christopher. 2000. *Complicity: Ethics and Law for a Collective Age*. Cambridge: Cambridge University Press.

Leder, Drew. 1990. *The Absent Body*. Chicago: University of Chicago Press.

Little, Margaret Olivia. 1997. "Suspect Norms of Appearance and the Ethics of Complicity." In *In the Eye of the Beholder: Ethics and Medical Change of Appearance*, edited by Inez de Beaufort, Medard Hilhorst, and Søren Holm, 151–167. Oslo: Scandinavian University Press.

Little, Margaret Olivia. 1998. "Cosmetic Surgery, Suspect Norms, and the Ethics of Complicity." In *Enhancing Human Traits: Ethical and Social Implications*, edited by Erik Parens, 162–176. Washington, DC: Georgetown University Press.

Malmqvist, Erik, and Kristin Zeiler. 2010. "Cultural Norms, the Phenomenology of Incorporation, and the Experience of Having a Child Born with Ambiguous Sex." *Social Theory and Practice* 36 (1): 133–156.

Merleau-Ponty, Maurice. 2002. *Phenomenology of Perception*, translated by Colin Smith. London: Routledge.

Parker, Lisa S. 1993. "Social Justice, Federal Paternalism, and Feminism: Breast Implants in the Cultural Context of Female Beauty." *Kennedy Institute of Ethics Journal* 3 (1): 57–76.

Talero, Maria. 2006. "Merleau-Ponty and the Bodily Subject of Learning." *International Philosophical Quarterly* 46 (2): 191–203.

Thürmer-Rohr, Christina. 1991. *Vagabonding: Feminist Thinking Cut Loose*, translated by Lise Weil. Boston, MA: Beacon Press.

Tong, Rosemarie, and Hilde Lindemann. 2006. "Beauty under the Knife: A Feminist Appraisal of Cosmetic Surgery." In *Cutting to the Core: Exploring the Ethics of Contested Surgeries*, edited by David Benatar, 183–193. Lanham, MD: Rowman & Littlefield.

Williams, Garrath. 2002. "'No Participation without Implication': Understanding the Wrongs We Do Together." *Res Publica* 8 (2): 201–210.

6

UNCOSMETIC SURGERIES IN AN AGE OF NORMATIVITY

GAIL WEISS

A Visit to the Dentist

I would like to begin with an anecdote from a rather unlikely setting, namely, a pediatric orthodontist's office in the United States
(Arlington, Virginia) where I spent a morning in the spring of 2011
with my son Simon, who had an appointment for what we were
told would be "minor dental surgery." Simon and his twin Colin had
been wearing braces for the previous couple of years, and Simon had
his removed once and for all about a month before this visit. Being
the usual harried working parent, I did not make specific inquiries
regarding this follow-up appointment, aside from clearing my morning schedule so I could be in attendance. I assumed that it involved a
routine post-braces procedure that was part of the standard course of
treatment. And, it turned out, that is exactly what it was, and yet it is
the very *routineness* of the nonmedically necessary, cosmetic surgery
that was performed that bears directly on the topic of this essay.

Wearing braces is itself a form of dental enhancement and so,
perhaps, I should not have been surprised that the orthodontist, Dr.
N., saw his task as not completed with the removal of the braces
but rather only finished once the teeth were as perfect as he and his
colleague, Dr. G, could make them. As background, Simon and his

brother Colin are missing their lateral incisors, the two upper teeth adjacent to the two front teeth and, based on the actual configuration of their teeth at an initial visit, Dr. N. recommended opposite forms of orthodontic treatment. Colin's braces have made the empty spaces even wider to accommodate the teeth implants he will eventually receive to replace the missing lateral incisors. Simon's braces closed the space between the missing teeth, hiding the fact that there are two less upper teeth in his mouth than there are supposed to be. His canine teeth have slid into the spot where his lateral incisors should have been and the rest of his upper teeth have been repositioned accordingly. To a layperson, the braces seemed to do the job just fine. There are no longer any extra spaces between Simon's perfectly aligned, upper front teeth, and you would have to have him open his mouth and count the teeth to know that any of them are missing. But to the orthodontist, it was crucial that the missing teeth look like they *were actually there*, and so the dental surgery Simon had performed was intended to make the two canine teeth take on the lateral incisors' physical appearance and not just their function. More specifically, this involved reshaping his two canine or cuspid teeth so that they would *visually* resemble the missing lateral incisors.

The routineness of the surgery was marked by the fact that we were never explicitly asked if we wanted to have the extra bonding and chiseling done to Simon's canine teeth to "transform them" into lateral incisors. No special permission forms were signed by us ahead of time, though the one-page handout we were given in advance, informing us that Simon shouldn't eat or drink for four hours before the scheduled surgery, briefly mentioned that insurance would cover everything but the nitrous oxide required to sedate Simon for the procedure. Despite the lack of advance information regarding exactly *what* was going to be done during the surgery and *why* it was being done, Dr. G., the pediatric orthodontist who did the dental surgery, did carefully explain what she was doing *as* she was doing it. The constant flow of information she provided, coupled with her warm, patient, and reassuring manner, were extremely effective in lulling any underlying anxiety either my son or I had about the procedure. I was abruptly jolted out of my complacency, however, by an offhand comment Dr. G. made as she was putting the finishing touches on his teeth, a comment that was totally lost upon my fourteen-year-old semi-conscious son reclining passively in the chair. Briefly interrupting her chiseling, Dr. G. suddenly looked over at me, cheerfully proclaiming: "square teeth are masculine and rounded teeth are feminine, so I am going to "man him up a little bit, ok?" The pride she took in her craft was unmistakable from her tone, but so too, were the gender presuppositions embodied in her words. Simon's soon-to-be squared teeth were like the icing on the cake, the final *pièce de résistance* that would subtly reinforce his masculinity every time he opened his mouth, without, I should add, most laypeople ever even realizing that this was being done. Indeed, by supplying me with this information, I felt like Dr. G. had just admitted me into a club of initiates, offering me knowledge from the dental world that was not readily available to those of us who occupy what Thomas Mann, in his bildungsroman *The Magic Mountain*, famously referred to as "the flatlands." Dr. G. did not know that my teaching and research centrally engages issues of gender, and so she had no idea that I found her casual comment to be absolutely stunning. Wow, I thought, here in this basement dental office Dr. G has just offered me, on a silver platter, not one of the gleaming instruments beneath her hand, ready to be put to work to complete the masculinization of my son's insufficiently gendered teeth, but the perfect opening for this essay.

The Three Ns: The Natural, the Normal, and the Normative

> It might be worthwhile, sometimes, to inquire what Nature is, and how men work to change her, and whether, in the enforced distortions so produced, it is not natural to be unnatural.
>
> —Charles Dickens, *Dombey and Son*

Dickens introduces this provocative remark in the midst of a description of the unnatural rigidity of personality that marks his title character, the wealthy businessman, Paul Dombey. Indeed, it is the very unnaturalness of Mr. Dombey's allegedly "natural" disposition that leads Dickens' omniscient narrator to question whether "it is not natural to be unnatural." "Alas!" the narrator continues, "are there so few things in the world about us, most unnatural, and yet most natural in being so?" (Dickens 2001, 684). The answer, it becomes clear, is a resounding "no." Indeed there turn out to be a plethora of both human and nonhuman phenomena that are "most unnatural and yet most natural in being so." More generally, Dickens challenges us to acknowledge that the unnatural can as readily be natural as the natural can be unnatural. By demonstrating their perverse interchangeability in so many of his characters, including his protagonist Paul Dombey, Dickens effectively deconstructs false presuppositions about what counts as natural and what counts as unnatural behavior.

This essay takes up Dickens' call to reexamine the "naturalness of the unnatural" and the "unnaturalness of the natural" through an inquiry into contemporary rhetorics of bodily enhancement. While substantial attention has been paid by scholars to the high demand for cosmetic plastic surgery procedures, most of which, in one way or another, promise to offer the client a more youthful, more attractive,[1] and, ultimately, more "normal" appearance, much less attention has been paid to the growing countermovement that embraces the same new medical technologies but seeks to use them to transform normative bodies in nonnormative ways,[2] that is, to produce what are commonly regarded as ugly, monstrous, and/or abnormal bodies.[3] Though it might be tempting to claim that these latter, "uncosmetic" surgeries are completely opposed in intention and kind to "cosmetic" surgeries, both appeal to notions of naturalness and normality and both utilize rhetorics of *enhancement* that require further exploration in their own right.

Cosmetic surgeries, no less than uncosmetic surgeries, alter accepted notions of normalcy and naturalness; both reveal how the very concepts of the normal and the natural are historically, socially, and increasingly medically constructed. As soon as both surgical and nonsurgical body modifications become culturally sanctioned possibilities,[4] the very distinction between the "normal" and the "abnormal" body, if it ever seemed clear to begin with, becomes irrevocably blurred. And, with respect to how this alters our view of Nature, Kathy Davis observes that with the rise of plastic surgery, the notion of Nature-as-the-ultimate-constraint is replaced by Nature-as-something-to-be-improved-upon. Whereas plastic surgery was formerly aimed at repairing bodily deficiencies that made a person notably different from the rest of the world, it has increasingly come to be seen as a normal intervention for essentially normal bodies. Bodies no longer have to be damaged or impaired to merit surgical alteration. Growing older, gaining or losing weight, or simply failing to meet the transitory cultural norms of beauty are now sufficient cause for surgical improvement. Cosmetic surgery, Davis asserts, allows us to transcend age, ethnicity, and even sex itself (Davis 1995, 18).

Though this is a topic for another investigation, I should note that I am suspicious of Davis' sweeping assertion that cosmetic surgery produces bodies that transcend age, ethnicity, and even sex itself. Her claim is rendered even more problematic by an accompanying footnote, where she states that this transcendence is "evidenced by recent strides in sex-change operations—the most radical form of cosmetic surgery," since it is not at all clear to me whether and how post-operative transsexuals transcend sex (Davis 1995, 182). Setting these important issues aside, what I would like to focus on instead is her suggestion that cosmetic surgery has become *normalized* in many contemporary societies. That is, despite the fact that cosmetic surgery attempts to produce a bodily *enhancement*, a quality or ability that body did not have before, such as the replacement of my son Simon's missing lateral incisors with newly reshaped, "appropriately" masculine teeth, these medical technologies have, as Davis notes, simultaneously come to be regarded "as a normal intervention for essentially normal bodies."

Focusing, in particular, on the intricate interconnections among what I call the 3 Ns—the normal, the natural, and the normative— I argue that, paradoxically, rapid *expansions* in medical technologies often function to reinforce and further entrench the *narrowness* of norms, thereby producing ever more restricted views of what counts as normal and natural. In addition, by collapsing the distinction between the real and the ideal, the growing number of "enhancement" surgeries available to the "average" American, European, and Asian consumer leads those individuals who refuse such "improvements" or those who, god forbid, actively seek to modify their bodies in nonnormative ways, to be regarded as not only *aesthetically deficient* but also *morally blameworthy*.

While traditional moral theory tends to concern itself with the normative implications of particular ethical positions, weighing which account offers the most intuitively compelling analysis of how and why human beings should act (or refrain from acting) in specific situations, Michel Foucault, in a Copernican turn prefigured by Nietzsche, emphasizes the various disciplinary mechanisms that societies have historically utilized to present the normative as both *normal* and *natural*. With Foucault, I maintain that ethical (as well as social and political) norms must be understood, first and foremost, as *corporeal* practices that change over time and across cultures; acknowledging this requires, moreover, that we attain a better understanding of why some bodies have historically been seen as making a greater moral claim upon us, insofar as they are regarded as being more normal and more natural than other bodies. More broadly, I would argue, it is precisely when we grasp that normativity, normalization, and naturalization are closely intertwined, fundamentally interdependent temporal, spatial, and embodied processes, that we can better assess their collective impact in shaping not only ethical but also medical, scientific, legal, economic, and religious conceptions of what it means to be human.

By deconstructing attempts to distinguish sharply between cosmetic and uncosmetic surgeries, this essay seeks to demonstrate how changes in accepted understandings of what is normal, natural, and normative reveal and intensify the interdependency of these three phenomena.[5] Although many people might readily agree that that which is viewed as normative by a given society almost always functions as the standard (even if it is acknowledged to be an ideal standard) for normality, there is perhaps less consensus about whether and how conceptions of the natural fit into the picture. If we attempt to separate the 3 Ns conceptually and understand normativity as primarily concerned with providing moral guidelines for how human beings should act in a given situation, normalization as operating in an entirely different sphere to distinguish the normal from the abnormal (often with serious medical and legal implications), and naturalization as a nonmoral process that is best explored scientifically, we end up with unsatisfying, "thin" accounts of very complex phenomena that work together in both visible and not so visible ways to establish the acceptable parameters of individual, social, and political life. My goal, by contrast, is to offer, through the lens of what I am calling "uncosmetic surgeries," a "thick" account of the often invisible yet remarkably pervasive framework normativity, normalization, and naturalization collectively provide for contemporary ethical theorizing and practice.

Drawing not only on Foucault but also on the work of phenomenologists, feminist theorists, critical race theorists, and disability theorists, I would like to call attention to a few of the many complex, yet often invisible ways in which normativity, normalization, and naturalization reinforce one another to produce bodily imperatives that are deemed socially and ethically acceptable.[6] With respect to nonnormative and even antinormative plastic surgeries, I argue that the simultaneous fascination and repulsion that accompanies these transgressive corporeal transformations is morally instructive, not least because these competing reactions express conflicting normative concerns about both the possibilities and the limits of embodied agency. These "uncosmetic" surgeries defy traditional views of surgery (i.e., to repair what is damaged) as well as culturally sanctioned standards of physical beauty, where the latter are viewed as something that we should all be striving to attain to the best of our abilities by maximization of our "god-given" or, increasingly, surgically enhanced, biological and genetic "assets." A central claim I am making is that these nonnormative surgeries, through the moral and aesthetic repulsion they induce, as well as the widespread social, political, and medical opposition they create, reveal the intensity of our corporeal, psychological, normative, and economic investments in the bodily enhancements our society defines as "normal."

The very distinction between cosmetic and uncosmetic surgeries clearly varies from one culture and time period to another (e.g., opposing views of female genital "cutting" is a contemporary case in point); indeed, sometimes the very same bodily transformation can be interpreted as enhancing one's normality in one cultural context while rendering one more abnormal in another. Significantly, to the extent that an individual's body is viewed as violating accepted norms, whether deliberately (e.g., through voluntarily sought out nonnormative body modifications) or through an unfortunate injury or accident, the response is often the same: that individual becomes a target of aesthetic and moral disapprobation, even if this is mixed with outrage in the former case or pity in the latter. Not uncommonly, social, political, and economic discrimination follows.

In order for these latter issues to be effectively addressed, however, we first need to arrive at a clearer understanding of the notion of enhancement itself; more specifically, we need to tease out some of the problematic, taken-for-granted assumptions that underlie what I call the "rhetorics of enhancement," discourses of corporeal perfection that permeate not only medical and popular literature regarding cosmetic surgery but also much of the work being done by contemporary analytic bioethicists on this topic. This, I believe, is a task that can best be performed through a phenomenological method of description, albeit one that is attuned, as Husserl's own phenomenology was not, to the complicated and intersecting roles gender,

race, class, age, ethnicity, nationality, and ability all play in determining both *how* a given phenomenon appears as well as the *meaning* of
its appearance.

Rhetorics of Enhancement in Contemporary Bioethics

In their introduction to a 2009 anthology entitled *Human Enhancement* that contains essays by several leading bioethicists and ethicists,
the coeditors, Julian Savulescu and Nick Bostrom, after duly noting
the vagueness of the very concept of enhancement, identify two challenges that they assert must be met satisfactorily for the term to be
morally useful. "First," they claim, "some account needs to be given
of what counts as an enhancement—an account that must be reason-
ably intelligible and non-arbitrary, capturing something that might
plausibly be thought of as a kind. Second, given such an account,
it needs to be shown that it tracks a morally relevant distinction"
(Savulescu and Bostrom 2009, 3). Savulescu and Bostrom next raise
a series of questions regarding several "contextual variables" that they
feel must be acknowledged and addressed to meet these two conditions: "Precisely what capacity is being enhanced in what ways? Who
has access? Who makes the decisions? Within what cultural and sociopolitical context? At what cost to competing priorities? With what
externalities?" (2009, 3). That they view these to be essential, moral
questions rather than contingent policy matters that can be safely set
aside until enhancement regulations are being implemented is reinforced by their insistence that "[j]ustifiable ethical verdicts may only
be attainable following a specification of these and other similarly
contextual variables" (Savulescu and Bostrom 2009, 3). Though these
questions themselves warrant further attention in their own right, I
am especially interested in the inference Savulescu and Bostrom draw
from the claim that these "contextual variables" must be included in
an account of the moral status of specific human enhancement procedures. "To accept this conclusion," they tell us, "is to accept a kind
of *normalization* of enhancement" (Savulescu and Bostrom 2009, 3–4).
Their point is that even asking, much less answering these questions
presupposes that bodily enhancement itself is a normal, and therefore,
acceptable goal for an individual (or even a society) to wish to pursue.
But is it? And if it is, what counts and fails to count as an enhancement in the first place?

While surgical "enhancements" may hold out the promise of
normalcy to those who are able and willing to pay the price, the
extraordinary medical and financial measures needed to realize this
promise make the normalization of enhancement, at a practical level
at least, an illusory fiction for most people in the world today. Moreover, even to talk about the normalization of enhancement requires
that we specify not only what we mean by enhancement but also
what we mean by normalization. Though it may seem obvious to
those of us who are theorists of embodiment that our bodies are
both normalizing and normalized, that is, constitutive of norms that
define normalcy and constituted by them, it is also evident that the
failure to live up to specific bodily norms for one's gender, race, class,
ethnicity, religion, age, and physical and cognitive ability consolidates
and reinforces these norms as much, if not more than, cases where
an individual satisfactorily upholds them. Uncosmetic surgeries, I
would argue, are a perfect case in point. Before one can critically
assess the normative presuppositions that are violated through specific
uncosmetic surgeries, however, it is necessary to respond to Savulescu
and Bostrom's challenge to provide an intelligible and nonarbitrary
account of what counts as an enhancement. This seems like an especially crucial task, moreover, precisely because many uncosmetic surgeries *are* often viewed as enhancements by those who seek them.
Indeed, it is readily evident that whether a particular plastic surgery is
viewed as cosmetic or uncosmetic is most often assessed through the
gaze of the beholder. To complicate matters further, there are not one
but many beholders. These latter include: 1) the doctors who perform
or assist with the procedure; 2) the patient her-/himself; 3) in the case
of minors, the parents or guardians who gave permission for the surgery; and 4) extended family, friends, colleagues, casual acquaintances,
and even strangers who bear witness to the procedure's transformative effects. In addition, I am arguing, these corporeal alterations are
never simply of aesthetic significance but also have specific psychological, economic, and moral effects that reverberate far beyond the
patient herself, reifying cultural norms even and precisely when these
latter are being defied by the patient and/or by the procedure.

Returning to the question of what should and should not be
considered an enhancement, we would seem to have a plethora of
resources to consult since contemporary literature on enhancement
has exploded in the late twentieth and early twenty-first centuries.
In many ways, this literature has been playing a "catch-up" role as it

vainly seeks to address the burgeoning number of thorny ethical issues arising out of the rapid development of new biotechnologies directed not only toward existing bodies but also to future bodies through increased opportunities for pre- and post-embryonic genetic modification. With too few exceptions, current debates about the possible uses and abuses of enhancement technologies have been dominated by analytic philosophers. Savulescu and Bostrom's groundbreaking 2009 anthology is a perfect example of this trend. Though the anthology includes some cross-cultural (primarily Asian) perspectives to balance out its strong Anglo and Anglo-American orientation, most of the contributors are well-known, contemporary analytic moral philosophers whose essays attempt to provide clear parameters to distinguish morally acceptable from unacceptable enhancement procedures. This is, no doubt, extremely important work and yet, the underlying, nagging question of what, exactly, counts as an enhancement and who decides remains, for the most part, unacknowledged and therefore untheorized. Instead, the common assumption in the majority of essays seems to be that we all "know" what is being referred to when we appeal to the term "enhancement," and thus the important issue is not what an enhancement even is but whether certain types of possible enhancements should or should not be permissible. And, in the case of both permissible and impermissible enhancements, there is a serious policy concern with who should play the regulatory role in allowing some and forbidding others.

Savulescu and Bostrom identify two main camps in the contemporary enhancement debates:

> the transhumanists on one side, who believe that a wide range of enhancements should be developed and that people should be free to use them to transform themselves in quite radical ways; and the bioconservatives on the other, who believe that we should not substantially alter human biology or the human condition. (2009, 1)

There are also, they add, some "miscellaneous groups who try to position themselves in between these poles, as the golden mean" (Savulescu and Bostrom 2009, 2). Bioconservatives, even if united in their opposition to specific enhancement procedures (e.g., genetic enhancements), are forced to draw a line in very murky waters, since, as Savulescu and Bostrom observe, "In one sense, *all* technology can be viewed as an enhancement of our native human capacities, enabling us to achieve certain effects that would otherwise require more effort or be altogether beyond our power" (2009, 2). The examples they provide to support this broadened conception of enhancement are both illuminating and provocative. "Are not" they ask,

> shoes a kind of foot enhancement, clothes an enhancement of our skin? A notepad, similarly, can be viewed as a memory enhancement—it being far from obvious how the fact that a phone number is stored in our pocket instead of our brain is supposed to matter once we abstract from contingent factors such as cost and convenience. (Savulescu and Bostrom 2009, 2)

These examples constitute a *reductio ad absurdum* argument against any hard-and-fast attempt to distinguish mundane, generally noncontroversial technological enhancements that are more or less readily available to the average consumer and that are intended to remedy bodily shortcomings, and, in the process, often accentuate and improve an individual's physical, cognitive, and/or aesthetic characteristics (and we might certainly add eyeglasses, colored contact lenses, hearing aids, and crutches to this list), from medical enhancements that can only be accomplished under the skilled hand of the surgeon or geneticist. While it is certainly plausible to argue on the basis of these types of examples that technologically enabled bodily enhancements themselves fall under a continuum, ranging from the common to the uncommon, from the mundane to the exotic, it nonetheless remains unclear whether a continuum model forecloses the possibility of drawing a morally compelling line between permissible and impermissible enhancements. An additional and, I think, more urgent problem is that a continuum model does not help us to solve the original question of what counts or does not count as an enhancement.

One reason why I believe this latter question so stubbornly resists resolution, whether one is a transhumanist, a bioconservative, or occupies a middle position, is because the analytic proclivities of the majority of ethicists and bioethicists working on these issues are not oriented toward identifying what turn out, upon close inspection, to be some surprisingly problematic presuppositions regarding the meaning of the basic term that underpins the debate, that is "enhancement." Instead, the primary concern seems to be how best to divide up the relevant field of actual and potential enhancements into conceptually and morally distinct categories.[7] A refreshing alternative to this dominant analytic trend that tends to sweep meta-questions about enhancement itself under the rug can readily be found in the work of several contemporary continental body theorists who utilize a variety of methodologies, including phenomenology, genealogy, feminist theory, critical race studies, deconstruction, and critical disability studies, to illuminate the dangers of focusing too heavily on the actual and possible outcomes of a given phenomenon (e.g., the personal, social, and medical *effects* of particular surgical enhancements) rather than seeking to provide a satisfactory, "thick" description of the phenomenon itself.

Rethinking Enhancement

As noted earlier, the question of what counts as an enhancement leads, inevitably, to the question of who gets to decide whether a particular body modification should, or should not, be viewed as an enhancement. In *Tattooed Bodies: Subjectivity, Textuality, Ethics, and Pleasure*, Nikki Sullivan makes the following claim in response to the dramatic shift in significance that an individual who has the letters H A T E inscribed across his knuckles associates with his tattoo, that is equally instructive, I would suggest, for a discussion of enhancements more generally:

> Insofar as the meaning of this tattoo has changed, at least for its bearer, whilst the graphic itself has remained the same, the implication is that tattoos neither contain nor represent a fixed referential reality, or, to put it another way, the relation between signifier and signified is unstable. It demonstrates that the tattoo is not simply reducible to a symbolic representation of the truth of the subject, but rather that the tattoo is inseparable from the subject and can be understood as a process (rather than an object) in and through which the ambiguous and open-ended character of identity and of meaning is constantly (re)negotiated in and through relations with others and with a world. (2001, 19)

By insisting "that tattoos neither contain nor represent a fixed referential reality," that a tattoo does not and cannot represent "the truth of the subject, but rather [. . .] a process in and through which the ambiguous and open-ended character of identity and of meaning is constantly (re)negotiated in and through relations with others and with a world," Sullivan offers us a dynamic model for understanding the complexity of the phenomenon of enhancement (as well as specific enhancement debates!) more generally. Resisting appeals to a "depth" model of the subject to account for the meanings and identities that emerge in and through both normative as well as nonnormative bodily modifications, she focuses outward upon the "systems of power/knowledge [that] constitute the very morphologies and potentialities of bodies" (Sullivan 2001, 72) with the goal, ultimately, of destabilizing these systems (as well as the bodies inscribed by them) to produce "a different economy of bodies and pleasures" (Sullivan 2001, 82).

Rather than viewing such a project as leaving the 3 Ns behind altogether, Sullivan is asking us to rethink the normalcy and naturalness of conventional economies of pleasure according to which specific normative standards are measured and justified. "Tattooed bodies," she suggests, "could be said to tell stories that provide a key to the decipherment of the social and personal significance of embodied being as it is lived in contemporary Western culture, and, at the same time, to articulate 'something else'" (Sullivan 2001, 171). Bearing in mind the indeterminacy of this "something else," which, I would argue, arises out of the tattooed body's surplus of meaning that exceeds and even has the potential to shatter cultural conventions in the very process of inscribing them, she maintains that "the stories they seemingly tell, are duplicitous" (Sullivan 2001, 177). The sources of this duplicitousness, moreover, do not arise solely from the tattooed bodies themselves.

In *Self-Transformations: Foucault, Ethics, and Normalized Bodies*, in the midst of a discussion of François Ewald's account of norms and normalization, Cressida Heyes argues that within the language/system of normalization "there are no absolute standards of good, perfection, or beauty, only relative measures within a local scale of meaning." "And," she tellingly adds, "if they prove inadequate to their assigned task, they can be altered without disloyalty to any deeper truth" (2007, 34). In a later chapter devoted to cosmetic surgery that uses as a case study the incredibly popular "reality TV" show *Extreme Make-over*, Heyes stresses that common rhetorics of enhancement includ-ing "taking charge of one's destiny, becoming the person one always wanted to be, or gaining a body that better represents the moral vir-tues one has developed, are all forms of working on the self within a regime of normalization" (2007, 105). Identifying the promise of that elusive "something else" that can emerge, as Sullivan implies, in the midst of even the most well-established cultural narratives, and contra the quote from Davis I cited earlier, Heyes declares that though it is impossible to transcend or live outside a "regime of normalization," there are nonetheless "practices of working on oneself as an embod-ied subject that refuse the habituated trajectories of normalization and gesture toward an art of living with greater embodied freedom" (2007, 112). Even if one rejects, or is at the very least suspicious of the Foucauldian terms in which Heyes presents this humanistic vision of "greater embodied freedom," the central insight that she, Sullivan, and many others, including Ladelle McWhorter and Margrit Shildrick, are pointing us toward, is that the nonnormative makes its appearance not outside of but at the very heart of the normative, and this is precisely why it has such transformative potential. Whether this "duplicitous story" is being told through McWhorter's examples of gardening and line-dancing in *Bodies and Pleasures: Foucault and the Politics of Normalization*, Heyes' example of yoga in *Self-Transfor-mations*, or even through Sullivan's many examples of tattooed bod-ies, this "something else" that simultaneously evokes and exceeds the normal, the natural, and the normative is precisely what keeps the question of enhancement and the 3 Ns themselves, open to new pos-sibilities and therefore, to new meanings.

Historically, as Shildrick in *Embodying the Monster: Encounters with the Vulnerable Self* and Rosemarie Garland Thomson in *Extraordinary Bodies: Figuring Physical Disability in American Culture and Literature* remind us, there is a widespread and diverse group of what Garland Thomson calls "extraordinary bodies," that is, nonnormative bodies that have been designated as unnatural, abnormal, and "monstrous." With blatant disregard for the crucial "contextual variables" identi-fied by Savulescu and Bostrom that can also include whether they are bodies people are born with, whether they are the product of surgical alteration or less invasive bodily modifications, and whether these bodies' nonnormativity accords with a person's own desires and intentions, their "aberrant corporeality," as Shildrick calls it, serves as the basis for lumping them together and finding them aesthetically, physically, sometimes mentally, and almost always morally "deficient." Precisely because of the undecidability that haunts the question of what is and is not monstrous, the concept of the monstrous, as Shildrick notes, "resist[s] closure of meaning." Calling upon us to view the "fissures, breaks, contradictions, and indeed unexpected continuities in the received meaning of the monstrous" not as "problems to be resolved, but opportunities to reconfigure first impressions," she argues that rationalist attempts to resolve the perennial controversy surrounding the category of the monstrous conceal "a far more complex process of contestation in which a whole range of modernist parameters of knowledge —truth and fiction, self and other, body and mind, inner and outer, normal and abnormal—are at stake" (Shildrick 2002, 27).

These processes of contestation are alive and well, as Heyes reveals through her discussions of weight-loss programs and cosmetic "makeovers," whether the goal is to embody normative, culturally sanctioned bodily ideals, whether one actively pursues body modifications that violate these norms altogether, or even if, as not uncommonly happens, one ends up doing the latter through trying to achieve the former! Returning to my son Simon's recent trip to the dentist, the question of whether or not "masculinized teeth" are indeed an "enhancement" clearly never occurred to Dr. G. Nor did the question of whether or not it is normal, natural, or even desirable to surgically "makeover" canine teeth into lateral incisors especially when the majority of us, who are not dentists, cannot identify the specific differences between them and, equally importantly, do not really care about them.

In order to avoid ceding contemporary debates about enhancement over to the analytic ethicists and bioethicists who are all too happy to keep dominating them, it is crucial that a more phenomenological approach be taken to the question of enhancement (both human and nonhuman), not to resolve the question once and for all, as they seek to do, but, on the contrary, to keep us open to the diverse historical, individual, social, political, economic, aesthetic, and moral meanings that testify to the destabilizing force of that indefinable "something else" that marks the perennial contestability of hard-and-fast distinctions between normative and nonnormative bodies.

Notes

1. It is important to note that youth and beauty are often presented as virtually synonymous in these contexts.
2. Two contemporary feminist cultural theorists, Nikki Sullivan and Margrit Shildrick, are notable exceptions in this regard.
3. These words frequently function synonymously as well, though each has a distinct etymology of its own.
4. And, as Kathy Davis notes, this actually occurred centuries ago; she cites Gabke and Vaubel who claim the first known plastic surgery took place in India in 1000 BC (Davis 1995, 14).
5. This essay forms part of a larger project, a monograph provisionally entitled *Normalizing Bodies*, that builds upon yet moves beyond Foucault's analysis of bodily disciplinarity by focusing on how specific racial, sexual, ethnic, able-bodied, and class differences have served to mark particular bodies as morally unworthy, aesthetically distasteful, and scientifically suspect.
6. The concept of a bodily imperative is introduced and discussed in depth in chapter 7 of my 1999 book *Body Images: Embodiment as Intercorporeality*.
7. Indeed, Savulescu's most recent coedited volume, *Enhancing Human Capacities* (Savulescu, Meulen, and Kahane 2011), attempts to remedy the lack of specificity regarding the notion of enhancement in this earlier volume with separate sections devoted to different types of enhancement including: cognitive enhancement, mood enhancement, physical enhancement, lifespan extension, and moral enhancement.

References

Davis, Kathy. 1995. *Reshaping the Female Body: The Dilemma of Cosmetic Surgery*. New York: Routledge.

Dickens, Charles. 2001. *Dombey and Son*, edited by Alan Horsman. Oxford: Oxford University Press.

Garland Thomson, Rosemarie. 1997. *Extraordinary Bodies: Figuring Physical Disability in American Culture and Literature*. New York: Columbia University Press.

Heyes, Cressida. 2007. *Self-Transformations: Foucault, Ethics, and Normalized Bodies*. Oxford: Oxford University Press.

McWhorter, Ladelle. 1999. *Bodies and Pleasures: Foucault and the Politics of Normalization.* Bloomington: Indiana University Press.

Savulescu, Julian, and Nick Bostrom. 2009. *Human Enhancement.* Oxford: Oxford University Press.

Savulescu, Julian, Ruud ter Meulen, and Guy Kahane. 2011. *Enhancing Human Capacities.* Oxford: Wiley Blackwell.

Shildrick, Margrit. 2002. *Embodying the Monster: Encounters with the Vulnerable Self.* London: Sage.

Sullivan, Nikki. 2001. *Tattooed Bodies: Subjectivity, Textuality, Ethics, and Pleasure.* Westport: Praeger.

Weiss, Gail. 1999. *Body Images: Embodiment as Intercorporeality.* New York: Routledge.

7

"BIID"?

Queer (Dis)Orientations and the Phenomenology of "Home"

NIKKI SULLIVAN

Over the last decade or so there has been increasing interest in the desire for the amputation of a healthy limb or limbs. Such desires, once held to be paraphilic, are now largely taken to be symptomatic of what psychiatrist Michael First calls Body Integrity Identity Disorder (BIID). As this diagnostic term suggests, the disorder thus named, is characterized primarily by a lack of bodily integrity, of a sense of wholeness. Indeed, those experiencing such desires often describe a feeling of disjunction between the selves they are and the bodies they have, and as a result, BIID is regularly posited as analogous to so-called Gender Identity Disorder (GID). The psychiatric construction of these experiences as "disordered" engenders a number of biopolitical effects that this chapter sets out to challenge. First, the lack of integrity felt by those desiring "nonnormative" morphologies is constituted as "disordered": the implication being that the bodies of these individuals are obviously "whole" and yet for some reason they fail to experience their corporeality as such. Second, wholeness is constituted not only as visibly self-evident, but more particularly, as the natural (and therefore ideal) bodily-state that all those who are not disordered simply have. Third, insofar as integrity is taken as fundamental to humanness, then the aim of medicine is to restore the ideal state that has been lost or compromised or is unable to be experienced as such. In short, then, BIID is constituted as an individual(ized) pathology that has little or nothing to do with one's being-in-the-world.

Rather than reproducing these ontological assumptions and the material effects they produce by debating who should have access to what forms of medical intervention and on what basis, this chapter takes a deconstructive approach to BIID, mapping the phenomenological effects of such nomenclature while simultaneously problematizing its presumed empirical status. In short, I wish to demonstrate that BIID is less the description of an empirical reality than a biopolitical somatechnology; one that establishes and polices boundaries and borders between "us" and "them," between proper and improper bodies—both individual and social—and evaluates their worth in terms that replicate (and naturalize) dominant idea(l)s about bodies, selves, and the relations between them.

In order to queer the somatechnics of abjection at work in and through BIID, I want to reorient debates about the desire(s) for amputation, and other forms of "nonnormative" embodiment, away from the question of integrity with which such debates are primarily concerned and toward a consideration of "orientation." The reason for this, as I explain in more detail later, is twofold. First, the focus on integrity is almost entirely confined to the figure of the person who suffers and does not include an analysis of those who evaluate the alleged lack of integrity and make clinical decisions—or, in the case of a more general public, moral judgments—on the basis of their perception of the "other" who suffers.[1] Second, and relatedly, this limited focus veils over the fact that all who are involved in any consideration of integrity, or, for that matter, in any intercorporeal encounter, are, as Haraway (2007, 3) notes, "consequent on a subject- and object-shaping dance of encounters." Given this, it is the dance that Haraway identifies that is of more interest to me than the notion of integrity per se, since the former is illustrative of the ways in which particular somatechnologies[2] of identity and difference operate such that some desires and morphologies are naturalized whereas others are constituted as abject(ed).

BIID: What's in a Name?

Body Integrity Identity Disorder (BIID) is, as I said, a diagnostic term for what is often described as the incessant and insufferable experience of a lack of "wholeness" or "bodily integrity." Researchers have been keen to determine from whence this experience of lack comes, particularly given that the integrity of a fully limbed and fully functional body is commonly taken to be visibly self-evident. But, as Wim Dekkers, Cor Hoffer, and Jean-Pierre Wils (2005, 179) note, "bodily integrity" is less an empirical fact than "an ambiguous notion" shaped by competing moral points of view. This is perhaps not surprising given that historically the term "integrity" has been used to refer not only to the state of being whole, complete, unimpaired, undiminished, untouched, perfect, and so on, but has also been linked etymologically to moral soundness or rectitude: to "uprightness" and/or "straightness"—a point I return to later in the chapter. What gives BIID (as a diagnostic category) its conceptual coherence is, of course, the unspoken (and unquestioned) assumption that the "ordered" individual, the ("normal") person not suffering from BIID (or some other such pathology) experiences his/her body, his/her "self" as "whole." Bodily integrity, as an idealized state, then, takes on the mantle of "the natural," and thus the morally desirable.

Before we consider how this particular understanding of bodily integrity operates in accounts of the desire for amputation, blindness, deafness, and so on, I want first to very briefly discuss its deployment in debates about other modificatory medical procedures. My aim in doing this is twofold: first, I want to (re)situate the body projects associated with "BIID" in the context of (trans)formative practices more generally,[3] and second, I want to critically examine what Dekkers, Hoffer, and Wils refer to as two different approaches to the question of bodily integrity, both of which rely on the notion of integrity as a natural given and a moral good. These they call the "person-oriented approach" and the "body-oriented approach."

The person-oriented approach to bodily integrity is one in which personal autonomy and control over one's body are perceived (and thus constituted) as fundamental human rights. On this neo-liberal model the individual's bodily integrity must be respected by others and protected (as far as is possible) by the State. Moreover, in circumstances where bodily integrity may, for various reasons, be lost or compromised, the individual is understood as having the right to access procedures designed to restore "wholeness." Think, for example, about discourses surrounding organ transplantation. Similarly, this approach undergirds arguments against "medically unnecessary" procedures that, when carried out without a person's consent—as, for example, in the case of infants—are said to violate bodily integrity and the associated right to bodily self-determination. This approach is commonly taken by opponents of neonatal circumcision. For example, the Declaration of Genital Integrity (adopted at the 1989 General Assembly of the First International Symposium on Circumcision) begins thus: "We recognize the inherent right of all human beings to an intact body. Without religious or racial prejudice, we affirm this basic human right" (cited in Dekkers, Hoffer, and Wils 2005, 180). From a person-oriented perspective, neonatal (or "involuntary") circumcision violates this right insofar as it involves the removal of tissue from the body of a person who has not consented to such a procedure. In the literature that takes this position, there is a distinction drawn between neonatal circumcision and what we might think of as an informed decision made by a consenting adult to undergo the removal of the foreskin. However, there are some "intactivists" who perceive "the human body itself [as] demonstrat[ing] a kind of integrity, wholeness or completeness" (Dekkers, Hoffer, and Wils 2005, 183), as having an inherent moral value that we should not allow to be overridden by claims to autonomy and self-determination (except, perhaps, in some exceptional circumstances).[4] From this perspective—which Dekkers, Hoffer, and Wils refer to as the "body-oriented approach"—circumcision would constitute a wrong regardless of whether or not the person undergoing the procedure consented to it.

Interestingly, then, while the "body-oriented approach" shares with the "person-oriented approach" a conception of bodily integrity as both naturally given and morally desirable, the conclusion the former draws from this premise is opposed to that arrived at by the latter. In short, from a body-oriented perspective, the body takes (moral) precedence over the person who temporarily inhabits it, whereas from the person-oriented perspective, the person takes (moral) precedence over the body he or she owns. What becomes clear here, and indeed what is apparent in most accounts of bodily integrity and/or its lack, is the (problematic) assumption (and reproduction) of a distinction between the body and the self or mind.

While there is much talk of a return to the body in contemporary Western culture, it is nevertheless the case that in the context of neoliberalism, what Dekkers, Hoffer, and Wils refer to as the "person-oriented approach" to bodily integrity is far more common than the "body-oriented approach." As Tamsin Wilton notes, for example, in accounts of and responses to transsexualism, "it is whatever *inhabits* the transsexual body that matters [. . .] The surgeon act[s] *on* the body to ease the pain of the dys/embodied self 'inside'" (cited in Davy 2011, 52). Similarly, so-called cosmetic procedures are more often than not justified on the basis that they furnish the person whose body is pre-operatively "wrong" and/or at odds with his/her sense of self with the integrity to which she/he allegedly has a natural right. But despite this commonplace privileging of the person over the body, of consciousness over what is constituted as little more than brute matter, the argument that the person suffering from BIID has a natural right to integrity (in the same way as does the cosmetic surgery recipient and/or the person with "gender dysphoria") has not, to date, resulted in access to surgical procedures that might engender a *restitution ad integrum*, that is, a restoration of intactness.

Elsewhere[5] I have argued that this asymmetry is largely an effect of the (generative) perception of bodies with less than four "full-length," "fully functioning" limbs, with eyes that do not see, as "disabled." And in the dominant imaginary "disability" is constituted as abject(ed), as the "zone of uninhabitability," the "site of dreaded identification against which—and by virtue of which—the domain of the subject [. . .] circumscribe[s] its own claim to autonomy and to life" (Butler 1999, 237).[6] Consequently, the desire for amputation (or for blindness, deafness, etc.) as a *restitution ad integrum* is most often perceived by those who do not experience such desires as a contradiction in terms, symptomatic of madness (psychopathology) and/or badness (perversion), and thus as evidence that the "wannabe"[7] lacks the capacity to make informed, rational decisions about his/her well-being and therefore does not have, or should not be accorded, the right to self-determination.[8] This privileging of the perception of bodily integrity as visibly self-evident over the experience of the person who, like Gregg Furth, desires to rid himself of a "foreign body" and thus to "become whole, not disabled" (cited in Dotinga 2000)[9] functions, I contend, to abject the wannabe from the domain of the subject and to overcome the disorienting experience of being faced with culturally unintelligible desires and morphologies.

One possible response to this sort of ontological stand-off might be to suggest, as Slatman and Widdershoven (2010) do in their work on organ transplantation, that given the seeming centrality of bodily integrity to individual well-being, we have a moral responsibility to articulate and support differential conceptions of "wholeness" (or lack thereof) that would justify diverse treatment protocols. Indeed, it is the belief that "being somebody, being a unique individual, presupposes a wholeness or unity, an *integrum*" (2010, 74) that motivates Slatman and Widdershoven's research into the "conditions for the successful integration of a new limb into one's identity" (2010, 74), such that the transplant recipient can once again "be the body they have" (2010, 80). Drawing on the significantly different experiences of two hand-transplant recipients, Clint Hallam and Denis Chatelier, the authors argue that while for the former (who eventually had the transplanted hand removed) the "transplant violated his bodily integrity instead of restoring it," for Chatelier, who "had lost his experience of embodied wholeness" after both his hands and forearms were blown apart when a firework he was carrying detonated, "the transplant restored it" (Slatman and Widdershoven 2010, 86).

Slatman and Widdershoven's phenomenological understanding of bodily integrity not as a given but as something one actively (although perhaps less than consciously) works to achieve in and through one's relations with others and with a world is clearly more sophisticated than the "person-oriented" and the "body-oriented" approaches (which rely on and reproduce a distinction between body and mind, self and other, and so on) discussed earlier. However, their project is, I want to suggest, problematic in the following way (or for the following reason). Despite acknowledging that integrity is not achievable (at least not in any absolute sense) and that in fact, as Diane Perpich notes, "it could be considered as a (violent) myth which may cause undesirable effects" (cited in Slatman and Widdershoven 2010, 88)— and the demonization of Chatelier makes this point painfully clear as I demonstrate in due course—they "still wish to defend the idea of integrity" (2010, 88). This desire leads them to make the moral claim that we should respect the other's bodily integrity (even if we cannot perceive it as such).

On the surface, this claim sounds reasonable enough, but what its authors fail to recognize is that the failure to perceive the other's integrity as such is in fact a structural effect of the myth of integrity (as something we have or do not have) that functions, to borrow a phrase from Sara Ahmed (2006, 121, 137), as a "straightening device." Margaret Shildrick is similarly critical of Slatman and Widdershoven's article, arguing that they seem to misunderstand (the import of) Jean-Luc Nancy's understanding of "disintegration as the condition of becoming" (Shildrick 2010, 14). Consequently, Slatman and Widdershoven's (2010, 88) assumption that "we can contribute to the making of decisions that will [. . .] respect [the other's] bodily integrity" results not only in the reaffirmation of integrity as a moral good but, by association, in a failure to critically interrogate the ways in which habituated orientations shape our perspective/perception such that our responses (to the other) are, as I show in my discussion of the Hallam case, at once, less than conscious,[10] profoundly affective, and, for the most part, normalizing.

The lack of critical attention paid by Slatman and Widdershoven to the negative responses to Clint Hallam's decision to have the transplanted hand removed is, I contend, both symptomatic and illustrative of the problem with their work that I have identified here. In the following section I elaborate this claim not with explicit reference to the notion of integrity but instead by turning to a phenomenological understanding of orientations. My decision to turn away from the notion of integrity is threefold. First, I am mindful of the fact that simply arguing that integrity is a myth does little or nothing for those whose orientation toward particular abjected morphologies is "blocked" and whose being-in-the-world is thus dominated by the experience of alienation, of suffering, and so on. Second, it seems to me that what is at stake in the dominant responses to Hallam and Chatelier, and to those desiring amputation, deafness, bigger breasts, thinness, longer legs, and so on, is not so much integrity, but rather, the position and the status of the "objects" (the morphologies) toward which such desires are oriented and thus, in turn, the status and position of the orientations themselves[11] and of the subjects thus oriented. Third, while I want to maintain a focus on the suffering experienced by those whose desires for or orientations toward amputation, deafness, and so on, are "blocked" I want, for ethicopolitical reasons that will become clearer in due course, to shift the focus of scrutiny away from these abjected morphologies and interrogate instead the invisible center, the "here," if you like, from which desires and/or morphologies arrive or are given (in and through particular historical orientations) as "other."

The Clint Hallam International Surgical Soap Opera[12]

In her book *Queer Phenomenology*, Sara Ahmed states that

the concept of "orientations" allows us to expose how life gets directed in some ways rather than others, through the very requirement that we follow what is already given to us. For a life to count as a good life, then it must return the debt of its life by taking on the direction promised as a social good. (2006, 21)

Orientations on this model are less natural inclinations than the performative effect of the work of inhabitance or dwelling-with; orientations shape and are shaped by our "bodily horizons" or "sedimented histories," and thus are necessarily morphological. However, as Butler, Merleau-Ponty, Ahmed, Heidegger, and others have noted, insofar as our orientations, the embodied place(s)/perspective from which we engage in and with others and the world are given to us, and become sedimented in and through repetition; they become "naturalized" such that the histories that "make us be" disappear from view. In and through this process of inhabit(u)ation certain things (i.e., "objects," ways of thinking, styles of being, bodily experiences, and so on) become available to us, while others are constituted as "a field of unreachable objects" (Ahmed 2006, 15), as abject(ed).[13] Thus, as Ahmed explains, "we do not have to consciously exclude those things that are not 'on line.' The direction we take excludes things for us" (2006, 15)—a point Slatman and Widdershoven appear to forget.

With these insights in mind, let us turn to the figure of Clint Hallam. But let me first stress that this turn to "Hallam" (as a discursive figure shaped by a range of somatechnologies that I discuss in due course) should not be read as suggesting that Clint Hallam ("the man") suffered from BIID. Rather, I am interested in the ways in which the somatechnologies at play across this figure—and in particular, Hallam's decision to have the grafted hand amputated—orient and are oriented by particular idea(l)s about bodies and bodily practices.

On the 13th of September 1998, Hallam, a New Zealander who had lost his right hand in a circular saw accident fourteen years earlier, became the first recipient of a human hand transplant. Shortly after the operation Dr. Jean-Michel Dubernard, one of the co-leaders of the surgical team who performed the transplant, is reported as saying, "Th[is] surgical breakthrough gives hope to millions of victims of workplace and domestic accidents, survivors of war or land mines, and individuals born with hereditary deformities" (cited in Campbell 2004, 450). In the popular imaginary, then, the hand transplant signaled the arrival of a time and place in which "anatomical incompleteness" need no longer exist, of a golden age in which all those unfortunate enough to suffer this particular "disability" might be remade whole. And of course, there was no question—at least not in the popular press—that this so-called advancement was anything but a common good. But this vision of an able-bodied futurity was sorely shaken when, in February 2001, the hand that had held out so much promise, was amputated.[14] However, as both the surgeons involved and the media were quick to point out, the amputation was by no means the result of a failure on medicine's behalf.

In the months following the amputation the international press was awash with stories that, in their attempt to render intelligible Hallam's rejection of "the hand," consistently painted a picture of the New Zealander as a disturbed and disturbing individual, a person whose body had been made "right" but whose being was entirely "wrong."[15] Interestingly, Hallam—who the medical team (allegedly) discovered after the transplant, had spent time in a New Zealand prison for fraud and had seemingly continued to be involved in criminal activities after the operation—is frequently referred to in newspaper reports as "a mercurial character"[16] ("Sleight of Hand" 2000), a "trickster,"[17] a liar:[18] as someone who cannot be pinned down, who refuses to stay in (his) place.[19] A report from *The Guardian*, for example, states, "What frustrates [. . .] the [. . .] doctors involved is [Hallam's] unpredictability, the mystery of his whereabouts, and his conviction that he knows what is best for his hand. He could be in Chicago. He could be in Las Vegas. He could be anywhere" (2000). As Professor Nadey Hakim, one of the doctors on Hallam's team, reported:

> Last time [I] spoke to him [he] was calling from Las Vegas. [. . . I] begged him to look after the hand, to take his medication, to travel—as he was supposed to—to a university in Chicago that had promised to pay him in exchange for being able to perform experiments on him. He [Hallam] said, "Yeah, yeah, I'm in charge of my arm" [says Hakim]. What does he mean? I don't know. It wasn't the ideal choice of patient. ("Sleight of Hand" 2000)

Later in the article Hakim returns to the latter point, lamenting the fact that the transplant team had not chosen a patient more like Denis Chatelier for the legendary "first hand transplant" since, claims

Hakim, "He [Chatelier] is a decent man. He stays in. He listens to his doctors' advice. He takes his medicine" (Hakim cited in "Sleight of Hand" 2000).

What most interests me about the vision of Hallam presented by (some) members of his surgical team is what it tells us about the investment in fixing, in stasis, in clear-cut and unchanging boundaries[20] that informs not only their perception of the "troublesome" New Zealander but also their bodily horizon(s), the place(s) from which they dwell, and the(ir) field of unreachable objects. "We gave him the chance of a lifetime," one surgeon told *The Times*, "and he ruined it [. . .] he was such a bad example" (cited in GK 2001, np).

From this privileged and institutionally authorized perspective, then, the surgeons (who could be said to metonymically stand in for "medicine") gave Hallam a world in which to dwell, a domain in which to be subject; they directed him toward a futurity known (to them) as "the good life," and yet he failed to follow their directions and thereby to reinscribe the familiar path that those coming after him could, in turn, follow. Drawing on Ahmed's work I want to suggest that selecting Hallam (as the candidate for the first hand transplant) and giving him a world in the shape of a hand—a hand that interestingly did not "fit"—constituted an "act of recruitment." Recruitment, writes Ahmed, restores the body of the institution, which depends on gathering bodies to cohere as a body. Becoming a "part" of an institution, which we can consider as the demand to share in it, or even have a share of it, hence requires not only that we inhabit its buildings, but also that we follow its line (Ahmed 2006, 133–134), that we become aligned with it.[21] And of course, Hallam did neither, instead eschewing the "straightening device[s] that function to *hold things in place*" (Ahmed 2006, 66).

Let me elaborate on this by turning to a comment made by the Australian surgeon Professor Earl Owen who co-led the team that performed the transplant, and later removed the hand. In response to the interviewer's question about Hallam's alleged failure to cooperate with doctors, Owen states,

> The first three months after the operation he was a good boy, if you like. He was a normal patient, he did his physiotherapy, he had his blood tests, he stayed close to the hospital, which he'd contracted to do, and he was fine, and then he suddenly

[. . .] went walkabout—that's an Australian expression—but it means he disappeared and he set the pattern of disappearing from then on. (Transplanted Hand Removed 2001)

As a fellow Australian I was struck by Owen's use of the colloquialism "walkabout" in this statement. "Walkabout," a term coined by early settlers to describe a little-understood "nomadic" practice (or set of practices) allegedly participated in by (some) indigenous Australians, is, I want to suggest, the product of a white Australian colonialist optics rather than an empirical reality. In the narratives of cultural difference that have, for the last two hundred years or so, circum-scribed not only social relations in Australia but also the materialities of those who make up the *socius* and those who are condemned to its margins, to the zone of uninhabitability, "walkabout" has played a significant role.

In an article entitled "The Walkabout Gene" (1976), American anthropologist Charlotte Epstein, who spent time in outback south-central Australia in the early 1970s, relates a series of disturbing encounters that poignantly illustrate this claim. In a discussion about academic achievement with a second-grade (nonindigenous) teacher in a school whose population was 20 percent Aboriginal or "mixed-race," the teacher assured Epstein that

> the Aboriginal children could never equal the European children, and that the reason for this was a basic genetic dif-ference that manifested itself in walkabout behavior. To illus-trate, she [the teacher] pointed to one [indigenous] child and told [Epstein] that last week he had gone walkabout [. . .] "He left in the middle of a new section in math[s] [said the teacher]. Now he'll never be able to catch up with the oth-ers. And this is characteristic of them." (Epstein 1976, 141)

Another (white) teacher, from a different school, told Epstein, "The Aborigine is very complicated." And he continued, "You see [. . .] he can't discipline himself the way we do. He does what needs doing today, but he won't do for tomorrow. And every few weeks, he goes walkabout" (Epstein 1976, 144).

In each of the encounters recounted here, a particular point of view—what we might think of as the "here" of "whiteness"—is taken as given, and from this "givenness" "the Aborigine" and/or the other who cannot inhabit whiteness (or take up the domain of the subject) acquires both a direction and an identity—abject and abjected to the zone of uninhabitability, or, if you like, "homelessness."[22] In "forgetting" the histories of dwelling-with that shape racial difference in this particular, situated way then, Owen's use of the term "walkabout" (re) enacts the labor of repetition that disappears through labor and thus renders the difference he perceives as such "natural." In other words, Owen's generative vision of walkabout puts the "nonwhite" other[23] in his place and functions to hold him there by fixing his difference, shaping what he can and cannot do. At the same time, the contours of "inhabitable space" are reinforced in and through this (coincident)[24] encounter such that Owen, his colleagues, and the institution of medicine are once again able to "feel at home," to be positioned and to take up the position of master of all that they survey.

Reconfiguring the Phenomenology of Home

As I said earlier, space, dwelling, and morphologies are coconstitutive: just as space and place, the "here" and the "there," the present, past, and future are shaped by the ways in which bodies are oriented in relation to them, so too, morphologies are constituted, formed and transformed, lived, if you like in and through their specific situatedness. But as we know, worlds unfold predominantly along (already given) lines of privilege that are the effect of sedimented histories. And, as Ahmed notes, and the outrage directed at Hallam shows, "following such lines is 'returned' by reward, status and recognition" whereas not following them, or not being able to follow them because their mode of operation, their "zero-point of orientation," necessarily excludes the body one is/has from inhabitable space, constitutes the lived experience of some modes of bodily being as "out of place" (Ahmed 2006, 183). In other words, the tauto-logic that produces the "exclusionary matrix" and is reproduced by it generatively effects what it claims to merely name, thus rendering particular morphologies structurally "out of reach," "naturally" undesirable, and naturalizing this particular (hegemonic) vision. Again, this claim is poignantly (and, I think, painfully) illustrated by another encounter Epstein relays in "The Walkabout Gene."

In a third school at which Epstein carried out her research, a fourth-grade teacher spoke proudly to the author of how the students (who were about 50 percent white and 50 percent indigenous) got along "Just beautifully [. . .] They see each other as all the same— no differences." When Epstein asked the teacher to explain what she meant by this, the teacher responded by showing Epstein some self-portraits the children had recently produced, all of which depicted white children with light-colored hair. Somewhat perplexed, Epstein asked the teacher if any of the children ever portrayed themselves as "dark skinned," to which the teacher replied "No" in a manner that suggested her to be

> comfortable in the rightness of things. Then a slight frown creased [. . .] [the teacher's] forehead and she leaned toward [Epstein] [. . .] lowered her voice, [and said] "Do you see that child there?" [. . .] indicating a very dark [skinned] Aboriginal child. "The other day, when I asked the children to draw themselves, he colored himself very dark. I asked him why, he'd never done that before. And he said to me I'm black, and I'm beautiful." (Epstein 1976, 144)

I realized, continued the teacher, "that someone must have said something to him and that he was upset. But we straightened it out, and he's fine now." "He draws himself white-skinned now?" asked Epstein (who had the recently produced "white" self-portraits in front of her). "Yes," answered the teacher. "He's quite alright now. It was just a temporary thing" (Epstein 1976, 144).

There is so much that could be said about this anecdote, but for reasons of brevity I confine my comments to one aspect of the situation, that is, the "seeing queerly" and the "straightening out" of the indigenous child as black *and* beautiful. In her discussion of the spatial experiments recounted by Merleau-Ponty in *Phenomenology of Perception*, Ahmed argues that "queer effects," that is, effects that disorient— such as, for example, when the "here" of whiteness is faced with a vision of the "nonwhite" body as beautiful, as inhabitable, as the site of an "I"—are overcome through the realignment of what Nirmal Puwar refers to as "matter out of place" (2004, 10) with the bodily horizon. This (re)alignment with lines of privilege depends, as Ahmed (2006, 66) notes, "on straightening devices that keep things in line, in part by 'holding' things in place." Given this, one might argue that the threat posed by the queer vision of the morphological other, the dark-skinned child, is overcome by the "straightening out" to which the teacher refers, that is, the realignment of the domain of the subject with whiteness, the putting of the indigenous other back in his place (i.e., the zone of uninhabitability), and the holding in place of the contours of difference by the repetition of privileged lines (i.e., the indigenous child once again depicts himself as white thus aligning himself with the dominant and naturalized ideals of the "here" of whiteness, which, ironically, he will never be able to inhabit as "home"). The "I'm black and I'm beautiful" moment is an important one not least because as Gayle Salamon writes, "questions of what we are cannot be extricated from questions of what we do, and if that doing sometimes disturbs presumptions of proper identity or proper place, perhaps that disturbance can be a means of forging hopeful new modes of knowledge and new methods of inquiry" (2009, 230). In much the same way that the idea that black is beautiful or that nonwhite morphologies might be habitable and therefore desirable seemed culturally unintelligible in the context of early 1970s white Australia, encounters with bodies without the so-called full complement of limbs, with hands that do not fit, with ears that do not hear, and so on, could in our current context, be said to produce queer effects, to disorient the lines of privilege that constitute certain morphological futures as necessarily excluded and to make visible lines that disappear from view at the point at which "the subject" emerges (Ahmed 2006, 15) and from which that subject apprehends a world.[25] If, then, as Ahmed claims, the question of orientation is about how we "find our way" and how we come to "feel at home," the question of disorientation is about how the encounter with the "unhomely" (the uncanny as the repudiated foundation of the subject's dwelling) queers or denaturalizes habituated modes of dwelling-with, such that "being-at-home" is recast as the contingent effect of ongoing labor that is never mine alone. Of course, as we have seen in the examples discussed throughout this chapter, queer disorientations can be, and often are, divested of their disruptive potential in and through the deployment of a range of straightening devices, one of which is pathologization. In perceiving, and thus naming, the diverse desires and morphologies currently associated with BIID as "disordered," both wrongness and suffering become firmly located in the individual in need of fixing, of straightening out, of realignment. What is

denied in this process is the fact that for (many) wannabes the source
of suffering lies not in the bodies they want but do not have, nor even
in the fact that they desire amputation, deafness, and so on. Rather,
suffering is engendered as an effect of a life lived "out of place," of
not being at-home-in-the-world or in the body that gives one a
world, a "here" from which to extend into phenomenal space and by
which to shape that space. Given this, the challenge, I want to suggest,
is to move away from the moral imperative to understand and/or
respect the others' desires, their morphological difference, and instead
to articulate an ethics of dwelling, a critical interrogation of "lines of
privilege" (Ahmed 2006, 183), those naturalized positions/perspec-
tives from which particular worlds unfold while others are abjected:[26]
"to trace the lines for a different genealogy, one that would embrace
the failure to inherit the family [or familiar] line as the condition of
possibility for another way of dwelling in the world" (Ahmed 2006
178), one that would admit or even embrace the inherent liminality
of "home," multiple evocations of home[27] as always in the making,
always (un)becoming-with, as something other, and something more,
than the exclusory effect of unexamined inhabit(u)ation. Perhaps,
after all, home is not a singular dwelling in which integrity naturally
reigns.

Notes

1. In this sense, my project is similar to that of critical whiteness
   scholars who, rather than focusing on the "racialized other,"
   interrogate instead the invisible center or organizing principle
   against which everything "other" is measured (and found want-
   ing), that is, whiteness.
2. The term "somatechnics" is derived from the Greek σῶμα
   (body) and τέχνη (craftsmanship). It is intended to highlight the
   inextricability of bodily being and the techniques (*dispositifs* and
   "hard technologies") in and through which morphologies are
   (trans)formed. For a more detailed explanation of the term, as
   well as work that critically deploys it, see Sullivan and Murray
   (2009).
3. For an extended discussion of this move see Sullivan (2009a).
4. For example, from a Kantian perspective, it may be acceptable to
   remove a part of the body in order to save the whole, whereas

for some religious conservatives any intervention is regarded as a violation of God's will since God is the owner of the body of the individual.

5. See Sullivan (2005).

6. "The disability rights movement has taught us that atypicality does not necessarily mean disorder" (Reis 2007, 538). See also Dekkers, Hoffer, and Wils' discussion of Diana DeVries regarding the fact that the so-called disabled body is not always experienced as lacking integrity.

7. This is a term that some people desiring the amputation of a healthy limb or limbs use to refer to themselves. It is often used in the same context as are the terms "pretender" and "devotee." The former—"pretender"—is used to refer to someone who performs the identity or bodily status that he or she wishes to attain. For example, someone who uses a wheelchair even though his or her legs are fully functional. A "devotee" is, in this context, someone who desires amputees. Wannabes can be, and often are, pretenders, and devotees are sometimes wannabes.

8. Müller (2009), for example, takes this position.

9. See Dotinga (2000).

10. What we have here, then, is the difference between positing tolerance as an ideal that each of us might consciously strive to attain and the kind of critical analysis that Jessica Cadwallader (2007, 2010) has undertaken of the performative (trans)formation of "bodily tolerances."

11. Why is it that so much time, energy, and money is put into the continuing search for the gay gene, the trans brain, and so on, while at the same time, there is not research—at least none that I am aware of—that is concerned with locating the source of "gender concordance" or heterosexuality or integrity. See also Richardson's critique of the work of Zucker. Think also of Ray Blanchard's account of "target location error." Both of these are about naming what we might think of as "queer (dis)orientations," or orientations that are "out of line" with the norm. Aversion therapy is clearly, as its name suggests, an attempt to reorient, to turn the patient away from the "wrong" object.

12. I borrow this phrase from Campbell (2004).

13. Sedgwick (1990, 8) makes a similar point when she says: "particular insights generate, are lived with, and at the same time are themselves structured by particular opacities." She also says:

"Ignorances, far from being pieces of the originary dark, are produced by and correspond to particular knowledges and circulate as part of particular regimes of truth" (1990, 8).

14. According to a BBC news report, the amputation was carried out in London after Hallam's request for the procedure was turned down by Dr. Dubernard, who co-led the surgical team on the grounds that the body was inviolable under French law. See http://news.bbc.co.uk/2/hi/europe/982817.stm. Accessed May 25, 2010.

15. One surgeon in an article in *The Times* says "we chose the wrong patient" (cited in GK 2001, np). Similarly, Professor Owen is cited as saying that Hallam was the "wrong choice."

16. At one point in *The Guardian* article the author describes Hallam (after the transplant and before the amputation) as "a man with two sets of fingerprints" ("Sleight of Hand"2000, np).

17. See Campbell (2004, 453).

18. Professor Earl Owen is cited as saying, "I mean this in the nicest way, but he is a liar of extraordinary talent" ("Sleight of Hand" 2000, np).

19. *The Guardian* report "Sleight of Hand" (2002, np), for example, refers to "Hallam's rootlessness."

20. The author of "Sleight of Hand" claims that Hallam's medical team "learned that a last-minute panic before Hallam left Australia for Lyon [where he was to undergo the transplant]—when he claimed to have forgotten to renew his passport and made a frantic appeal for emergency travel documents—was in fact due to his having surrendered his passport to an Australian court during investigations into his alleged involvement in a fuel racket." This is an interesting detail in its focus on Hallam's "illegal" border-crossings.

21. For a similar account of the relationship between integrity and integration, see Stryker and Sullivan (2009).

22. The myth of *terra nullius*—of "no man's land"—enabled white settlers to "make" a home (whose making was then forgotten) in "Australia" and literally denied indigenous peoples a home. The concept of *terra nullius* became a major issue in Australian politics when in 1992, during an Aboriginal rights case known as *Mabo*, the High Court of Australia issued a judgment that was a direct overturning of *terra nullius*. For more detailed analyses of this myth and its effects, see Watson (2002) and Kercher (2002).

23. It is probably worth reiterating here that Hallam is a New Zealander, while Owen is Australian. Historically, New Zealand has been position by Australia(ns) as its sort of "poor cousin," its other, if you like. New Zealand is also often represented in the Australian imaginary as marginal to Australia, not only geographically, but in a whole range of ways. In making this claim and/or discussing the incidents related by Epstein it is not my intention to conflate the position of "Hallam" and that of "indigenous Australians," or to suggest that the mechanisms of abjection operate in exactly the same way in both cases. Rather, my aim is to bring to light some of the somatechnologies of identity and difference that simultaneously naturalize some morphologies and desires, some ways of knowing, seeing, and being and constitute others as abject(ed).

24. I use this term in the Husserlian sense.

25. Again, I'd like to stress the fact that I am not implying that these examples are reducible to one another, merely that they are structurally connected, and that recognizing this can be useful to any attempt to think through an ethics of dwelling or of intercorporeality.

26. In this, my project is in keeping with the aims of queer theory, critical whiteness studies, and critical disability studies—at least as I understand them—none of which is concerned with calling for respect for, understanding of, or tolerance toward racialized, sexualized or pathologized others. Instead, all three deploy deconstructive methodologies that call into question that which is structurally invisiblized in and through dominant somatechnologies (for example, "heterosexuality," "whiteness," and "normalcy" or "able-bodiedness" as institutions or structuring devices).

27. I borrow this phrase from Fortier (2001).

References

Ahmed, Sara. 2006. *Queer Phenomenology: Orientations, Objects, Others.* Durham and London: Duke University Press.

Butler, Judith. 1999. "Bodies That Matter." In *Feminist Theory and the Body: A Reader*, edited by J. Proce and M. Shildrick, 235–232. Edinburgh: Edinburgh University Press.

Cadwallader, Jessica. 2007. "Suffering Difference: Normalisation and Power." *Social Semiotics* 17 (3): 375–394.

Cadwallader, Jessica. 2010. "Archiving Gifts." *Australian Feminist Studies* 25 (64): 121–132.

Campbell, Fiona Kumari. 2004. "The Case of Clint Hallam's Wayward Hand: Print Media Representations of the 'Uncooperative' Disabled Patient." *Continuum: Journal of Media & Cultural Studies* 18 (3): 443–458.

Davy, Zowie. 2011. *Recognizing Transsexuals: Personal, Political and Medicolegal Embodiment*. Farnham, UK: Ashgate.

Dekkers, Wim, Cor Hoffer, and Jean-Pierre Wils. 2005. "Bodily Integrity and Male and Female Circumcision." *Medicine, Health Care and Philosophy* 8: 179–191.

Diprose, Rosalyn. 1994. *The Bodies of Women: Ethics, Embodiment and Sexual Difference*. New York: Routledge.

Dotinga, Randy. 2000. "Out on a Limb." http://www.salon.com. Accessed March 25, 2005.

Dreger, Alice. 2005. *One of Us: Conjoined Twins and the Future of Normal*. Cambridge, MA: Harvard University Press.

Epstein, Charlotte. 1976. "The Walkabout Gene." *The Urban Review* 9 (2): 141–144.

First, Michael. 2005. "Desire for Amputation of a Limb: Paraphilia, Psychosis, or a New Type of Identity Disorder." *Psychological Medicine* 35: 919–928.

Fortier, Anne-Marie. 2001. "'Coming Home': Queer Migrations and Multiple Evocations of Home." *European Journal of Cultural Studies* 4 (4): 405–424.

GK. 2011. "Hand Transplant Recipient Throws in the Towel." *Hastings Center Report*. http://findarticles.com/p/articles/mi_go2103/is_1_31/ai_n28827853/.

Haraway, Donna. 2007. *When Species Meet*. Minneapolis: University of Minnesota Press.

Jacobsen, Kristen. 2009. "A Developed Nature: A Phenomenological Account of the Experience of Home." *Continental Philosophy Review* 42: 355–373.

Kercher, Bruce. 2002. "Native Title in the Shadows: The Origins of the Myth of *Terra Nullius* in New South Wales Courts." In *Colonialism and the Modern World: Selected Studies*, edited by G. Blue, M. P. Bunton, and R. C. Croizier, 100–119. New York: M. E. Sharpe.

Lawrence, Ann. 2006. "Clinical and Theoretical Parallels between Desire for Limb Amputation and Gender Identity Disorder." *Archives of Sexual Behavior* 35: 263–278.

Loeb, Elizabeth. 2008. "Cutting It Off: Bodily Integrity, Identity Disorders, and the Sovereign States of Corporeal Desire in U.S. Law." *WSQ: Women's Studies Quarterly* 36: 44–63.

Merleau-Ponty, Maurice. 1962. *Phenomenology of Perception*, translated by Colin Smith. New York: Routledge & Keegan Paul.

Müller, Sabine. 2009. "Body Integrity Identity Disorder (BIID): Is the Amputation of Healthy Limbs Ethically Justified?" *American Journal of Bioethics* 9: 36–43.

Perpich, Diane. 2005. *Corpus Meum*: Disintegrating Bodies and the Ideal of Integrity. *Hypatia* 20 (3): 75–91.

Puwar, Nirmal. 2004. *Space Invaders: Race, Gender and Bodies Out of Place*. Oxford: Berg Publisher.

Reis, Elizabeth. 2007. "Divergence or Disorder? The Politics of Naming Intersex." *Perspectives in Biology and Medicine* 50: 535–543.

Richardson, Justin. 1999. "Response: Finding the Disorder in Gender Identity Disorder." *Harvard Review of Psychiatry* 7: 43–50.

Salamon, Gayle. 2009. "Justification and Queer Method, or Leaving Philosophy." *Hypatia* 24 (1): 225–230.

Sedgwick, Eve. 1990. *Epistemology of the Closet*. Berkeley: University of California Press.

Shildrick, Margrit. 2010. "Some Reflections on the Socio-Cultural and Bioscientific Limits of Bodily Integrity." *Body & Society* 16 (3): 11–22.

Slatman, Jenny, and Guy Widdershoven. 2010. "Hand Transplants and Bodily Integrity." *Body & Society* 16 (3): 69–92.

"Sleight of Hand." 2000. *The Guardian*, Tuesday, May 30. http://www.guardian.co.uk/g2/story/0,3604,320016,00.html.

Steinbock, Anthony. 1995. *Home and Beyond: Generative Phenomenology after Husserl*. Evanston, IL: Northwestern University Press.

Stryker, Susan, and Nikki Sullivan. 2009. "King's Member, Queen's Body: Transsexual Surgery, Self-Demand Amputation, and the Somatechnics of Sovereign Power." In *Somatechnics: Queering the Technologisation of Bodies*, edited by S. Murray and N. Sullivan, 49–64. Farnham, UK: Ashgate.

Sullivan, Nikki. 2005. "Integrity, Mayhem, and the Question of Self-Demand Amputation." *Continuum: Journal of Media and Cultural Studies* 19 (3): 325–333.

Sullivan, Nikki. 2007. "'The price we pay for our common good?' Genital Modification and the Somatechnics of Cultural (In)Difference." *Social Semiotics* 17 (3): 395–409.

Sullivan, Nikki. 2008. "The Role of Medicine in the (Trans)Formation of 'Wrong' Bodies." *Body & Society* 14 (1): 103–114.

Sullivan, Nikki. 2009a. "Transsomatechnics and the Matter of 'Genital Modifications.'" *Australian Feminist Studies* 24 (60): 275–286.

Sullivan, Nikki. 2009b. "Queering the Somatechnics of BIID." In *Body Integrity Identity Disorder: Psychological, Neurobiological, Ethical and Legal Aspects*, edited by A. Stirn, A. Thiel, and S. Oddo, 187–198. Lengeritch, Germany: Pabst.

Sullivan, Nikki, and Samantha Murray (eds.). (2009) *Somatechnics: Queering the Technologisation of Bodies*. Farnham, UK: Ashgate.

Watson, Irene. 2002. "Aboriginal Law and the Sovereignty of *Terra Nullius*." *Borderlands* 1 (2). http://www.borderlands.net.au/vol1no2_2002/watson_laws.html.

The World Today Archive. 2001. Monday, February 5.. http://www.abc.net.au/worldtoday/stories/s242198.htm.

"Transplanted Hand Removed." 2001. The World Today Archive, Monday, February 5. http://www.abc.net.au/worldtoday/stories/s242198.htm.

8

SEXED EMBODIMENT IN ATYPICAL PUBERTAL DEVELOPMENT

Intersubjectivity, Excorporation, and the Importance of Making Space for Difference

KRISTIN ZEILER AND LISA GUNTRAM

The doctor said: "You might not have one." But I just thought he was joking really, so I just laughed. I really thought "No, but that's not possible, that's kind of like saying that you don't have a heart."

—Joanna

Introduction

For many teenagers, puberty is a time of transition. For some teenage girls, this time of transition into womanhood may also be a time when they come to know that they have no womb and no vagina or that they have no womb and what medical professionals refer to as a "small" vagina. For some, such as Joanna in the quote above, this may be incredible. It can also be a shocking experience. It can make the young woman's body stand forth to her, temporary, in a disruptive mode that affects her bodily self-awareness as well as her relations to others—even if the experience is likely to vary depending on the sociocultural context in which the woman lives.

Importantly, as time goes by, these young women may also find new ways of making sense of their female embodiment. They may emphasize that everyone is different and that is normal to be different or that their bodies fit with sociocultural norms about female bodies in other ways than in terms of these specific body parts.

This chapter offers a phenomenological explication of three phenomena that recurred in interviews with young Swedish women who in their teens have come to know that they have no womb and no vagina or a "small" vagina:[1] a changed bodily self-awareness, attendance to sociocultural norms about female bodies and how this can affect interaction, and expressions of sexed embodiment as both "normal" and "different."

The interviewed women also emphasized the importance of sharing their experiences so that other young women in similar situations would know that they are not alone, and other others may reflect on how to support women in this situation. It is our hope that this chapter will contribute in this regard by highlighting that there is not only one mode of female embodiment but many and by bringing forth the ethical dimension of intersubjective meaning-making when a young woman is told that she has no womb and no vagina or a "small" vagina.

The chapter intertwines the philosophical discussion with examples from the interviews, and is divided into three parts. First, the chapter addresses how the vagina and the womb may be phenomenologically present in their absence, and painfully so, when the young woman is told that she has not these body-parts. Second, it examines how gendered patterns of behavior, including expectations and norms about female and male bodies, can form embodied agency via the phenomenological concepts of incorporation and excorporation. The concept of excorporation, as a reverse incorporation, has been developed elsewhere (Malmqvist and Zeiler 2010) as has the issue of how the subject may live a continuous excorporation for longer periods of time and how this may feed into the subject's bodily alienation (Zeiler 2013). Here, we elaborate on the concept of excorporation via phenomenological work on the body as expression, on bodily expression as taking place between self and other, and on emotions as bodily expressions that shape bodies and align some bodies with and against other bodies (Ahmed 2004; Käll 2009; Merleau-Ponty 2006). Finally, we shift focus to young women's ways of handling their new bodily knowledge and their body-world relations, when they have come to know that they have no womb and no vagina or a "small" vagina. We discuss sexed embodiment as a style of being (see Heinä-maa 1999) and emphasize that such a conceptualization preferably should be combined with an analysis of asymmetrical relations that make some changes in one's style of being more difficult than others. This combination highlights the ethical dimension of our reasoning. Because of the way self and other are intrinsically related to each other, we are all already implicated in processes of shared meaning-making and the formation of social space—where some bodies more so than others are given room.

Some words are needed about the situation and treatment when young women learn that they have no womb or vagina, or only parts of a so-called normal-sized vagina. Uterine and vaginal agenesis, that is, a congenital absence of the womb (uterus) and of the entire or parts of the vagina occurs in about one in four thousand to one in ten thousand women (ACOG 2002). The affected women will not menstruate or be able to gestate and conceive and may have difficulties in performing penile-vaginal intercourse. However, neither sex chromosomes nor ovaries are affected, and the women develop "normal" secondary sex characteristics (Morgan and Quint 2006). While there as yet has been no success in transplanting a uterus, a neo-vagina can be created through surgery or by stretching the vaginal dimple either by using dilators gradually increasing in size or through penetrative intercourse. A surgically created vagina will moreover most often require subsequent dilation or penetrative intercourse in order to maintain its size (Edmonds 2003). Dilation is, however, often a painful and demanding procedure that requires a lot of effort and time on the women's part—and penetrative intercourse may also be painful (Guntram 2013; Liao et al. 2006). Nevertheless, in an international consensus statement on the management of intersex conditions it is stated that the absent "or inadequate vagina (with rare exceptions) *requires* a vaginoplasty performed in adolescence" (Lee et al. 2006, 492; emphasis added). The interviewees' mainly present the interventions as making "normal" sex possible.[2]

Female Bodily Self-Awareness Reconsidered

Maurice Merleau-Ponty's (2006) *Phenomenology of Perception* provides a valuable starting point for an analysis of embodied subjectivity and agency. In this perspective, body and mind are intrinsically bound together, and it is our bodies that open up the world to us and allow the world to be for us at all. This is conceptualized via the notion of the lived body. The lived body is the lived relationship to a world immersed in meaning that we constantly interpret and make meaningful to ourselves through interaction with others.

This is also the starting point in Drew Leder's (1990) examination of how our bodies, or parts of our bodies, can recede from reflective awareness in everyday interaction with others. When going for a walk in the forest with a friend, we may be relatively unaware of our back muscles and our feet. These body parts can "dis-appear" from our reflective awareness while enabling our activity of walking (Leder 1990, 24–25). They may also "dys-appear" if we for some reason stumble and fall: the hurting body part now stands forth as a hindrance; we cannot continue the walk and the return trip may appear to be long. Dys-appearance takes place when the body appears to the subject as "ill" or "bad" (Leder 1990, 84), and this is often the case when we experience pain or illness.[3]

On the one hand, this can be helpful as a starting point in order better to understand young women's experiences of coming to know that they have no womb and no vagina or a "small" part of the vagina. As exemplified by Joanna quoted in the epigraph to this chapter, some women described being told that they had no womb and no vagina or a "small" part of the vagina as an experience that was difficult to grasp. When being examined by the doctor and told that she might not have a womb, Joanna explained that she just laughed. To her that could not be possible. It was as unimaginable as saying that she didn't have a heart. Others described how they reacted differently; one woman recalled how she fainted when being told that she did not have a womb. Afterward, she said, she felt that she did not want to live anymore. As a third example, a woman, here called Patricia, described how the doctor at first kept on talking but then grew quiet as the examination continued. "Shit!" Patricia recalled herself thinking and added that her heart started throbbing, "Something isn't right." Patricia described how she felt stressed. In her view, not even the doctor seemed to know how to explain what she saw.

These are examples of a theme that recurred in the interviews (Guntram 2013): the women's initial shock and disbelief when being given this new information about one's body. In phenomenological language, being told that one had no womb and no vagina or a "small" vagina seems to result in a changed mode of bodily existence. If the woman previously lived her body as the taken-for-granted center of existence, the tacit bodily taken-for-grantedness now dissolves. Her body can instead dys-appear, in Leder's sense of the term, whereas it previously could dis-appear from her attention. This matters for the young woman's very mode of being in the world, and a supportive clinical encounter—sensitive to the particular situation of the young woman—needs to take this into account.

On the other hand, these young women's experiences involve more than dis-appearance shifting into dys-appearance. At stake is the future function that the young women may have attributed to these particular organs, the womb and the vagina, before being told that they did not have these organs.

Leder (1990) differentiates between three ways in which one's own body can dis-appear from one's attention (focal, background, and depth disappearance), and the case of depth disappearance is relevant for the present discussion as a starting point.[4] Organs that depth disappear, *pace* Leder, typically resist both reflective attention and control; such as is the case for viscera. This may also be the case for the womb for girls before puberty, and yet this description is inadequate. In cases where a young woman has assumed that she may one day experience pregnancy and childbirth, her assumed present womb has been a part of her corporeal field of future possibilities in another way than, for example, her liver or spleen. Expectancy becomes important here, since certain organs are not only expected to be there (as is also the case with the liver and pancreas) but also expected to allow for certain future actions and experiences for the girl. A similar reasoning can be applied to the assumed present vagina. While this body-part has been and is physically more accessible to her, and in this way potentially more present to her, it may likewise primarily have been present to her—before puberty—as a part of her corporeal field of future possibilities, if she has assumed that she may one day want to experience vaginal intercourse.

This calls for a nuanced analysis of female bodily self-awareness in order to understand more precisely the experience of coming to know that one has no womb and no vagina or a "small" vagina. Whereas the womb is not part of these young women's bodily engagement with others and the world in the same way as are their hands, eyes, or legs in movement or visual perception (and neither focal nor background disappearance is therefore applicable), yet it neither depth disappears in the way of the liver or spleen. Still, coming to know that one does not have womb and vagina, as a young woman, highlights that one lacks abilities that often are assumed to be part of female embodiment. If this is the case, the corporeal field of expected future possibilities may be disrupted. This also points at the intersubjective dimension of that which stand forth as expected and desired corporeal possibilities in the first place. Indeed, some of the young interviewed women underline that they long for "typical" female bodily experiences. As one such example, the young woman Elsa described the womb as a great part of "all this that you have to have in order to have children and all; for all that which makes you a woman." Elsa had been told that she should feel lucky that she did not have to care about painful menstruations, but she said that she would rather have them. She would like to know what it really feels like, "this which is typically female," and she described her bodily situation as "terrible."

These stories indicate a bodily absence that is painfully present. Moreover, the absence resembles the way the body or a body part may dys-appear by standing forth as a thematic object of attention that is hurting, ill, or bad in experiences of pain or illness. This time, however, body parts that stand forth in a *dys* state are those the subject now has come to know that she has never had. Furthermore, the womb and vagina are attributed strong symbolic value in these stories. In one way, these women seemed to long for a bodily dys-appearance that other women may experience in menstruation, because sharing *this* particular dys-appearance would make one's own body less dys-appearing in another sense: it would no longer appear as different from the assumed "typical" female body.

This sheds light on some dimensions of the experience of coming to know that one has no womb or no vagina or a "small" vagina. However, we will now discuss how the phenomenological concepts of incorporation and excorporation can enable an understanding of the intersubjective dimension of this experience. Whereas the concept of dys-appearance highlights a mode of being in which the body stands forth as a thematic object of attention, the concept of excorporation allows an examination of disruptive experiences where gendered patterns of behavior, including expectations and norms about female and male bodies, no longer can reside on prereflective and practical levels of existence and coexistence.

Incorporation, Excorporation, and Emotions in Shared Space

Merleau-Ponty mainly discusses incorporation as a process through which physical objects or skills come to be experienced as integrated parts of the subject's lived body. This also means that the subject's bodily grasp on the world is extended. The reasoning can be further explained with the use of the concept of the body schema, which denotes the dynamic and organizing structure that enables body-world relations. The body schema provides us with tacit know-how of our own bodies, their relation to space and the position of body parts. It refers to the way the body relates to and opens onto the world of possibilities in terms of "I can," that is, in terms of what possibilities are open to me as a specific lived body. As a dynamic structure, it may be diminished as when we fall ill or be expanded as when we learn new skills. Irrespective, the changed body schema will matter for the world that it opens up to us.

The reasoning is often exemplified with Merleau-Ponty's (Merleau-Ponty 2006, 165) discussion of the blind man who learns to use the stick, but many more examples can be given. Incorporation can take place when someone learns to bike, write, play an instrument, or sail. Through repeated action and habituation, through the "motor grasping of a motor skill," the subject's body schema, his or her system of sensorimotor capabilities, can be transformed and the transformed lived body opens up the world to the subject in new ways (Merleau-Ponty 2006, 165). New skills are incorporated, recede to prereflective and bodily levels of existence, and enable smooth and seamless engagements with others and the world. In the case of the blind man, he comes to experience the stick as an integrated and extended part of his bodily existence that allows him to find his way easier than before. The point is that the transformed lived body opens up the world to the subject in new ways; new skills are incorporated, and once incorporated, they typically recede to prereflective and bodily levels of existence. This enables smooth and seamless engagements with others and the world.

Now, this reasoning has been applied to other patterns of behavior that are repeated through motor actions over time, such as those involved in the learning of gendered behavior and in the habitual and corporeal enactment/expression of expectations and norms about sexed bodies (Malmqvist and Zeiler 2010; Zeiler 2013). Such a learning of gendered patterns of behavior can take place if the little child, in close interactions with others, learns to appropriate (more or less) gender-specific patterns of behavior, gendered expectations and norms, through repeated action and habituation. This incorporation of gendered body-world relations does not require that young children tell themselves "this is what girls/boys look like, should look like, move their bodies, this is how they should behave." Whereas the child may ask questions about differences between girls and boys (and arguably, this is how many expectations and norms are given and reinforced), this is not what matters most for incorporation. Crucial, instead, is the idea that patterns of behavior can become integrated parts of someone's lived body through repeated action and that such behavior can be gendered. Furthermore, once gendered patterns of behavior have been incorporated into the lived body, they can recede from the subject's reflective awareness. In this way, and for a young woman, the processes of incorporation can explain how culturally shared, bodily enacted or expressed gendered behavior including expectations and norms about female embodiment can recede from reflective attention and become what she "just" does. Whereas the woman may be implicitly aware of the cluster of patterns of gendered behavior and expectations and norms about sexed bodies as a cluster that *she* enacts, she may not be explicitly aware of them except when asked to explain or justify her behavior. Instead, they become taken-for-granted parts of her bodily existence and coexistence through which she can engage with others and the world, in everyday activities and interactions.

However, this taken-for-granted bodily engagement with others and the world typically changes when a young woman is told that she has no womb and no vagina or a "small" part of the vagina. In the interviews, one woman recalled that she started to cry as she was told about her condition. When she entered the waiting room, where her friend was waiting, she screamed out loud. Another woman described how she thought that the doctor was lying. "This could not be me. This is not me, this, this is not me," she explained that she repeated in her head as the doctor drew a picture to illustrate her ovaries and the absent uterus.

The concept of excorporation can shed light on this experience. Excorporation implies that something that has been part of the subject's lived body on a prereflective and practical level becomes a thematic object of one's attention: one cannot but attend to it. That which previously was incorporated no longer enables smooth and seamless interaction with others and the world because it now fails to "extend" the lived body in the way that previously was possible. Transparency is lost, and this is typically an unwanted experience.

Also excorporation can be explained with the example of the blind man with the stick. This time, however, let us assume that this time the stick breaks into two parts in the man's activity of walking. This being the case, the blind man can no longer engage with others and the world as smoothly as before. The man's lived body-world relation is (at least temporarily) disrupted, and he cannot but attend to that which is now broken—the stick. In the language of incorporation and excorporation, the stick has previously been incorporated in the blind man's lived body, but it now becomes excorporated. It can no longer function as an extension of his lived body nor enable him to find his way when walking.[6]

Again, there are differences between the case of a stick and gendered behaviour, expectations and norms (discussed elsewhere, see Zeiler 2013; Malmqvist and Zeiler 2010). There are also similarities: in both cases, excorporation implies that that which previously was lived as parts of who the subject's being-in-the-world, up until now, no longer can function in this way. Whereas she previously lived gendered patterns of behavior, expectations, and norms about female bodies, prereflectively and practically, she cannot continue doing so as before. This new information about her body makes her attend to that which she previously lived in a direct and non-thematized manner, such as assumptions that women have wombs and vaginas and that these organs will enable certain activities and experiences. Her previously taken-for-granted gendered body-world relation becomes at least temporarily shattered, when these expectations and norms stand forth as thematic objects of attention.

So far, this reasoning on excorporation has focused on intentionality and action. In order to further elaborate on this concept, we suggest a shift in focus to Merleau-Ponty's discussion on how *affectivity forms bodily existence together with others*. For Merleau-Ponty, the lived body is more than a point of view of the world, an instrument for certain activities or a mediator of the experiencing self. The lived body is "our expression in the world, the visible form of our intentions" (Merleau-Ponty 2006, 5). Because of this, the subject's bodily expressions, including emotions, are typically not hidden from others.

The affective dimension lay at the heart of relations between self and others. Though emotions may be subtle, they are commonly felt by both self and other in shared space. Even if we at times try to not visibly express an emotion, it makes sense to think of emotions as neither neatly kept "within" the subject nor only accessible to the subject. Because they can saturate shared space and form both self and other, they can "'make' and 'shape' bodies" and align individuals with each other (Ahmed 2004, 31). This can be put even stronger: bodily expression, including emotions, can be seen as happening *between* individuals in shared space, as forming both self and other— and as located in shared space rather than as located in the subject (Käll 2009; Ahmed 2004).

This matters for the discussion of both incorporation and excorporation. Incorporated culturally shared norms are corporeally expressed, and individuals not only appropriate certain culturally shared bodily enacted or expressed norms through bodily praxis: these norms are also *communicated* in such praxis, in the intersubjective space between self and other. Here, however, we focus on how bodily expressions in shared space can form processes of excorporation.

The reasoning on bodily expressions as located in shared space allow an analysis of what emotions *do*, *how* they shape bodies when they saturate shared space between the young women, their families and friends, and sometimes also medical professionals. In situations of excorporation, emotions in shared space may alleviate the pain that excorporation often implies. They may also aggravate the experience.

Furthermore, emotional expressions in the communicative space between self and other can be shaped by "longer histories of contact" in terms of past interactions, expressions, and historicity (Ahmed 2004). In the case of the young women, the contact between self and others seemed often to be shaped by specific histories about how female bodies should look and what actions they should enable, and when such histories of the "typical" female body did not "fit" with the young women's bodies, both self and others could react in strong emotional ways. This was the case in some women's stories of how they told their close ones, families, and friends about their condition and how these persons broke into tears and started to sob. Other examples contained descriptions of experiences of shame and self-disgust. This was the case for Maria, who said that she was angry but also that she felt ashamed and vulnerable. Maria explained that she was disgusted with her body and that she broke up with her boyfriend, even though he declared that it was her heart that mattered and not other parts of her body. "I didn't want anyone to touch me," she explained, "I didn't want him to touch me. That was very much my feeling."

Situations such as these can be understood in terms of an emotional forming and reforming of one's lived body and one's bodily space in relation to bodies and spaces of others. The affective intensity between bodies aligns some bodies (as the young woman's body) against other bodies (other women's and men's bodies). In this way, if others respond to the young woman's bodily situation by crying, and as a reason for crying, it can hardly be surprising if this (in)forms her lived bodily self. Indeed, these others' response to the subject's bodily expression—the way their eyes burn with tears as a response to the young woman's story— is likely to inform her very experience of sadness or anger (see Käll 2009). Likewise, the example of Maria indicates how the emotion of shame can make the self turn away from others toward itself.

Let us now return to excorporation. Whereas excorporation often is suddenly initiated, it can also continue over time and be aggravated over time. This can take place if the subject *lives the disruptive movement that breaks the lived body apart in excorporation for longer periods of time* (Zeiler 2013). To this we add a dimension: if emotions form bodies in shared space as suggested above, then certain forms of emotional forming and reforming of bodies can *further aggravate excorporation by deepening the way the young woman's body stands forth to her as a hindrance for action and, perhaps, as shameful.* Such a deepened experience of excorporation may lead to bodily alienation. Still, and most importantly, there are ways to resist this and there is an ethical dimension to this resistance.

Sexed Style of Being: Rethinking Female Embodiment

In the following, we do not wish to go into reasoning on female bodily subjectivity that boils down to discussions about what qualifies as "typical" for female bodily existence, since this can reinforce normative dichotomous thinking on embodiment that we want to avoid. An examination of how sociocultural, historical, and individual differences can form the subject's *sexed and unique* bodily being-in-the-world is more promising for the point we want to make. Importantly, this examination needs to be combined with a critical discussion of asymmetrical relations that make some modes of bodily existence more difficult than others. As will soon be discussed, this matters for how difficult it can be to resist alienation when one has come to know that one has no womb and no vagina or a "small" vagina.

Merleau-Ponty's (2006) conception of human bodily existence as a *style of being* is a useful starting point in this regard. A style of being refers to a certain manner of engaging with others and the world, which emerges from the body's capacities, from habituated expressive postures, ways of feeling, thinking, acting, and responding to others. It is the result of a habitual mode of being that gradually feeds into our bodily existence and "acquires a favoured status for us" (Merleau-Ponty 2006, 513, 469, 382). This is the case for the man who has built his life upon an inferiority complex for many years; he has made a dwelling place in certain attitudes and patterns of action and being, and this can form perception, emotion, and action—and because of this he may come to see certain social situations as intimidating, feel intimidated by and shy away from them.

A style of being gives the subject's bodily existence stability without stagnation and integrates affective, sensorimotor, and perceptive dimensions of it. In this sense, having a style is a matter of "being a body and having a history," as put by Linda Singer (1981, 161). Our style of being puts some restrictions on us in terms of what actions, gestures, and so forth, will be easy for us. At the same time, there is no determinism in a style of being, and we may act unexpectedly, contrary to that style even if this is less probable. There is freedom, but this freedom needs to be understood against the backdrop of the idea that we are born into a world already constituted with meaning; the subject's freedom is bound up with her or his bodily existence and coexistence. In this sense, a style of being is not static, though changes are likely to take time.

The concept of a style of being is promising for rethinking sexed embodiment, as suggested by Sara Heinämaa (1999). She points out that it makes no sense merely to look at singular events in a woman's life, or organs in her body, in order to understand the lived experience of female embodiment. Instead, womanhood can preferably be understood as a style of being that cannot be grasped through searches of a common form or source, but should rather be understood as a way of acting that "runs through one's whole life like a melody" (Heinämaa 1997, 27). And just as in the case of a melody, in which certain tunes will be more likely to follow than others in order for there to be a melody, so is it with female embodied being-in-the-world.

Heinämaa suggests that this is the view that lay at the heart of Simone de Beauvoir's *The Second Sex*. In her reading, Beauvoir sees female and male bodies as "different variations of human embodiment: they both realize and recreate 'in their different ways' the human condition, which is characterised by fundamental ambiguity" (Heinämaa 1999, 123). Whereas both woman and man can experience their bodies as that which they are and that which they have, sometimes as subject and sometimes as object, there is also a difference between female and male embodiment. The specificity of female embodiment lay in "its mode of changing," (Heinämaa 1999, 124), in the temporal structure of alien vitality that forms "a continuous cyclic vein in the flow of her experience (Heinämaa 2003, 81).

This can be seen as implying a focus on *a* female tune of embodiment, but if so, this is not the only possible interpretation of what sexed embodiment as a style of being can imply. Indeed, in analogy with the case of music, certain tunes are more likely to follow than others in a melody, but there is also a wide variety in how a melody may run, and female tunes need not be understood in contrast to, for example, male tunes of embodiment.

One more thing is noteworthy. When Heinämaa discusses sexual identity as a stylized identity, in relation to Husserl's discussion of the concept of style, she suggests that one's sexual identity runs through one's whole life as a way or manner in which lived experiences and acts follow each other, continue, and change. And when this manner of changing itself changes—for example, in childhood, adolescence, sickness, or old age—then it "does so in a characteristic way, such that a unitary style manifests itself once more" (Heinämaa 2011, 47). Perhaps a key to this reasoning lay in Heinämaa's suggestion in relation to this quote, that sensuous experience is fundamental for sexual identity. Arguably, some dimensions of sensuous experience—exemplified with sensation, motility, and sense perception—will remain the same over time also when we experience changes in our very manner of changing.

However, even if the young women's sensuous experience remain the same also after they have come to know that certain future corporeal possibilities will not be there for them, they now know that their bodies will not be able to follow all the expected changes in the manner of changing that they themselves may see as characteristic for them as women. And such stability at a time when one expects change can result in a changed bodily self-awareness and a temporary rupture in one's habitual manner of engaging with others and the world as a sexed and unique bodily subject, that is, in one's sexed style of being.[7]

We will now focus on the intersubjective dimension to this reasoning. Just as a bodily style of being is informed by past interactions with others and past ways of responding to others' actions, gestures, and expressions in Merleau-Ponty's work, so is it with sexed embodiment as a style of being. Someone's sexed style of being will be informed by expectations and norms about what a particular sexed embodiment means and should mean that others have expressed in past interaction, by her or his own past and present ways of responding to these others, by her or his own bodily existence. It is thus pointless to enter a discussion of what is "mine" or what comes from "others" in my sexed style of being: these dimensions are intrinsically interwoven. Furthermore, this reasoning highlights that someone's sexed style of being is not a matter of the subject's own choice in any simple sense.

With this in mind, re-creation of one's sexed bodily style of being can be ongoing but not without continuity with the past, and it can be more or less difficult depending on one's own and others' bodily existence. Indeed, the re-creation that may take place after the aforementioned rupture in one's sexed style of being can take time and involve harder work than that involved in changes of one's sexed style of being that many other teenagers experience when they undergo puberty. And how hard work this might be partly depends on the social asymmetry of bodies.

Phenomenologists commonly agree that others have already inhabited and shaped the world, and others make the world familiar to us, in our early years and in continuous interactions. In this way, human being-in-the-world is characterized by thorough intersubjective meaning-making, where others "give" the world to us by making it familiar to us, and where we also "give" the world as meaningful to others. We can also "give" bodily habits, postures, and expressions to each other in close interactions with others, as discussed for example by Rosalyn Diprose (2002), and we may "give" corporeally enacted and expressed expectations and norms to each other as discussed in relation to the phenomenon of incorporation and excorporation.

Such giving—if this term is used—need not be harmonious, and it certainly need not imply an equal distribution of time, space, and ability to make the world a familiar place.

This becomes relevant when rethinking sexed subjectivity via the concept of style of being. Cultural beliefs and norms about bodies matter for how some bodies are given attendance and space, and other bodies are seen as odd; this discrimination operates through bodies and impacts them. This matters for how difficult or easy it is to express oneself, as a bodily being, when one's body is different from that of others in unexpected ways. As long as one's body "fits" these cultural beliefs and norms, it can be easy to "forget"—or rather take for granted—the strong cultural process where only some bodies are given space (see Diprose 2002, 170–175). This highlights that it is not enough to say that freedom lays in the way that the subject can corporeally engage with and alter the meaning and significance of the past that has shaped her or his bodily existence. We need also to examine how asymmetrical valuation of bodies can make some changes in the subject's sexed style of being more difficult than others.

Let us once more return to the stories of the young women in our previous research but this time to their descriptions of how they try to conceptualize their own existence in terms of difference. Whereas it may be difficult to express oneself in other ways than those dominant in one's cultural setting, these women commonly opt for one of two strategies to do so: either by conceiving one's bodily self as *differently normal* or *normally different* in relation to assumptions and beliefs about female embodiment (Guntram forthcoming).

The first is the case when some women downplay the importance of these particular organs and emphasize that they share other bodily features that are considered typically female by them, such as ovaries and XX chromosomes. The effect of this narrative strategy is supportive: the interviewee is just slightly different from other women. This is also the effect of the second approach, when women explain that, after all, "everyone is different." Being different, then, is normal, since there are *multiple ways* in which sexual difference is experienced and contextually made meaningful.

Irrespective of which route is taken, these can be seen as routes to not continue living a continuous excorporation (that may eventually lead to bodily alienation). The routes may be more or less successful and difficult, partly depending on whether others have already created space for being different and what *kind* of space others have created. In keeping with the analogy of music, experiences such as these may make the subject reflectively seek new, potentially very different, ways to continue the melody. Furthermore, some women explained that it was much "worse" not to have a vagina than not to have a womb. This was the case for Joanna, who said that finding out that her vagina could not be stretched to a "normal" size and that she "had to" have surgery was even worse than finding out about the womb. As a teenager, and particularly in interactions with friends, Joanna found that the inability to have intercourse was a greater issue than pregnancy. There may be different reasons for this discrepancy, but in keeping with the analogy of melody, women described it as easier to find ways to continue melodies of infertility in their own unique way than to find melodies relating to the absent vagina. The tune, pitch, and structure of their own melody did not resemble those melodies the women, and others, have heard before.

This way of thinking sexed embodiment highlights that there is not only or primarily *one* tune of female being-in-the-world. Furthermore, and importantly, this also highlights the close intersubjective and, indeed, intercorporeal relation between self and other. It shows that we all are involved in processes of giving of sexed bodily styles of being and of making some sexed bodily styles of being more difficult to express than others. And there is a crucial ethical dimension to this reasoning. Because of the way self and other are intrinsically related to each other—as seen in the discussion of incorporation, excorporation, and affectivity that form both self and other—we are all already implicated in processes of shared meaning-making and the formation of social space, and it does matter, ethically, how we engage in such meaning-making and space formation.

Acknowledgments

We would like to express our deep gratitude to the interviewees who shared their experiences. We also thank Linda Fisher and other participants at the conference Feminist Phenomenology and Medicine for helpful remark on a previous version of this text.

Notes

1. Our main concern is conceptual development, and we will discuss specific empirical examples that invite us to engage with conceptual development in new ways. See Guntram (forthcoming) for

a detailed analysis of semi-structured interviews with ten young women as regards their experiences of medical treatment.

2. An analysis of the women's narratives about medical interventions, normality, heteronormativity, and resistance is further discussed by Guntram (2013).

3. This can be contrasted with the way the body "eu-appears" when standing forth, to the subject, as strong or pleasurable (Zeiler 2010).

4. My hands may disappear from my reflective awareness when I write (focal disappearance), and this is different from the way my legs may disappear in the same activity (background disappearance). Whereas my hands disappear because they form the origin of the actional field of writing, my legs may slip to the margin of my consciousness because they have a merely supportive role in my engagement with the world in this situation. Depth disappearing body parts are typically not involved in the intentional, sensorimotor engagement that connects subject and world.

5. Only one interviewee explicitly mentions that she had realized that her vagina was smaller than what she considered "normal" before she had her first appointment with a gynecologist. However, this need not mean that the women have not explored their bodies before receiving the diagnosis. Rather it could point to norms concerning female masturbation, women's possibilities to speak about exploring one's genitals, and level of report between interviewer and interviewee. Noteworthy also is that a couple of the women describe that they had had intercourse before being diagnosed, but that this did not make them aware of their vagina being "small." This may highlight beliefs about the "normal" levels of pain involved when a woman has intercourse for the first time and that what is considered a "too" small vagina always is a matter of interpretation and negotiation, for example, in relation to norms and beliefs about the vagina's purpose, sexual practice, and sexual partners.

6. Please note that the blind man's bodily mode of being in the world is thoroughly shaped by the stick, and even when broken or absent, it will continue to form his bodily being in terms of him not being able to engage with others and the world as easily as before without it. In parallel, expectations and norms about sexual difference are unlikely to become objects of attention in the same way as any other object because of us—as bodily beings—being so thoroughly formed by them (see Zeiler 2013).

The phenomenon of excorporation has also been illustrated via Martin Heidegger's example of how the hammer, as a tool for hammering with a purposeful in-order-to structure, makes the carpenter not explicitly attend to it when engaged in the activity of hammering (Malmqvist and Zeiler 2010).

7. The new knowledge about the body matters for woman's experience of her body and her bodily sensations. For instance, this becomes clear as some women describe their fear of what a sexual partner might think of their body and how this fear may inform their bodily sensations in the sexual encounter.

References

American College of Obstetricians and Gynecologists. 2002. "ACOG Committee Opinion No. 247, July 2002. Nonsurgical Diagnosis and Management of Vaginal Agenesis." *International Journal of Gynaecology & Obstetrics* 79 (2): 167–170.

Ahmed, Sara. 2004. *The Cultural Politics of Emotion.* Edinburgh: Edinburgh University Press.

David, Noela. 2009. "New Materialism and Feminism's Anti-Biologism: A Response to Sarah Ahmed." *European Journal of Women's Studies* 16 (1): 67–80.

Diprose, Rosalyn. 2002. *Corporeal Generosity: On Giving with Nietzsche, Merleau-Ponty, and Levinas.* Albany: State University of New York Press.

Edmonds, D. Keith. 2003. Congenital Malformations of the Genital Tract and Their Management. *Best Practice & Research Clinical Obstetrics & Gynaecology* 17 (1):19–40.

Guntram, Lisa. 2013. "Creating, Maintaining and Questioning (Hetero)relational Normality in Narratives about Vaginal Reconstruction." *Feminist Theory* 14 (1): 101–121.

Guntram, Lisa. Forthcoming. "Negotiations of Normality and the Meaning of a Diagnosis: Exploring Women's Experiences of Atypical Pubertal Development." Submitted.

Heinämaa, Sara. 1997. "What Is a Woman? Butler and Beauvoir on the Foundations of the Sexual Difference." *Hypatia* 12 (1): 20.

Heinämaa, Sara. 1999. Simone de Beauvoir's Phenomenology of Sexual Difference. *Hypatia.*14 (4): 114–132.

Heinämaa, Sara. 2003. "The Body as Instrument and as Expression." In *The Cambridge Companion to Simone de Beauvoir*, edited by Claudia Card, 66–86. Cambridge: Cambridge University Press.

Heinämaa, Sara. 2011. "A Phenomenology of Sexual Difference: Types, Styles, and Persons." In *Feminist Metaphysics: Explorations in the Ontology of Sex, Gender and the Self*, edited by Charlotte Witt, 131–155. Dordrecht: Springer.

Käll, Lisa Folkmarson. 2009. "Expression between Self and Other." *Idealistic Studies: An Interdisciplinary Journal of Philosophy* 39 (1/3): 71–86.

Leder, Drew. 1990. *The Absent Body*. Chicago: University of Chicago Press.

Lee, Peter A., Christopher P. Houk, S. Faisal Ahmed, and Ieuan A. Hughes. 2006. "Consensus Statement on Management of Intersex Disorders." *Pediatrics* 118 (2): 488–500.

Liao, Lih Mei, Jacqueline Doyle, Naomi S. Crouch, and Sarah M. Creighton. 2006. "Dilation as Treatment for Vaginal Agenesis and Hypoplasia: A Pilot Exploration of Benefits and Barriers as Perceived by Patients." *Journal of Obstetrics and Gynaecology: The Journal of the Institute of Obstetrics and Gynaecology* 26 (2): 144–148.

Malmqvist, Erik, and Kristin Zeiler. 2010. "Cultural Norms, the Phenomenology of Incorporation, and the Experience of Having a Child Born with Ambiguous Sex." *Social Theory & Practice* 36 (1): 133–156.

Merleau-Ponty, Maurice. 2006. *Phenomenology of Perception*. London: Routledge.

Morgan, Elisabeth M., and Elisabeth H. Quint. 2006. "Assessment of Sexual Functioning, Mental Health, and Life Goals in Women with Vaginal Agenesis." *Archives of Sexual Behavior* 35 (5): 607–618.

Singer, Linda. 1981. "Merleau-Ponty on the Concept of Style." *Man and World* 14: 153–163.

Zeiler, Kristin. 2010. "A Phenomenological Analysis of Bodily Self-Awareness in the Experience of Pain and Pleasure: On Dys-Appearance and Eu-Appearance." *Medicine, Health Care and Philosophy* 13 (3): 333–342.

Zeiler, Kristin. 2013. "Phenomenology of Excorporation, Bodily Alienation and Resistance: Rethinking Sexed and Racialized Embodiment." *Hypatia: A Journal of Feminist Phenomenology* 28 (1): 69–84.

9

REASSIGNING AMBIGUITY

Intersex, Biomedicine, and the Question of Harm

ELLEN K. FEDER

> To be born is both to be born of the world and to be born into the
> world. The world is already constituted, but also never completely con-
> stituted; in the first case we are acted upon, in the second we are open to
> an infinite number of possibilities. But this analysis is still abstract, for we
> exist in both ways *at once.*
>
> —Maurice Merleau-Ponty, *Phenomenology of Perception*
> (emphasis in original)

Surgical management came to define the standard of care for children born with ambiguous genitalia beginning in the 1950s.
Because intersex conditions were in the main unknown to parents
of affected children and to society at large, an important element of
medical management was the education of parents in these conditions. While information regarding a given condition and the nature
of the treatment was frequently and by design partial or misleading,
the intention of physicians working in this area was to ensure an
unambiguous gender identity for the child and his parents.

Some key elements of the medical management of atypical sex in
children have changed in the last ten years. Adults with intersex conditions and their parents have spoken out about how the standard of
care has affected their lives, and their stories have been powerful testament to the physical and emotional damage wrought by the standard

of care. Increasing numbers of pediatric specialists today reaffirm the good intentions that motivated earlier practices but also acknowledge the clinical ignorance, even arrogance, that governed care—especially their failure to convey to parents what one group of practitioners describes as the potential "side-effects" of surgery, including the likelihood of damaging of erotic sensation (e.g., Dayner, Lee, and Houk 2004; see also Lee and Houk 2010, 1). More recently researchers have also reported on the lack of certainty or confidence among physicians themselves with regard to the standard of care (Karkazis, Tamar-Mattis, and Kon 2010). Today, specialists in the treatment of intersex conditions or what are now called "disorders of sex development" (DSD) have embraced informed consent as a new model of "shared decision making" (Dreger, Sandberg, and Feder 2010) is coming to the fore.

These are indisputably important changes. And yet, it does not appear that there has been a significant reduction in normalizing surgery, particularly in the United States. Where in the past, surgery was undertaken by physicians who understood themselves to be responding to a "social emergency," today these surgeries are performed in response to "what parents want" (e.g., Rebelo, Szabo, and Pitcher 2008).[1] Physicians are facilitating normalizing procedures to satisfy not only the parents' wishes, however; physicians claim that without surgery, parents will be unable to bond with their child. The child's good depends on the parents' love and acceptance (e.g., Eugster 2004, 428). If the condition of that love is the normalization of the appearance of atypical sex, then, these physicians seem to agree, surgery is indicated. But what if the performance of these surgeries has the opposite effect? What if it turns out that normalizing surgeries impede the love they are meant to facilitate?

Parents of children with atypical sex are described in the literature as confused or frustrated (Malmqvist and Zeiler 2010, 133), anxious or disoriented (Gough et al. 2008, 503–504). Of course, these are characterizations that may obtain with respect to any number of medical conditions that occur in the neonatal period. Confusion or frustration would be a likely result if a child is experiencing trouble breathing or has an irregular heartbeat that cannot easily be explained. If there has been no indication of a problem during pregnancy, and one's child is suddenly removed to a neonatal intensive care unit, there is every reason to expect new parents will experience anxiety and disorientation. Indeed, a recent study of stress in mothers with children with DSD demonstrated they had levels of stress comparable with those mothers of children with type 1 diabetes (Kirk et al. 2010). Acknowledging the stress that parents experience, however, cannot justify a standard of care exceptional in medicine, organized as it is around the relief of the parents rather than the care of the child. This is not to say that relief of parental distress has no place in medical management of DSD; indeed, advocates and critics of the standard of care would agree that attending to parents' distress at the birth of a child with unusual anatomy is of critical importance both for ensuring the care of the child in their charge and for the well-being of a parent whose own sense of self may be deeply unsettled. "Parents of children born with unusual anatomies," Alice Dreger writes,

> may suddenly find themselves unsure about their *own* social and familial role. How are they supposed to act? What are they supposed to think, feel, do, say? They know only how normal parents are supposed to behave, but they can't be normal parents if they don't have a normal child. They seek surgical "reconstruction" of a normal child in part because they feel like they will know how to be a parent to that child, whereas they often feel uncertain how to be a parent to this one. (2004, 57; emphasis in original)

This matter of parental responses to a child's anatomy merits more sustained consideration than is reflected in the current approach, focused on "erasing" the problem of atypical sex. When physicians say that surgery is "what parents want," we should ask, specifically, what it is parents really want, that is, what they mean ultimately to achieve, and whether surgery will in fact satisfy parents' aims. If what "normal parents" want is the best chance for their child to flourish, we should not take for granted that normalized appearance guarantees flourishing. The limited evidence that exists suggests that normalizing genital surgery does not provide parents relief or reassurance in the long term.[2] My aim in this chapter is to examine the nature of the harm that results from the prevailing model of medical management insofar as it focuses on relieving parental discomfort.

Evidence of the harm caused by the most prominent features of medical management since its beginnings in the 1950s has been substantial: physical and psychosocial injury caused by clitorectomy in girls with clitoromegaly, castration and sex reassignment in boys with micropenis, performance of uncomfortable vaginal dilation in young children following vaginoplasty or the creation of a neovagina, psychosocial damage that the early emphasis on maintaining the secrecy of a child's sexual ambiguity from the child and extended family, trauma provoked by genital exams and medical photography: these are among the accepted practices that appear to have changed dramatically in the last ten years. That change must be credited to the adults as well as their parents who have given voice to the suffering they have endured,[3] together with the recognition that the standard of care entailed violations of accepted principles of bioethics, most obviously those concerning informed consent and the avoidance of paternalism.

But there is a harm of another kind, the prevention of which may not be recognized within the terms of accepted principles of bioethics. It is damage that occurs at the level of what Maurice Merleau-Ponty describes by the term "body schema" in *Phenomenology of Perception* (1962). In what follows, I propose a framework for understanding the particular harm that normalizing genital surgery in infancy and early childhood may entail in phenomenological terms. Merleau-Ponty's work provides valuable resources for understanding this harm, even as his failure to attend to gender difference, and his adoption of a masculinist notion of subjectivity, may present obstacles for its elaboration. Such problems may be resolved with Merleau-Ponty's account, I propose, if we integrate his notion of the body schema with his reflections on human emergence appearing in his engagement with Malebranche in lectures he delivered in 1947–1948 for students preparing for the *agrégation* in philosophy (Merleau-Ponty [1968] 2001). Jacques Lacan's account of the mirror stage complements Merleau-Ponty's reflections by providing a ground for recognizing the particular harms that normalizing surgeries can effect given that they are generally performed during the period (between the ages of six and eighteen months) that Lacan identifies as the critical inauguration of this process of subject formation.[4] Bringing this account into conversation with Merleau-Ponty's engagement with Malebranche provides important insight into a kind of harm that physicians and perhaps even those who experience it may not be fully able to name, identify, or understand. Located at the junction of the corporeal and the psychic, it is neither precisely corporeal nor psychic, making it difficult to describe what may be at stake for the child—and for the family as a whole—in parents' decisions to normalize a child's sex anatomy.

In the second part of the chapter I turn to the narrative of a man who underwent sex reassignment and normalizing surgery as an infant. When I got to know him more than ten years ago, I knew him as Kristi, a young, funny, and engaging lesbian and intersex activist. What I relay here is the result of a conversation we had in 2010, after I had become reacquainted with him as Jim. Still young, funny, and engaging, and now a straight man, Jim agreed to help me consider this problem of harm through reflecting on his own experience. His story captures what, following Suzanne Kessler (1990), we may take to be a characteristic episode in the history of medical management. It also offers insight into the lasting effects of early normalizing surgeries that remain part of the standard of care, revealing the material and symbolic harms that prevalent forms of evidence in this field inadequately capture. While some may see in his story only the terrible consequences of a gross medical error in judgment, something that better-informed physicians would never have committed, much of his treatment, and the motivations for his treatment, are continuous with the standard of care today that makes of atypical sex a condition "like no other." Attending to these harms, I conclude, speaks to the need in medicine for another kind of moral framework—what Gail Weiss (1999) calls an "embodied ethics"—that may provide better guidance for parents and physicians in caring for children with unusual anatomies.

The Body Schema and Its "I Can"

The concept of the body schema grounds Merleau-Ponty's (1962, 198, 236–237) distinctive ontological claim that who and what we are as embodied subjects is "ambiguous": subject and object, perceiver and perceived. This ambiguity denotes the irreducibly "dynamic" (Merleau-Ponty 1962, 100) space that makes experience possible. Recognizing this dynamic, we must reckon with the fact that our bodies themselves cannot be objectified for an "I think" (Merleau-Ponty 1962, 153):

> My awareness of [my body] is not a thought, that is to say, I cannot take it to pieces and reform it to make a clear idea. Its unity is always implicit and vague. It is always something other than what it is, always sexuality and at the same time

> freedom, rooted in nature at the very moment when it is
> transformed by cultural influences, never hermetically sealed
> and never left behind. Whether it is a question of another's
> body or my own, I have no means of knowing the human
> body other than that of living it, which means taking up on
> my own account the drama which is being played out in it,
> and losing myself in it. (Merleau-Ponty 1962, 198)

This is to say, "I *am* my body" (Merleau-Ponty 1962, 198; emphasis added). Taylor Carman summarizes this point nicely when he
explains that for Merleau-Ponty, the body schema "is not a product but a condition of cognition, for only by being embodied am
I a subject in the world at all: 'I am conscious of my body via the
world,' [. . .] just as 'I am conscious of the world through the medium
of my body'" (Carman 1999, 220, citing Merleau-Ponty 1962, 82).
Consciousness understood in phenomenological terms cannot then
be understood as "a matter of 'I think that' but of 'I can'" (Merleau-
Ponty 1962, 137).

Even as feminist readers have found a rich theoretical framework in Merleau-Ponty's phenomenology, they have commented on
ways that the gender neutrality of his account of subjectivity finally
"reduces the specifically intersubjective experience of the body manifest in an encounter with another embodied person to the corporeal dynamic operative with the body proper (*le corps propre*)," and
so neglects the "gender-specific experience" of this body (Stawarska
2006, 92; see also Weiss 1999, 2). Famously beginning with Iris Marion Young's landmark "Throwing Like a Girl" ([1980] 2005), feminist
criticism of this problem has revealed how Merleau-Ponty's treatment
covers over the kinds of objectification of women that inhibits the "I
canness" of the body, the way its flesh opens onto, is always already
constitutive of, the world. The sense of the "I can" Merleau-Ponty
describes cannot be understood in terms of conventional conceptions
of the autonomous subject, and the meaning of the intentions that
issue from this subject. Acknowledging how possibilities for engagement may be forestalled by an inhibiting "self-consciousness of the
feminine relation to her body" (Young 2005, 44), the objectification
she makes her own, is important for understanding the particular
harm I want to identify in the medical management of DSD. Feminists' critical appropriation of Merleau-Ponty's phenomenology provides challenging resources for exploring the losses that can occur as

a consequence of normalizing genital surgeries in infancy and early childhood. But appreciation of those losses requires attending more closely to Merleau-Ponty's understanding of the development of human subjectivity.

Being Seen, Being Loved:
Conditions of Human Emergence

In his lectures on Malebranche (1947–1948) that closely follow the publication of *Phenomenology of Perception*, Merleau-Ponty provides a corrective to the limiting notion of the "body proper" on which his published work focuses. In her essay "Merleau-Ponty and the Touch of Malebranche," Judith Butler (2005, 204) provides a compelling reading of these lectures that offers an unexpected and moving consideration of "the primary conditions for human emergence" that enriches our understanding of Merleau-Ponty's account of subjectivity. Merleau-Ponty's engagement with Malebranche focuses mainly on the "point of departure for sentience itself, the obscurity and priority of its animating condition" (Butler 2005, 194). "On one hand," Butler writes,

> this is a theological investigation for Malebranche. It is not only that I cannot feel anything but what touches me, but that I cannot love without first being loved, cannot see without being seen, and that in some fundamental way, the act of seeing and loving are made possible by—and are coextensive with—being seen and being loved. [. . .] But Malebranche in the hands of Merleau-Ponty—Malebranche, as it were, transformed by the touch of Merleau-Ponty—becomes something different and something more. For here, Merleau-Ponty asks after the conditions by which the subject is animated into being. (2005, 195; emphasis added)

Butler suggests that the "fundamental inquiry into the animating conditions of human ontology" that occurs here may supplement (and perhaps complete) the important work on "The Intertwining— The Chiasm" that remained unfinished at Merleau-Ponty's death. "This chiasm," she explains, "is the name for the obscure basis of our self-understanding, and the obscure basis of our understanding of everything that is not ourselves" (Butler 2005, 198). That obscurity is resolved for Malebranche in the mystery of divinity that mediates the subject's "passage through alterity which makes any and all contact of the soul with itself necessarily obscure" (Butler 2005, 199). This connection between human and God as He manifests Himself in this obscurity also shapes what Merleau-Ponty called the "I can" in *Phenomenology of Perception*, for, it "is by virtue of this connection, which I cannot fully know, between sentience and God, that I understand myself to be a free being, one whose actions are not fully determined in advance, for whom action appears as a certain vacillating prospect" (Merleau-Ponty 1962, 199). Human freedom—that is to say, one's possibilities for becoming—remains mysterious; it is not located "in" the subject, and yet its animating conditions, beyond the subject, exceed her ability fully to objectify them.

At the end of her essay Butler (2005, 203) suggests that we might understand these lectures to constitute Merleau-Ponty's recasting of "psychoanalysis as a seventeenth-century theology": while the "material needs of infancy are not quite the same as the scene that Malebranche outlines for us as the primary touch of the divine," she writes, "we can see that his theology gives us a way to consider not only the primary conditions for human emergence but the requirement for alterity, the satisfaction of which paves the way for the emergence of the human itself" (Butler, 2005, 204). Because their early childhood experience can put into relief the sorts of pivotal interactive moments with their parents that might otherwise be taken for granted, accounts of those individuals who have undergone normalizing genital surgeries provide a privileged opportunity to examine the conditions that "pave the way" for this emergence and the conditions that impede it.

Criticisms of the standard of care of intersex conditions that focus on the suffering caused by past treatment speak evocatively to "the requirement for alterity"—the need for the "seeing" and "loving" (m)other. But to the extent that such criticisms are recognized by most pediatric specialists who continue to recommend, or present normalizing surgery as an "option" (Parisi et al. 2007, 355), they persist in seeing normalizing surgery as the means of securing parents' love of their children. The problems of the past—which many physicians report they relay to parents faced with decisions about normalizing surgery today (Parisi et al. 2007, 355)—are understood to be the result of inadequate surgical techniques of the past (e.g., Leslie,

Cain, and Rink 2009). Reducing these problems to technical matters, however, precludes consideration of what may be more consequential questions concerning the effects of normalizing surgery per se.

Lacan's account of the mirror stage provides an explicit psycho-analytic account of human emergence that Butler sees as implicit in Merleau-Ponty's reading of Malebranche. During the first few months of life, before the process of individuation begins, the infant relates to its body and the body of its mother in terms of its parts: the fist, foot, or nipple it finds in its mouth. The mirror stage marks the beginning of a process of identity formation in which the infant, at about six months of age, encounters its own unified image. This is, Lacan remarks, a joyful moment, arousing so much interest that the baby works to surmount the challenges of its inability to stand, devis-ing the means to prolong its first recognition of itself as a whole body (Lacan [1966] 1977, 2). But the "flutter of jubilant activity" evident at this moment is not only the delight in the image of the child's own body but also of the "persons and things" around him (Lacan 1977, 1), including the animated gaze and recognition of the mother the baby also sees reflected in the mirror.[5]

Many writings on the mirror stage emphasize the alienation that the recognition of one's body, distinct from other bodies, brings. As Merleau-Ponty writes, the "objectification of his own body discloses to the child his difference, his 'insularity,' and, correlatively, that of others" (Merleau-Ponty [1960] 1964, 119; cf. 129). At least at the beginning of his exposition of the mirror stage, however, Lacan does not emphasize alienation[6] so much as the vulnerability of the baby, the observation that its joyful (mis)recognition of a unified image of itself comes at the moment when the baby is "still sunk in his [. . .] motor incapacity and nursling dependence" (Lacan 1977, 2).

In *The Imaginary Domain*, Drucilla Cornell (1995, 38) argues that the "Lacanian account allows us to understand just how fragile the achievement of individuation is, and how easily it can be under-mined, if not altogether destroyed, by either a physical or symbolic assault on the projection of bodily integrity." The fragility of this achievement is owing to the dependency of the infant on the other, first because the other enables the infant to repeat the experience of encountering its mirror image, the experience that conveys its sense of bodily integrity vital to the child's developing sense of self. Cornell (1995, 39) explains that

in this way, the sight of another human being, including
the infant's actual image in the mirror, or in the eyes of the
mother or primary caretaker, is crucial for shaping identity.
This other, who, in turn, both appears as whole and confirms
the infant in its projected and anticipated coherence by mirroring him or her as a self, becomes the matrix of a sense of
continuity and coherence which the child's present state of
bodily disorganization would belie.[7]

Given the importance of the other's role in this founding moment
of subject formation, we must ask what the implications of normalizing genital surgery during this process of mirroring could entail.
What effect might the changing of the body's appearance have for
the child? How might the pain postsurgical recovery brings figure in
what is, from a psychoanalytic perspective, a critical period in development? What changes might occur in the ways those significant
"others"—those whose eyes serve as mirrors to the infant—relate to
him?

If we are discouraged from asking such questions because of the
paucity of good "evidence" we can gather from such an investigation, we should recall that it is precisely because of the fear that a
parent will not relate well, that is, will not serve as a good mirror, to
a child with an unusual sex anatomy that normalizing genital surgery
remains the standard of care. But granting that the sort of evidence
most everyone wants is not forthcoming should not (as it largely
has to this point) justify the unchecked performance of normalizing surgery in children too young to consent to these procedures.
It isn't that physicians do not see cautionary tales in the experiences
of those whose surgeries occurred ten or twenty or thirty years ago;
they evidently see in these stories errors or inadequacies of technique.
Though today physicians may less frequently promote these surgeries
as a means of improving sexual or reproductive functioning, the questions they ask remain technical. They do not challenge their assumptions that these interventions promote affective, social functioning. In
the experiences of those able to articulate their experience as adults,
we find challenging responses to the recommendations of physicians
to normalize a child's appearance, and parents' agreement—or sometimes urging—to do so.

Jim's Story

Jim did not know anything about his sex reassignment until he was twelve years old. Company had already arrived one evening at the house, and Jim was with his mother in her bedroom while she finished getting ready. "I don't know why she chose then but she told me that I was born a hermaphrodite and that I'd have to take pills to look like all the other girls." Jim—then called Kristi—recounts that the news, not that he would need to take hormone replacement, which he did not really understand, but of his ambiguous sex, brought feelings of excitement, fear, and exhilaration. It was for him a kind of affirmation, a "recognition that there was something wrong with me, that there was a reason I was unhappy and riddled with anxiety." It wasn't that Jim always "knew" he was born male, he says; he describes instead a sense of distance from his body, an "ineffable" sense of being out of place that was beyond his grasp[8] but brought nearer by his mother's revelation. Perhaps it remained just out of his reach because his mother never told him about the two surgeries he had had, first at about thirteen months, and then, when he was three and a half, to remove a smaller-than-normal penis and undescended testes.

Jim's recounting of his childhood is an account of two different bodies. One was a model of athletic prowess. An accomplished soccer player despite the physical disadvantage entailed by not having hormone-producing gonads, he remembers how the soccer field was where he was "truly happy," where he felt "very much in [his] body." But as he got older, even that experience took on what he describes as the "grayness" that characterized his life off the field: "All the girls around me started to change, to look more like women, and more beautiful. [. . .] I had to go to the doctor to have my change take place." The exhilaration Jim felt at twelve, when his sense of his difference from his peers was affirmed, flattened in later adolescence when he learned that "I would need to take all these pills and put on weight, and develop these breasts." Even so, he remembers, "I experienced my body as a success on the field. It didn't come easily. The older I got, the more I was surrounded by girls who were better and better." On the field, Jim's body was fluent in the "conversation of gestures" (Mead [1934] 1962, 181) that organized it. There, all the players "were encouraged to behave the way that I behaved naturally, which was aggressive, and focused [. . .] thinking about the game."

Despite or maybe because of the dull unhappiness he felt off the field, the resentment that he felt toward his teammates who were as conversant in the feminine gestures solicited off the field as they were those—athletic, unmarked, masculine—gestures on it, Jim did not resist the vaginoplasty his mother presented him as "a matter of course" when he turned eighteen. From his narrative, it does not seem that he saw vaginoplasty as a means of joining the girls in being the women they seemed effortlessly to become; rather, it seems that his assent was a measure of his indifference to his body, to what happened to his body, when it was not engaged athletically. Presented as "what would happen," it did.

Cornell remarks that the mirror stage "is not a stage in the traditional sense, because one never completes it" (Cornell 1995, 39; cf. Merleau-Ponty 1964, 119). That is to say, the "coherence" that passing through the stage is supposed to secure is never finally achieved, and yet it is this sense of coherence, or imagined coherence, that grounds one's identity, one's sense of self. That is to say, the "self" the infant sees in the mirror is not "already 'there' [. . .]. Instead, the self is constituted in and through the mirroring process as other to its reality of bodily disorganization, and by having itself mirrored by others as a whole" (Cornell 1995, 39). Jim's description of a secure sense of self, of bodily integrity on the soccer field, reflects what he describes as the consistent approval he received, particularly from his father. But when he was not in training, when he was not playing, the disorganization, the "grayness," returned. In his account, the despised vaginoplasty was a somatic insult that provoked a deeper discontent, an inability to forget his body as he had previously done. It was also an obstacle to intimate relationships, and, he would learn later when he consulted with a physician, it could pose a threat to his life: The type of vaginoplasty he had, had proven especially prone to cancerous growth (Schober 2006, 605–606). About a year after the surgery, Jim would seek his medical records and find out what had been taken from him.

It would take a few more years before Jim would seek medical help. No longer taking the female hormones he was prescribed as a teenager, his body consequently weakened with osteopenia and the onset of osteoporosis, his anger competing with his depression, Jim found a knowledgeable and compassionate physician and began a trial of testosterone therapy. He did so with some trepidation, not because he feared transition, he explains, but because the therapy might not have any effect: "I was worried because when I was born, my genitals didn't fully develop, the [doctor's] concern was that my body didn't respond to testosterone." If hormone therapy was not effective, Jim was afraid that he would be truly, as he put it, "up a creek." But it did work. The wonder in Jim's voice is evident when he recalls that his "body really sucked it in, absorbed every bit, like it was hungry for it. It was magical." It was magical because everything changed—his body, first, and then the ways that others related to him. Recovered fully from the osteopenia, "demedicalized," as his doctor proclaimed him, he sought removal of the vaginoplasty. Jim was a new man.

A New Man, the Same Kid

Jim's triumphant re-creation of himself is a remarkable testament to Merleau-Ponty's observation of the way that a body's sense of being "geared onto the world" is marked by the ways that one's body and its intentions may be welcomed by the world. Jim describes the experience of what Merleau-Ponty characterizes as "a certain possession of the world by [his] body, a certain gearing of [his] body to the world"; for the first time, at least off a soccer field, his intentions "receive the response they expect from the world" (Merleau-Ponty 1962, 250). In stores, at work, his interactions with people demonstrated a marked difference; he experienced an unfamiliar ease as he related to and among others as a man for the first time.

But his experience also confirms Merleau-Ponty's (1962, 393) claim that our existence "always carries forward its past, whether it be by accepting or disclaiming it." Those who knew Jim as Kristi see the same person. It is not that he has not changed, or that his friends, family, and longtime acquaintances were "really" seeing Jim all along; nor is it that he is still Kristi. When people—those who knew him as a child or young adult and his relieved mother—marvel that Jim is "the same kid," or remark that he "hasn't changed at all," they are speaking to a continuity in the sense of the person they know and love, his humor and gentle compassion, his resilience and edge. For those who knew Kristi and now encounter Jim, Merleau-Ponty's observations about our experience of the present and its relation to the past come to life:

> With the arrival of every moment, its predecessor under-
> goes a change: I still have it in hand and it is still there, but
> already it is sinking away below the level of presents; in order
> to retain it, I need to reach through a thin layer of time. It is
> still the preceding moment, and I have the power to rejoin it
> as it was just now; I am not cut off from it, but still it would
> not belong to the past unless something had altered, unless
> it were beginning to outline itself, or project itself upon, my
> present, whereas a moment ago it *was* my present. (Merleau-
> Ponty 1962, 416–417; emphasis in original)

The way that the meaning of one's past can be changed by the present, a past that paradoxically retains its integrity, conditions the possibility for the "reinvention" Jim has effected.

It may be helpful here to draw on Merleau-Ponty's use of the
image of "sedimentation" to understand how this is possible. One
might imagine one's experiences as accumulated layers of sediment,
forming a foundation for the stream of understanding that is ongoing. Merleau-Ponty cautions us not to see sediment as "an inert mass
in the depths of our consciousness," but a ground that also conditions
the possibility for the "spontaneity" that create for Merleau-Ponty the
"world-structure [. . .] at the core of consciousness" (Merleau-Ponty
1962, 130). Newly acquired thoughts or ways of seeing "draw their
sustenance from my present thought, they offer me a meaning, but I
give it back to them" (Merleau-Ponty 1962, 130). New thoughts or
understandings of our experience can provide surprising new directions for consciousness and create new layers of sediment. Following Merleau-Ponty's metaphor through to understand the effect of a
change such as Jim's, one might consider the effect that a particularly
heavy rain or disturbance at some point in a river could have on its
flow: its appearance and movement may be dramatically reshaped;
and yet its new appearance and direction would remain continuous
with its previous incarnation. This notion of sedimentation provides
a way to understand how an individual experiences oneself and one's
body as it becomes "habituated" to itself and its environment and
also speaks to the ways that intersubjective experience—the ways
that we make sense of one another in gesture and speech—figures in
"individual" experience. The impression that Jim is the "same person"
speaks phenomenologically to the ways that the continuity that Jim

and those who knew him as Kristi, coexists with—and not despite—the significant change he has undergone.

Jim's transition to living as a man[9] is not the first time he has experienced a significant shift in his view of his own past, however. When his mother told him that he had been born different, "special," as she said, he saw his previous experience with "new eyes," a different perspective that changed his understanding of the past as he lived it in the present, laying down new possibilities for the future. When he finally learned years later that being born special as he was had prompted his castration and the removal of his penis, there was another shift, one that complicates his evident attachment to and love for his parents. Jim recounts that "I never had any doubt that my parents loved me; I also never had a doubt that they were riddled with multiple prejudices about me and I [. . .] wished they were smarter and filled with less fear than they were." Learning of the surgery brought a still different perspective on himself and his world. But understanding, as his parents and all those who care about him would come to understand, the consequences of his sex reassignment, they were also able to see—and to mirror—this new man, "the same" lovable kid before them.

Toward an Embodied Ethics

I began this chapter by discussing the motivation for normalizing surgery in children with atypical sex anatomies. Jim's story provides an entrée for understanding the consequences of a treatment rationale grounded in satisfying parents' or society's, rather than children's, needs. In making the aim of treatment the relief of the suffering of the parents, and seeking to resolve or diminish that suffering by altering the child's body, of making it tolerable, the child, I would suggest, *is not seen*. Making the love of parents for a child conditional on the child's appearance puts that love in question; however good the intention, "the effect may be otherwise" (Dreger 2006, 261). Indeed, as Adrienne Asch puts it: "By undertaking [cosmetic] surgery before children can voice feelings about their bodies and their lives, the most loving parent can unwittingly undermine the child's confidence that she is lovable and loved. It is confidence in that love and lovableness that provides the foundation for dealing with what life brings" (2006,

229). The confidence in one's parents' love that Asch sees as vital to a child's flourishing also participates in the kind of enigmatic becoming-human with which Merleau-Ponty grapples in his thinking with Malebranche. This confidence may be understood as a condition of the possibility of the embodied "I can," the place where the body's materiality and consciousness "meet" and engage in the world and with others.

The exploration of an "embodied ethics" I have begun here must concern not only the status of the child as subject but the parents' subjectivity, as well. As Gail Weiss describes it, an embodied ethics is "grounded in the dynamic, bodily imperatives that emerge out of our intercorporeal exchanges and which in turn transform our own body [schemas], investing and reinvesting them with moral significance" (Weiss 1999, 158). Jim's transition is possible not only, or perhaps not primarily, because he finds acceptance and acknowledgment of his experience in his family and longtime friends, but because his family and longtime friends themselves change in response to this acknowledgment. This is the philosophical gloss on what Alice Dreger writes in her *Psychology Today* blog:

> If you want to be a parent, start getting used to the fact that your children will change you as much as you change them. I now know far more than I ever thought I would about trains, airplanes, and Australian native species thanks to my son. I am also more patient, more organized, more disorganized, more sleep deprived, and more in love with him than I ever thought I'd be. If you would not have your child explicitly manipulate your identity as a condition of loving you, do not begin your relationship with your child by doing the same. (Dreger 2010)

The ethical imperative articulated here—an embodied ethical imperative—should perhaps be understood as an essential supplement to, rather than replacement of, conventional approaches to bioethics. The imperative to which Dreger points is not one of "unconditional love"; it is instead an acknowledgment that parents' love, together with the caring work that constitutes parenting, should be understood to shape not only the child but the parents themselves. Were an "embodied ethics" to be taken seriously, it seems evident that the standard of care would change radically; its objects of intervention would shift from an exclusive focus on "the patient" to include also those who care for him. Such an ethics is not easily reduced to rules, or assessed via indicators of "quality care." Further investigation is required here, and the kind of phenomenological interrogation toward which Merleau-Ponty directs us offers rich resources for its elaboration.

Acknowledgments

Material from this chapter will also appear in Ellen K. Feder, *Making Sense of Intersex: Changing Ethical Perspectives in Biomedicine*, forthcoming from Indiana University Press, 2014.

There are a number of people without whose encouragement and advice this chapter would not have been possible. I am grateful to Lisa Folkmarson Käll and Kristin Zeiler for their invitation to the conference Feminist Phenomenology and Medicine that prompted the development of this analysis. Jim's generosity in sharing his experience and helping me to think through the problems I examine was absolutely essential for my thinking through the problem of the harm effected by the standard of care. Sincere thanks to Debra Bergoffen, Wilfried Ver Eecke, and Mary Rawlinson, whose early conversations about this essay got the analysis off the ground. Repeated thanks to Kristin, who provided insightful and incisive commentary with Lisa Guntram, as well as to all the other smart and supportive participants in the conference. Thanks are due also to Carolyn Betensky, Alice Dreger, Karmen MacKendrick, Shelley Harshe, Andrea Tschemplik, and Gail Weiss, who read and commented on earlier versions of this chapter.

Notes

1. Physicians' justifying surgery as fulfilling parents' wishes is not new, though its salience in these decisions appears novel. In an essay first published 1998, Cheryl Chase recounts a conversation with an endocrinologist that "he had never in his career seen a good cosmetic result in intersex genital reconstructions, but 'what can you do? The parents demand it'" ([1998] 1999, 150).
2. Laura Hermer (2002) points to the work of Slijper et al. (1998) to suggest that parents who have consented to normalizing surgery

for their children have not been satisfied, though she concludes that surgery may nevertheless be in children's best interest to secure parents' love (cited in Tamar-Mattis 2006, 90n226).

3. See, for example, narratives in Dreger 1999; Preves 2003; and Karkazis 2008.

4. For example, "In females with classic 21-OHD CAH who are virilized at birth, feminizing genitoplasty may be performed to remove the redundant erectile tissue while preserving the sexually sensitive glans clitoris and to provide a normal vaginal orifice that functions adequately for menstruation, intromission, and delivery. Clitoroplasty is typically performed in early childhood (*preferably at age 6–18 months*)" (New and Nimkarn [2002] 2006, 12; emphasis added). More recent recommendations indicate that surgery between three and six months is preferable. See, for example, Cornell University 2010.

5. I thank Wilfried Ver Eecke for emphasizing this important point. Interestingly, in following the reading of Henri Wallon, whose work predates Lacan's, Merleau-Ponty emphasizes the role of the other in this stage but in the form of the father (see Merleau-Ponty 1964, 127–128).

6. The notion of alienation, taken up in existentialist-psychoanalytic terms, carries a different valence in Merleau-Ponty's work that casts "alienation" as an integral moment of intersubjectivity. In "The Child's Relation with Others," Merleau-Ponty writes that it "is this transfer of my intentions to the other's body and of his intentions to my own, my alienation of the other and his alienation of me, that makes possible the perception of others" (Merleau-Ponty 1964, 118).

7. African American musician Ysaye Maria Barnwell's celebration of her grandmother in "There Were No Mirrors in My Nana's House" here comes to mind. When she sings, "the beauty that I saw in everything [. . .] was in her eyes/So I never knew that my skin was too Black [. . .] that my nose was too flat [. . .] that my clothes didn't fit" (Barnwell 1993), she acknowledges the affirmative "mirroring" that also protected her from racist denigrations of her body, of her self.

8. Merleau-Ponty (1962, 238) might characterize Jim's as a kind of "latent knowledge."

9. Some might ask, not unreasonably, whether Jim was going "back" to an original identity when he began to live as a man. A

phenomenological analysis would recast that question in terms of the somatic experience and the "sense" (*sens*) of which the experience is made in the world. The experience of injecting testosterone, for example, supplies a somatic experience, the available meaning for which is marked as "male" in our world, one that cannot be disentangled from history and culture. We should recall Merleau-Ponty's claim that "it is impossible to establish a cleavage between what will be 'natural' [. . .] and what [. . .] acquired. In reality the two orders are not distinct; they are part and parcel of a global phenomenon" (Merleau-Ponty 1964, 108). For a contemporary treatment of this issue that draws explicitly on the case of intersex, see Rosario 2009).

References

Asch, Adrienne. 2006. "Appearance-Altering Surgery, Children's Sense of Self, and Parental Love." In *Surgically Shaping Children: Technology, Ethics, and the Pursuit of Normality*, edited by Erik Parens, 227–252. Baltimore: Johns Hopkins University Press.

Barnwell, Ysaye Maria. 1993. "There Were No Mirrors in My Nana's House." In *Sweet Honey in the Rock: Still on the Journey*. Redway, CA: EarthBeat! Records.

Butler, Judith. 2005. "Merleau-Ponty and the Touch of Malebranche." In *The Cambridge Companion to Merleau-Ponty*, edited by Taylor Carman and Mark B. N. Hansen, 181–205. New York: Cambridge University Press.

Carman, Taylor. 1999. "The Body in Husserl and Merleau-Ponty." *Philosophical Topics* 27 (2): 205–226.

Chase, Cheryl. [1998] 1999. "Surgical Progress Is Not the Answer." In *Intersex in the Age of Ethics*, edited by Alice Domurat Dreger, 146–159. Hagerstown, MD: University Publishing Group.

Cornell, Drucilla. 1995. *The Imaginary Domain: Abortion, Pornography and Sexual Harassment*. New York: Routledge.

Cornell University. 2010. "Surgical Management of Congenital Adrenal Hyperplasia." Weill-Cornell Medical Center. http://www.cornellurology.com/uro/cornell/pediatrics/genitoplasty.shtml#technique.

Dayner, Jennifer, Peter A. Lee, and Christopher P. Houk. 2004. "Medical Treatment of Intersex: Parental Perspectives." *The Journal of Urology* 172: 1762–1765.

Dreger, Alice Domurat (ed.). 1999. *Intersex in the Age of Ethics*. Hagerstown, MD: University Publishing Group.

Dreger, Alice Domurat. 2004. *One of Us: Conjoined Twins and the Future of Normal*. Cambridge: Harvard University Press.

Dreger, Alice Domurat. 2006. "What to Expect When You Have the Child You Weren't Expecting." In *Surgically Shaping Children: Technology, Ethics, and the Pursuit of Normality*, edited by Erik Parens, 253–266. Baltimore: Johns Hopkins University Press.

Dreger, Alice Domurat. 2010. "To Have Is to Hold." In *Psychology Today* blog. http://www.psychologytoday.com/blog/fetishes-i-dont-get/201006/have-is-hold-0.

Dreger, Alice, David Sandberg, and Ellen K. Feder. 2010. "From Principles to Process in Disorders of Sex Development Care." *Hormone Research in Paediatrics* 74 (6): 419–420.

Eugster, Erica A. 2004. "Reality vs. Recommendations in the Care of Infants with Intersex Conditions." *Archives of Pediatric Medicine* 158: 428–429.

Gough, Brendan, Nicky Weyman, Julie Alderson, Gary Butler, and Mandy Stoner. 2008. "'They did not have a word': The Parental Quest to Locate a 'True Sex' for Their Intersex Children." *Psychology and Health* 23 (4): 493–507.

Hermer, Laura. 2002. "Paradigms Revised: Intersex Children, Bioethics and the Law." *Annals of Health Law* 11: 195–236.

Karkazis, Katrina. 2008. *Fixing Sex: Intersex, Medical Authority, and Lived Experience*. Durham, NC: Duke University Press.

Karkazis, Katrina, Anne Tamar-Mattis, and Alexander A. Kon. 2010. "Genital Surgery for Disorders of Sex Development: Implementing a Shared Decision-Making Approach." *Journal of Pediatric Endocrinology and Metabolism* 23: 789–806.

Kessler, Suzanne J. 1990. "The Medical Construction of Gender: Case Management of Intersexed Infants." *Signs: Journal of Women in Culture and Society* 16 (1): 3–26.

Kirk, Katherine D., et al. 2010. "Parenting Characteristics of Female Caregivers of Children Affected by Chronic Endocrine Conditions: A Comparison between Disorders of Sex Development and Type 1 Diabetes Mellitus." *Journal of Pediatric Nursing*. http://www.ncbi.nlm.nih.gov/pmc/articles/PMC2902038/?tool=pubmed.

Lacan, Jacques. [1966] 1977. "The Mirror Stage as Formative of the

Function of the I." In *Écrits: A Selection*, translated by Alan Sheridan, 1–7. New York: W. W. Norton & Company.

Lee, Peter A., and Christopher P. Houk. 2010. "The Role of Support Groups, Advocacy Groups, and Other Interested Parties in Improving the Care of Patients with Congenital Adrenal Hyperplasia: Pleas and Warnings." *International Journal of Pediatric Endocrinology*. http://www.hindawi.com/journals/ijpe/2010/563640/.

Leslie, Jeffrey A., Mark Patrick Cain, and Richard Carlos Rink. 2009. "Feminizing Genital Reconstruction in Congenital Adrenal Hyperplasia." *Indian Journal of Urology* 25 (1): 17–26. http://www.ncbi.nlm.nih.gov/pmc/articles/PMC2684317/.

Malmqvist, Erik, and Kristin Zeiler. 2010. "Cultural Norms, the Phenomenology of Incorporation and the Experience of Having a Child Born with Ambiguous Sex." *Social Theory and Practice* 36 (1): 133–156.

Mead, George Herbert. [1934] 1962. *Mind, Self, and Society from the Standpoint of a Social Behaviorist*, edited by Charles W. Morris. Chicago: University of Chicago Press.

Merleau-Ponty, Maurice. 1962. *Phenomenology of Perception*, translated by Colin Smith. New York: Routledge & Kegan Paul.

Merleau-Ponty, Maurice. [1960] 1964. "The Child's Relation with Others," translated by William Cobb. In *The Primacy of Perception*, edited by Jim M. Edie, 96–155. Evanston: Northwestern University Press.

Merleau-Ponty, Maurice. [1968] 2001. *The Incarnate Subject: Malebranche, Biran, and Bergson on the Union of Body and Soul*, translated by Paul B. Milan, edited by Andrew G. Bjelland Jr. and Patrick Burke. Amherst, NY: Humanity Books.

New, Maria I., and Saroj Nimkarn. [2002] 2006. "21-Hydroxylase-Deficient Congenital Adrenal Hyperplasia." *GeneReviews*. Seattle: University of Washington. http://www.ncbi.nlm.nih.gov/sites/GeneTests/review?db=genetests.

Parisi, Melissa A., et al. 2007. "A Gender Assignment Team: Experience with 250 Patients Over a Period of 25 Years." *Genetics and Medicine* 9 (6): 348–357.

Preves, Sharon E. 2003. *Intersex and Identity: The Contested Self*. New Brunswick: Rutgers University Press.

Rebelo, Ethelwyn, Christopher P. Szabo, and Grame Pitcher. 2008. "Gender Assignment Surgery on Children with Disorders of Sex

Development: A Case Report and Discussion from South Africa."
Journal of Child Health Care 12 (1): 49–59.

Rosario, Vernon. 2009. "Quantum Sex: Intersex and the Molecular Deconstruction of Sex." *GLQ: Intersex and After* 15 (2): 267–284.

Schober, Justice. 2006. "Feminization (Surgical Aspects)." In *Pediatric Surgery and Urology: Long-Term Outcomes*, 2nd ed., edited by Mark D. Stringer, Keith T. Oldham, and Pierre D. E. Mouriquand, 595–609. Cambridge, England: Cambridge University Press.

Slijper, Froukje M. E., Stenvert L. S. Drop, Jan C. Molenaar, and Sabine M. P. F. de Muinck Keizer-Schrama. 1998. "Long-Term Psychological Evaluation of Intersex Children." *Archives of Sexual Behavior* 27: 125–144.

Stawarska, Beata. 2006. "From the Body Proper to Flesh: Merleau-Ponty on Intersubjectivity." In *Feminist Interpretations of Merleau-Ponty*, edited by Dorothea Olkowski and Gail Weiss, 91–106. State College: Pennsylvania State University Press.

Tamar-Mattis, Anne. 2006. "Exceptions to the Rule: Curing the Law's Failure to Protect Intersex Infants." *Berkeley Journal of Gender, Law and Justice* 21: 59–110.

Weiss, Gail. 1999. *Body Images: Embodiment as Intercorporeality*. New York: Routledge.

Young, Iris Marion. [1980] 2005. "Throwing Like a Girl: A Phenomenology of Feminine Body Comportment, Motility, and Spatiality." In *On Female Body Experience: "Throwing Like a Girl" and Other Essays*, 27–45. Oxford: Oxford University Press.

Zeiler, Kristin, and Anette Wickström. 2009. "Why Do 'We' Perform Surgery on Newborn Intersexed Children?" *Feminist Theory* 10 (3): 359–377.

10

FEMINISM, PHENOMENOLOGY, AND HORMONES

LANEI M. RODEMEYER

The position that gender, and possibly also sex, is constructed is generally accepted by many theorists, especially those working in feminist or queer theory. For several decades, this argument actually followed two complementary tracks, one in the humanities, and the other in the sciences (broadly construed to include biology, medicine, psychology, and related areas). This parallel was fostered by a study by psychologist John Money, who claimed to have shown that a biologically born male could be successfully raised as a female, under the right conditions. Money gained fame through his revolutionary book *Man and Woman, Boy and Girl* (1973), especially through his claim that environment was *the* key factor in what determined whether a person grew up as a boy or a girl. His quintessential case study was David Reimer, born a boy but raised as a girl, following an accident during a circumcision operation.[1] Money was involved in the transformation of the baby boy to a girl (carried out through preliminary operations and social conditioning) and broadcast the case as evidence that "nurture" clearly won out over "nature." He was subsequently cited by feminists, sociologists, psychologists, and even medical personnel, and the case was pointed to as confirming evidence that our tendencies toward masculinity or femininity are determined not by our bodies but by our surroundings. As John Colapinto (2000, 69) writes, in his book presenting the story of the child,

The significance of the case was not lost on the then-burgeoning women's movement, which had been arguing against a biological basis for sex differences for decades. Money's own papers from the 1950s on the psychosexual neutrality of newborns had already been used as one of the main foundations of modern feminism.[2]

This agreement between the sciences and the humanities on the original gender-neutrality of humans was enjoyed for around three decades, culminating, one might argue, in Judith Butler's theoretical arguments that not only gender, but also sex, is constructed through coercive performative practices. Butler's argument, based on an analysis of the workings of language, psychoanalysis, philosophy, and culture, showed that what we identify as "real" (especially with regard to bodies) arises out of repetitive practices, coercions, and exclusions, both individually and culturally. We "see" gender as masculine/feminine and heterosexual/homosexual, and sex as male/female, because that is what has already been circumscribed by acceptable discourse and by what is performed. Further, we have no recourse to a "pure" body to which we can turn for evidence nor to a "prior" psychological existence that might offer a source of possibilities beyond these dichotomies, because these very notions of the "pure" and the "prior" are themselves constructed through our reference to them. As she says in her introduction to *Gender Trouble*: "To the extent the gender norms [. . .] establish what will and will not be intelligibly human, what will and will not be considered to be 'real,' they establish the ontological field in which bodies may be given legitimate expression" (Butler 1999, xxiii). And in her *Bodies That Matter*:

> If the body signified as prior to signification is an effect of signification, then the mimetic or representational status of language, which claims that signs follow bodies as their necessary mirrors, is not mimetic at all. On the contrary, it is productive, constitutive, one might even argue *performative*, inasmuch as this signifying act delimits and contours the body that it then claims to find prior to any and all signification. (Butler 1993, 30)

Language (or discourse), then, limits or guides how bodies appear.[3]

But Money's quintessential case study was not as successful as he originally thought, and made it out, to be. Simply put, the young "girl" did not socialize well as a girl, and she suffered in many aspects of her life: She fell behind in school, she had very few friends, and she had very low self-esteem. She was miserable and sometimes even violent. At the age of fourteen—shortly after having been told what happened to her—she decided to return to being male. The young man (who chose the name David), therefore, was hardly a success story for nurture over nature.

Interestingly, the failure of this case study was complemented by certain conclusions drawn in endocrinology, around the same time as this case study, but separate from it. Contrary to Money's position, endocrinologists, including Milton Diamond, found evidence in their studies of hormones that the overflow of certain hormones at a specific point in fetal development would result in certain types of sexual behaviors later on in young adult mammals (in this case, rats). Regardless of genitals, the grown rats could be found to exhibit certain "masculine" or "feminine" behaviors, depending on the wash of hormones that passed through the uterus during their fetal development. The possible importance of hormones to human development was ignored for a long time, especially given the weight and popularity of Money's case. However, a couple of decades later it was made clear, not only through subsequent studies and tests in endocrinology but also through a follow-up study on David, the young "girl" returned to "young man," that Money might have played a bit fast and loose with the early evidence. One effect for feminists was that "some feminist scholars quietly dropped the [. . .] case from new editions of their women's studies textbooks" (Colapinto 2000, 176).

So we are faced with an important question: What should feminism do if scientific studies do not seem to support important and/ or well-established feminist claims (or seem to oppose them)? This is *not* to claim that either 1) there is no collaborative work being done between science and feminism, or 2) that feminism *requires* a foundation in the sciences. Nevertheless, I believe the question is valid: If both of these areas hope or claim to be coming to conclusions that are true, or to have universal value (or even a widespread value), what should be done when their conclusions dramatically appear to conflict?

Judith Butler responds to this challenge, and to this specific case, in her *Undoing Gender* (2004). Taking up the same case study of David Reimer, Butler points out that both positions (the extreme positions being gender essentialism and social construction),[4] when enforced, are "unnatural" in their very attempts to achieve what is "normal" or "natural." In fact, they both require a certain amount of violence to achieve their ends: "Importantly [. . .] the malleability of gender construction, which is part of [Money's] thesis, turns out to require a forceful application. And the 'nature' that the endocrinologists defend also needs a certain assistance through surgical and hormonal means" (Butler 2004, 66). Thus, both positions ascribe to a certain presumption about the normal and/or natural, but in order to fulfill these categories, they prescribe surgical and hormonal alterations of the bodies that don't fit. In addition, Butler details that David Reimer, in his descriptions of his own experiences of his body—how it never felt right to be a girl or to become a woman—was only able to express these experiences through specific, limited discourses that presume a "normal" and/or "natural."[5] These discourses insist upon a dichotomy between man and woman as well as connections between certain types of bodies and certain types of behaviors (as well as likes and dislikes, tendencies toward clothing, and so on)—connections also usually presumed by both biologists and social constructionists. Further, Butler recognizes that David spent his childhood being seen through these discourses, such that he might not have been able to see himself in any other way. "[David] seems clear that the norms are external to him, but what if the norms have become the means by which he sees, the frame for his own seeing, his way of seeing himself?" (Butler 2004, 70)

However, for Butler, David is not doomed simply to express the discourses at hand; rather, by virtue of his situation, he has an opportunity to see them critically. With this view, he argues that he is more than his sexual parts, that he is lovable for more than the body that he is. While David's argument could be seen to fall under other discursive themes (discourse about personhood or the soul, for example), Butler (2004, 74) identifies him as pointing out an existence at the limits of those discourses:

> [David] emerges at the limits of intelligibility, offering a perspective on the variable ways in which norms can circumscribe the human. It is precisely because we understand,

without quite grasping, that he has another reason, that he *is*, as it were, another reason, that we see the limits to the discourse of intelligibility that would decide his fate.

In this way, for Butler, David is hardly a champion for a return to gender essentialism. Rather, the very discourse he used to describe how the category of female did not seem to fit him—evidence, for some, *against* social construction—is actually evidence *for* the pervasiveness of discourse.[6]

But how, then, do we address scientific studies, such as those of Diamond and his colleagues, that show a link between prenatal hormone exposure and postnatal sexual or gender-related behavior?[7] What should feminism—or, at least, feminist perspectives that argue the forcefulness of social construction—do about hormones?[8] Anne Fausto-Sterling (2000) examines the dialogue of empirical science with our understanding of gender, recognizing *both* that scientists integrate their own belief systems into their questions, studies, approaches, and conclusions (an accusation by feminists), *and* that science and scientific studies can identify certain grounds from which human experience is built (a claim by scientists):

> The dialectic of medical argument is to be read neither as evil technological conspiracy nor as story of sexual openmindedness illumined by the light of modern scientific knowledge. [. . .] Knowledge about the embryology and endocrinology of sexual development, gained during the nineteenth and twentieth centuries, enables us to understand that human males and females all begin life with the same structures; complete maleness and complete femaleness represent the extreme ends of a spectrum of possible body types. That these extreme ends are the most frequent has lent credence to the idea that they are not only natural [. . .] but [also] normal [. . .]. Knowledge of biological variation, however, allows us to conceptualize the less frequent middle spaces as natural, although statistically unusual. (Fausto-Sterling 2000, 76)

Fausto-Sterling points out that, while some scientific studies have been used to proclaim a narrow determinism based on biology—and these usually fall in line with certain societal belief structures—other studies reveal the variety of possibilities already apparent in "nature." That we acknowledge only a few of these variants, or that we call some of them "normal" and others "abnormal" or "unnatural," is not necessarily a result of biology but more often a result of social norms. Given this, biology can actually be used to *challenge* social norms as much as to substantiate them. So where does the body lie in this tension between biology and discourse?

The question might turn us first to the issue of discursive limits: The performative and discursive understanding of gender (as well as "social construction," broadly understood) identifies the limitations that discourses and performativities impose upon our bodies, and it reveals extremely well how we modify our lived experiences—or rather, how our lived experiences are modified for us—so that we fit within the discursive limitations that have been set. This position also shows a possibility for subversion, especially in the manipulation of discourses, the performing of the subversive, and the manifestation of marginal modes of existence (in discourse). In fact, the body, understood as performative, can be seen as the source of certain expressions of subversion in that it resists or undermines specific hegemonic discourses. (For example, as Butler has argued, the body subverts hegemonic discourse in drag performance as well as in its existence as a marginalized type.) Thus discourse/performativity is, on the one hand, limiting, and on the other, open to the subversion of its own limits. The body, seen as discursive, is that which is limited and, on occasion, is that which can subvert limits. However, if the body is discursive, and if discourses establish limits, then the body itself should also be able to posit certain limitations (as other discourses do). And if the body as discursive can be limited, then other discourses should also be restricted (or restrict-able) as the body is. In other words, if we understand the body as discourse—as opposed to there being merely discourses about "the body"—then the body should be able to establish limits and restrict other discourses just as certain discourses are seen to do to the body. The body should act like discourse, if it is discourse. Butler sees examples of this in the lived existence of marginalized groups, whose very embodied presence poses a challenge to hegemonic discourses. Such embodiments "draw the lines" of discourse, of what is intelligible and of what is beyond intelligible. In doing so, though, the body seems to exceed discourse in some way. In cases such as this, where the body exemplifies the margins or demonstrates that which has been excluded, it stands both within and without discourse at once.

I want to focus on the body "without" discourse—both in the sense of "outside" (the opposite of "within") and of "not having" discourse. Can the body also provide resistance that is somehow beyond discourse? Does it offer us any experiences that we can recognize as beyond the necessary lens of discourse—introducing possibilities for new discourses? Is there anything to the visceral, guttural, upheaving body itself? More generally, can there be limits to discourse other than its own subversion of itself? I would like to suggest, without denying all of the evidence that the body is discursive, that the body is also more than discourse. It acts like discourse—it is discursive—but it has its own density as well, a density that sometimes can rupture discourse. Of course, when we introduce this possibility, we face the danger of returning to some form of biological determinism. Even more threatening is the possibility of a return to a prefeminist restriction of women (and other groups) on the basis of certain interpretations of biology (for example, biological determinism interwoven with misogyny or racism)—a bit of a slippery slope, and one of which we, as feminists, must remain rigorously aware. Nevertheless, there are times, I would argue, when the body simply challenges certain discourses, occasionally *all* discourses—and it does this regardless of whether it has a discursive avenue with which to "express" this resistance. Granted, this resistance is almost always immediately taken up within discourse, becoming a named counterexample, a verbal challenge, among other things, which points to "the body" (now discursively understood) as the source of the challenge. However, the *motivation* for a new discursive counterposition comes, on occasion, from beyond the discursive realm, from fundamental, *lived embodied experience*.

The term "motivation" and my reference to "lived embodied experience" hearken us to phenomenology, and I believe it is through phenomenology and feminist phenomenology that we can better negotiate some of these tensions. Although certain phenomenologists are more often employed for feminist projects—Merleau-Ponty, Beauvoir, even Heidegger—I would like to introduce a few concepts by Husserl as a way to work through these issues. In a later work (*Analyses Concerning Passive and Active Synthesis*[9]), Husserl introduces the term "affectivity," which is the draw an object can have on me, its call to me to bring it into my attention. When the object affects me, calls to me, and I turn toward it, new affectivities can continue to pull me, drawing me in to examine the object more closely or with regard to certain determinations over others. Now, an object's affectivity can be socially motivated, such that I am called to notice things that are greatly meaningful in dominant discourses. This can even apply to the notion of race or gender. We are drawn to notice certain bodily parts and phenotypes because they have been rendered socially meaningful. But affectivity can also happen beyond discourse, such that I am called to notice something that contrasts largely with its surroundings (Husserl's main focus with regard to this term), or something that simply stands out for me. Infants, for example, notice visual contrast, and even subtle changes in their environments, well before they are integrated into language, and when I am looking for my wallet, it may jump out for me, even when it blends into the colors of the sofa.

Affectivity also applies to the body, although here we would understand the body through Husserl's two (rather well-known) terms for the body: The first is *Leib*, which is the body as sensory experience, as my lived, embodied experience. The other is *Körper*, which is the body as causal object, subject to laws of physics as well as intersubjective appropriation.[10] Clearly, these two notions of the body, *Leib* and *Körper*, overlap. A physical object falls on my hand, and I feel pain. My body releases a surge of hormones, and I feel sexual urges. Most often, the body as *Körper* and the body as *Leib* resonate with one another: I look like a woman to others, and I also feel like a woman. Often also, though, my experience of my *Leib* is enforced by how my *Körper* is given (back) to me: I look like a woman to others, and I am made to feel like a heterosexual woman: Through a variety of discourses, any feelings that exceed the heterosexual expression of my body are subdued, repressed, excised, and/or ignored. Sometimes my experience of my *Leib* resists such conditioning, and thus my body expresses itself differently than expected in hegemonic discourse. The *Leib* in such cases does not resonate with the *Körper* as an intersubjective object. And this dissonance, in some situations, can be the motivation for new discourses or new formulations of old discourses.

The difficulty we encounter when gender essentialist explanations contradict social constructionist explanations stems from the fact that both are taking up the notion of *Körper* in different ways— the one as a *physical* reality (genitals, chromosomes, hormones) and the other as a *social* reality (result of social conditioning, discourse, performance). Both presume or argue that the other understanding of *Körper* is subsumed or secondary to their own position. Both, further, insist that these *Körper*-realities either express or influence a person's experience as *Leib* in a more or less totalizing way. Neither considers at length whether my body as *Leib* might be its own "reality," that I can have feelings beyond the causal nexus as described by each position. But the *Leib* can have its own "voice," as it were. It is a voice not only of sensations, but also of vaguer, "gut" feelings of well-being, discomfort, disgust, euphoria, among others. Husserl described these all as "sensings" in his *Ideas II*, and they are mine, as perceived only by me. And while discourse may teach us to ignore or reinterpret some sensings (while using others as the basis for value judgments), we find them present when we are able to destabilize such discourses—and we find them to have been there already. In fact, sometimes these sensings can be the very source of destabilization; they can motivate a challenge of discourses.[11]

However, we now have three senses of body in play: the physical *Körper*, the social *Körper*, and the sensory *Leib*. Often, all of these senses resonate with one another. Sometimes they do not. When they do not resonate, the situation at hand determines how the differing voices will negotiate with one another; in some cases, one voice may be much more insistent than the others. Given what we have determined with regard to the *Leib*, we can analyze, phenomenologically, how the *Leib* might be experienced and how it might be affective—where the affectivity of the *Leib*'s sensings is what I am calling its "voice." To speak first in general, my *Leib* is experienced as having a certain heaviness or lightness (which can change depending on my circumstances); as having abilities to move, and not move, in definite ways; as having pains and pleasures related to itself and to other objects and people; as being sexual and gendered in certain ways (including asexual); and so on. Of course, this experience is in dialogue with the experience of my body as *Körper*, in both senses of the term. Deeper analysis would show how my *Leib*-body as heavy or light, as gendered, as having pain and pleasure, and so on, is filtered and/or modified by the physical and social senses of my embodiment—and many fine analyses have already been done. On those occasions when the experience of my body contradicts, challenges, or seems to exist outside of the realms dictated by the social and physical senses of the body, though, then we have affective evidence of *Leib*

as its own ground. Here, situations such as David's, that of the intersexual, and that of the transsexual can provide productive insights,
because in such cases, the three senses of physical *Körper*, social *Körper*,
and *Leib* begin to distinguish themselves from one another.[12]

So the *Leib* as its own ground can have an affective pull, and
we will turn to some specific examples in a moment. In general, an
affective pull can be anywhere on the spectrum from very strong to
terribly weak (Husserl 2001, 197, 202). One could argue that the
body as *Leib* would only be sensed on its own when its affective pull
is extremely strong, for otherwise, that pull might be nullified by the
discursive and physical senses of the *Körper*-body. Further, when the
body as *Leib* agrees with the other senses of the body, then its affective pull would not be noticed for itself, since all senses of the body
would be "pulling in the same direction," as it were. But there are
cases, as I have been arguing, when the body as *Leib* calls to me in
specific ways, such that I cannot live in agreement with certain discourses or physical senses of my body.[13]

Let us return to the situation of David, and the argument that
the hormonal wash through his fetal body determined his embodied
sense of being male. According to this argument, that crucial moment
of development "hardwired" David as male, such that even the injec-
tion of hormones later on would not be sufficient to counteract
his deep-set sense as male. The physical structure of his body, now
understood through endocrinology, had provided very specific limits
wherein David was able to experience his embodiment. For this reason, neither the social conditioning of therapy, nor the discourses of
his "femaleness" or "womanhood," nor the preliminary operations on
his genitalia to create female embodiment, nor the ingestion of estrogen were able to counteract this prenatal conditioning. Given the
terminology set out earlier, we could say that David's physical-*Körper*
was the ground for, and in alignment with, his sensings as *Leib*. This
physical ground, established prenatally, informed David's experience
of his body, and it expressed itself through the "voice" of his body—
how his body "felt" in relation to specific discourses and to himself.
Thus, in David's case, the physical-*Körper* provided the structural basis
for his embodied experience and expression as *Leib*, and this affective
voice would ultimately contradict the specific discourses that told
David he was a girl or that he was to become a woman. Here, phys-
ical-*Körper* and *Leib* were intertwined at some level, giving grounds

to David's challenge of the discourses (social-*Körper*) that said he was a woman.

David's story has often been compared to the situation of the intersexual, in spite of the obvious difference that David was born unambiguously male. And there are certain similarities: In cases where surgeries have been performed on intersexed infants (as surgeries were performed on David), those persons, in adulthood, often find that the sex to which they were surgically assigned does not fit how they feel: "These [intersex] individuals seemed to be listening to some inner voice that said that everyone in authority surrounding h/her was wrong. Doctors and parents might have insisted that they were female, removed their testes, injected them with estrogen, and surgically provided them with a vagina, but still, they *knew* they were really males" (Fausto-Sterling, 2000, 68–69). However, with further examination, we see significant differences. Here we have at least three manifestations of the physical-*Körper*: the anatomical body at birth (intersexed), the surgically altered body sometime later (either male or female), and the prenatal body infused by hormones. The sensing voice of *Leib*, however, may not resonate with any of these aspects of the physical-*Körper*, nor with the discourses at hand (the social-*Körper*). In other words, the intersexed person may have *Leib*-sensations that are neither male, nor female, nor strictly "intersexed" (as in a mixture of male and female). Rather that person may sense the body as a- or nonsexual, as fluid or queer, or as having many sexual expressions beyond male and female. This "inner voice"—or whatever it may be—seems to arise from a certain mode of existence of the body that is not being expressed, and finds no resonance, in either the discourses or the physical body at hand. Thus, regardless of anatomical manifestation at birth, or of probable hormonal influx during fetal development, or of surgical and hormonal "therapy," the physical-*Körper* does not always correspond with an individual's *Leib* (as it did in the case of David). In this case, the *Leib* seems to challenge both the physical-*Körper* (in its several manifestations) and the social-*Körper* understandings of the body. It stands, as it were, in a triangular relation of the three different positions.

Interestingly, David's situation is also often cited as parallel to that of the transsexual—even though it is repeatedly acknowledged that David was not a transsexual. The transsexual has a remarkably strong embodied sense (gender identity) that goes against the physical sense of the body, where, in this case, the anatomical body at birth and the hormonal wash *in utero* were unambiguously male or female. This voice of the *Leib* also goes against dominant discourses that correlate anatomical appearance with how one fits and feels in one's body. Thus, the transsexual's experience of sensing a difference from how his body appears anatomically *must* arise from his *Leib*. It is from the *Leib* as ground that the transsexual argues that her physical body, as well as the discourse(s) about it, is out of alignment with how she senses her *Leib*. Here the *Leib* stands its own ground against the physical-*Körper* and the social-*Körper*. In fact, in the case of the transsexual, these two notions of *Körper* are actually rather in alignment with one another, unlike in the cases examined previously. Therefore, the situation of the transsexual best exemplifies how the "voice" of the body, as *Leib*, expresses itself—against all other "meanings" of the body. It is a "voice," a sensing, that is grounded neither in physical descriptions nor social explanations—although this is not to say that it is not in dialogue with them, or that there are no influences in either direction. However, given what we see here, the *Leib* as its own ground can be the motivation for a variety of challenges to discursive limitations of the body as well as physical limits—even when the latter appear to agree with one another.

So we return to our thematic question: What should feminism do about hormones? While hormones appear to fall under the auspices of the *Körper* as physical body, as seen in the case of David, it is also the case that they can be intertwined with how I feel my own body. Thus hormones are in play with some senses of my body as *Leib* as well as the physical-*Körper*. In addition, of course, the discourse of hormones shows that this notion is also prominent in our experience of the body as social-*Körper*. A feminist phenomenology, developing on the terminology suggested here, can provide a more nuanced description and explanation of our embodied experiences. Structural limitations can arise from the physical- or the social/discursive-*Körper*, and the *Leib* can voice its own challenges. We can work through how these different senses of the body blend with one another, or how they challenge and contradict one another, depending on the individual and/or situation. Allowing for various types of experience of the body makes it possible for us to acknowledge— and to describe more fully—the experience of the transsexual, when everything in and on the body appears "normal"; or of the (surgically altered) intersex person who "knows" that something happened, other than what has been told to her; or of David, who knew that the assignment of female did not belong to him and that further feminizing sexual surgery would be wrong. These experiences remain valid, and they can be taken up rigorously in a phenomenological setting, giving the body its "voice"—in a variety of ways.

Acknowledgments

I would like to thank the editors of this volume (who were also the organizers of the conference Feminist Phenomenology and Medicine, Uppsala University, Sweden, May 18–21, 2011) for supporting my work on this project. I would also like to thank Fredrik Svenaeus for his comments on the essay, as well as conference attendees for their feedback. An earlier version of this essay was presented at the Bodily Phenomenology conference (Södertörn University, Sweden, May 19–21, 2010), and I am grateful to the organizers and attendees of that conference for their support and feedback.

Notes

1. The case of David Reimer has been used—overused, one could even say—as an analogy and/or argument for many positions regarding the body, gender, and experience. I do not wish to engage that literature here, other than my engagement with Butler's and Fausto-Sterling's references to the Reimer case. More importantly, I wish to argue that phenomenological terminology helps to reveal the *distinction* between a case like Reimer's and those for whom he has acted as analogy or "allegory," that is, the transsexual and the intersexual.
2. The "John/Joan case" took place in the late 1960s and 1970s.
3. The notion of discourse, especially for Butler, extends beyond the notion of language to gestures, actions, performance. Butler's argument is partially built upon Foucault's work on the body. Given the parameters of this essay, though, I do not introduce Foucault into my analysis.
4. Butler (2004, 66–67) sets up these extremes of "social construction" and "gender essentialism" as she seeks a position that neither confirms nor denies either of them.

5. Different disciplines, in their presumptions of the "normal" and/ or "natural," may actually have very different understandings in mind. While psychological "normal" may refer to an ability to cope successfully with one's own surroundings, medical "normal" refers to certain statistical and numerical parameters (which often change over time, such as the standard for "normal" weight). Unfortunately, this tension cannot be analyzed here.

6. Butler seems to imply that David's discussion of how he was lovable in spite of his body or genitalia is evidence for his being on the "limits of intelligibility." However, the discourse of being lovable for more than, or in spite of, one's body is actually a predominant discourse, a theme not only in religious discourses but also in popular parlance. Nevertheless, Butler's point may be that David's very existence is on the "limits of intelligibility," thus forcing him to take on other discourses, ones that emphasize the soul or the self over the body.

7. Butler's references to Milton Diamond's position actually misrepresent him on a key point. In Diamond's article, to which Butler refers, he argues (with his coauthor, Keith Sigmundson) in his concluding paragraph that immediate surgery on intersexed infants should be avoided or postponed, and instead, parents and family members should be referred to long-term counseling. While he does recommend raising any such infants with an XY chromosome as a boy, his final emphasis is on the complexity of the situation and on avoiding immediate surgery (Diamond and Sigmundson 1997, 303). This point is also made clear by Colapinto (who had interviewed Diamond) in his book on David Reimer's story, to which Butler also refers (Colapinto 2000, 210). Yet Butler portrays Diamond in this chapter as advocating immediate sexual reassignment surgery (see especially Butler 2004, 63–65), and on the basis of this, refers to him and his coauthor, Sigmundson, sharply as "purveyors of natural and normative gender" (Butler 2004, 66). While Butler's analysis of the difficulty of this situation still stands, and although she may have needed to place Diamond in the position representing biological determinism in order to carry out her own analysis, her portrayal of him is rather unfair.

8. Butler herself evades this issue in the particular chapter to which I am referring. Instead, she turns to the "discourse of self-reporting and self-understanding" (Butler 2004, 67) that takes place in

the case study of David Reimer, as detailed earlier. In the following chapter of the same book, she addresses the situation of transsexuality, especially with regard to its pathologization, and whether this ascription of pathology is strategically necessary in order to make the desired transition. Here, too, her focus turns to the language of the *DSM IV*, as well as to the motifs of autonomy, freedom, and liberty.

9. The *Analyses Concerning Passive and Active Synthesis* were presented as lectures in the 1920s and published in the *Husserliana* complete works as volume 11 in 1966. The English translation was published in 2001.

10. These terms, especially *Leib*, are developed most thoroughly in Husserl's *Ideas II* (published in the *Husserliana* series as volume 4). In this chapter, I divide the notion of *Körper* into two senses, the physical and the intersubjective. Husserl does not make this division explicitly, although it can be interpreted from his argument that it is only through the intersubjective view of my body as objective that I can see my own body objectively (see, for example, pp. 86 and 95), as well as his distinction between the phenomenological attitude (which yields the experience of *Leib*), the personalistic attitude (which turns us toward the human person and intersubjectivity), and the naturalistic attitude (which takes up the world and the body as physical nature) (see pp. 183ff.). However, Husserl does indicate a division within the notion of *Leib*: the *Leib*-body as sensing itself (through movement, weight, pain, pleasure, etc.) and as sensory experience of objects in the world. A discussion of this distinction within the notion of *Leib*, as well as Husserl's discussion of the different attitudes we can take on the body, is beyond the purview of this chapter.

11. While the notion of voice leads one to think of the spoken voice, it is clear that the voice emits many other expressions and sounds, and that it manifests a certain ambiguity between lived sensory embodiment and expressive world. For this reason, I have chosen the metaphor of the voice of the body—a "voice" that emits "expressions" and sometimes only "sounds," that "ex-presses" the body's fundamental experiences and experiential ground. For this analysis, the "voice" of the body, while also metaphorical, finds its expression through what I refer to as Husserl's notion of "sensings," described in his *Ideas II*, especially §39.

12. Justifiable complaints have been rendered for "using" the experiences of David Reimer, the intersexual, and/or the transsexual for various theoretical purposes. I acknowledge and agree with this criticism. My goal here is not to develop theory on the basis of these experiences, but rather, to introduce phenomenological terminology *for* these experiences. In other words, I suggest that certain phenomenological terminology, as I work with it here, can assist persons with differing types of embodied experiences to express their experiences more clearly.

13. That this disagreement between the different senses of the body causes turmoil is clear. Butler shows (as do others) how discursive enforcement results not only in the physical abuse of those who do not "fit" the hegemonic discourse but also in those individuals' struggling with their very sense of existence and of self. Perhaps understanding the body through these different senses can provide those who live their bodies as oppositional with a new way to describe their experiences, thus opening up an avenue to agreement between *Leib* and *Körper* (in both senses), if that is desired.

References

Benjamin, Harry, M. D. 1966. *The Transsexual Phenomenon.* New York: The Julian Press.

Butler, Judith. 1993. *Bodies That Matter: On the Discursive Limits of "Sex."* New York, London: Routledge.

Butler, Judith. 1999. *Gender Trouble: Feminism and the Subversion of Identity.* New York, London: Routledge.

Butler, Judith. 2004. *Undoing Gender.* New York, London: Routledge.

Colapinto, John. 2000. *As Nature Made Him: The Boy Who Was Raised as a Girl.* New York: HarperCollins.

Diamond, Milton, and Keith Sigmundson. 1997. "Sex Reassignment at Birth: A Long-Term Review and Clinical Implications." *Archives of Pediatrics and Adolescent Medicine* 151 (March): 298–304.

Fausto-Sterling, Anne. 2000. *Sexing the Body: Gender Politics and the Construction of Sexuality.* New York: Basic.

Foucault, Michel. 1980. *The History of Sexuality. Volume I: An Introduction,* translated by Robert Hurley. New York: Vintage Books/Random House.

Husserl, Edmund. 1989. *Ideas Pertaining to a Pure Phenomenology and to a Phenomenological Philosophy Second Book [Ideas II]*, translated by Richard Rojcewicz and André Schuwer. Dordrecht, Boston, London: Kluwer.

Husserl, Edmund. 2001. *Analyses Concerning Passive and Active Synthesis: Lectures on Transcendental Logic*, translated by Anthony J. Steinbock. Dordrecht: Kluwer.

Money, John. 1973. *Man and Woman, Boy and Girl: Differentiation and Dimorphism of Gender Identity from Conception to Maturity*. Baltimore: Johns Hopkins University Press.

11

THE BODY UNCANNY

Alienation, Illness, and Anorexia Nervosa

FREDRIK SVENAEUS

In this chapter I attempt a phenomenological analysis of some different ways in which the body may show up as *other* to its owner: various types of somatic illness and the case of anorexia nervosa. While illness forms the common thread of these ways of bodily alienation, the last example has been chosen also to introduce the thematic of gender politics and personal identity. There are many additional examples of bodily "otherness" that would be fruitful to explore that would make my analysis of the uncanny body more comprehensive, such as pregnancy, obesity, other mental disorders than anorexia such as depression or body dysmorphic disorder, different forms of plastic surgery, and organ transplantation, just to mention a few. All of these examples introduce the issue of living with a body that is in some sense no longer only unproblematically mine but also other to its owner. By invoking the issue of ownership here, I do not intend to subscribe to any liberal metaphysics of self-ownership. I am simply referring to the experience of being *as* a body, what the phenomenologist refers to as the "lived body," in contrast to the body appearing as an object visible and touchable to others, and to the person in question (Merleau-Ponty 1962).

The Alien Body

When the body reveals a life of its own, this is in many cases an *alienating* experience for the person to whom the body belongs. Illness, as we will see, is a major example of this, but it must be stressed already at this point that when the body displays a life of its own, this is not *necessarily* an alienating experience. Pregnancy is a clear example of the opposite (at least in some cases), as are other everyday situations when we find ourselves at the will of the body but do not suffer or feel alienated as a result of this: think of cases when the body reacts or performs on its own when we are faced with a demanding situation, such as fleeing in the face of danger or fighting off a disease. In such situations, we have an experience of the body taking command of the happenings, and it does so for our own good, so to speak. Similarly, we can allow the body to take over in activities that demand coordination and control that we are not able to execute by way of will and consciousness only: think of playing tennis or driving a car.

What does it mean to be bodily alienated in addition to having an experience of the own body as something the ways of which I do not fully control? I would say that it means that the body is experienced not only as not only mine (other) but also as *foreign* and *strange* to me. In my becoming bodily alienated, the foreignness of the body reminds me of a state of being at home with it that is no longer present and that I desire to have reinstated. The body is my basic home-being, and therefore alienation within the bodily domain is a particularly *uncanny* experience, compared to other ways of being alienated. Alienation is usually portrayed as an experience of becoming foreign to one's life in terms of the things one does and thinks (e.g., Marxist or existentialist frameworks of the authentic life),[1] but it can also be an experience of foreignness within the domains of embodiment.

The 1979 science fiction film *Alien*, directed by Ridley Scott, offers the archetypal example of the horrors of bodily alienation through being possessed and taken over by something foreign hiding itself in the body. After landing on an unexplored planet, from which the towing spaceship *Nostromo* has received strange transmission signals, a member of the crew is infected by an alien, parasitic creature, which lays its eggs in him by attaching itself to his face. Officer Kane (John Hurt) is taken on board and recovers as *Nostromo* takes off from the planet to continue its journey. He is, however, far from healthy, as the crew will soon find out. The scene in which, during a meal, Officer Kane begins to choke and convulse until an alien creature bursts from his chest, killing him and escaping into the labyrinths of the ship, is already famous in horror film history. A war begins between the creature and the remaining crewmembers, who are killed by the alien, one after the other in the creepy environment of the ship. In the last scene, Officer Ripley (Sigourney Weaver), the last survivor of the crew, has managed to flee the ship in a shuttle after blowing the creature to pieces, but she still has the crew's cat with her, and who knows what is hiding itself in its intestines? The Alien certainly survived to be the main figure of many succeeding movies, reminding us of the severe uncanniness of bodily parasitic possession, which, in real life, is limited to smaller creatures like worms, bacteria, or viruses.

Bodily alienation is an uncanny experience. The word uncanny actually hides the meaning of "alien" within itself, at least if we investigate the German etymological origins. The German word *unheimlich* (uncanny) has the double meaning of something being hidden and fearful (*heimlich*) and not being at home, that is: alienated (*unheimisch*). Sigmund Freud brings this out in his essay "The Uncanny," which rests heavily on early-nineteenth-century horror fiction, such as E. T. A. Hoffmann's story, *The Sandman* (Freud 1959). Freud's main hypothesis in the essay is that we experience something as uncanny when we find ourselves in doubt about whether it is dead or alive, as in the case of encountering automata or ghosts. What is uncanny in these examples is not the experience of the own body, but the experience of the body of something that (or someone who) is other than me and whose status with regard to being alive is uncertain. Freud, however, also gives a lot of other examples in the essay that describe the uncanny character of being controlled by something foreign that is nevertheless a part of oneself (the unconscious) and links this to the development of the ego as a separation from the mother and the father. His topic in these cases, however, is not bodily but rather psychic alienation:

> The uncanny effect of epilepsy and of madness has the same origin. The ordinary person sees in them the workings of forces hitherto unsuspected in his fellow-man but which at the same time he is dimly aware of in a remote corner of his own being. The Middle Ages therefore ascribed all such maladies to daemonic influences, and in this they were

psychologically almost correct. Indeed, I should not be surprised to hear that psycho-analysis, which is concerned with laying bare these hidden forces, has itself become uncanny to many people for that very reason. (Freud 1959, 397)

Neither Scott nor Freud brings up the fundamental alienation of the own body that occurs not through possession by any foreign powers, be it by ghosts, parasites, or humans, but through the ways of the body itself. As I pointed out earlier, the body has a life of its own, the ways of which can run counter to my wills and wishes. As Richard Zaner writes in his study, *The Context of Self*, in the chapter entitled "The Body Uncanny":

> If there is a sense in which my own-body is "intimately mine," there is furthermore, an equally decisive sense in which *I belong to it*—in which I am at its disposal or mercy, if you will. My body, like the world in which I live, has its own nature, functions, structures, and biological conditions; since it embodies me, I thus *experience myself as implicated* by my body and these various conditions, functions, etc. *I* am exposed to whatever can influence, threaten, inhibit, alter, or benefit my biological organism. Under certain conditions, it can fail me (more or less), not be capable of fulfilling my wants or desires, or even thoughts, forcing me to turn away from what I may want to do and attend to my own body: because of fatigue, hunger, thirst, disease, injury, pain, or even itches, I am forced at times to tend and attend to it, regardless, it may be, of what may well seem more urgent at the moment. (1981, 52)

The body is, indeed, not a thing that I am accidentally hooked up with and can chose to disregard, as a dualist, or, indeed, materialist, perspective might fool us into assuming.[2] The body is *me*, my fundamental way of existing and making myself at home in the world. This is why becoming a victim of the autonomous "will" of the body can be such an *uncanny* experience: at the heart of my home territory, foreignness now makes itself known.[3] The body, consequently, does not belong to me in the same way that I claim right of ownership to other things in the world, like clothes, books, a car, or a house. Not only can I experience my own body as an *object* of my experience—when I feel it or touch it or look at it in the mirror—but the body also harbors, on the subjective side of experience, the schemas that make a person's experiences possible in the first place. The body is my zero-place in the world—the place where I am which moves with me—that makes space and the place of things that I encounter possible to begin with.[4] This is why the experience of this very body as something painful and foreign becomes an uncanny experience: what was and indeed remains the cornerstone of me turns out to be not (only) me.

Drew Leder, in his important book *The Absent Body* (1990), draws our attention, in the same way Zaner does in the previous quote, to how the subjective body might appear as something that hurts and resists the will of its owner. Leder names this the "dys-appearance" of the body, indicating that the body can sometimes lose its transparent qualities and show up as a hindrance and obstacle for the person living it (1990, 69). In contrast to this, the "me-like" showing of the body is most often a *not* letting itself appear to me of the body. The body normally *disappears* to allow the things of the world that I encounter and create in my activities to show up (Leder 1990, 25). When I write these words on my computer, to offer a nearby example, my hands and eyes do not appear to me, and neither does the rest of my body, sitting on the chair and leaning on the table; they rather make my thoughts appear to me on the computer screen.

But that the body disappears does not mean that it ceases to exist. Through the attunements that penetrate my different ways of being-in-the-world, the body is *prereflectively* present to me exactly as my very way of being (Zahavi 1999), a fact that has been explored not only by phenomenologists but also by brain scientists (Damasio 1999). This prereflective, non-thematized appearance of the body is most often nonappealing in character, but just as the body might "dys-appear" in hurting and resisting our actions, it can also "eu-appear" when we enjoy the things we do, in both cases without attaining any object-like quality, as Kristin Zeiler has recently pointed out (2010).

The homelike being of the own body harbors processes beyond my control: notably, the autonomic functions of our visceral life that are controlled by subconscious processes of the brain stem. These processes, however, as has been pointed out, are normally not a source of uncanniness. We do not feel controlled in any foreign or bad way by the fact that we breathe air and digest food without having to think about it all the time; quite the contrary, it would be a very demanding and frightening experience to constantly have to support these life-sustaining processes by way of will and thought. Nevertheless, at the moment when the automatic functions of breathing and digestion become disturbed, they will (dys)appear to me. Sometimes the causes of dysfunction can be found in foreign disease agents conquering the body (bringing us back to the *Alien* example), but most often the changed appearance of the body is rather an imbalance of the lived body itself with multiple causes.

The books by Zaner and Leder are important since they, in contrast to most earlier works by phenomenologists, display an open and penetrating interest in the otherness of the lived body that dwells at the heart of its homelike being. Whereas Edmund Husserl and Maurice Merleau-Ponty were busy showing how the body is first and foremost not an object encountered by the person but the basic form of subjectivity itself (Zahavi 1999), Zaner and Leder attempt to give a fuller account of how the body as this basic form of subjectivity is also other, and sometimes alien, to its subject.

Phenomenology of Illness

It is important to understand the fundamental difference between a phenomenological illness concept and the concept of disease as it is usually understood. I have tried in earlier works to characterize and to a certain extent delineate the borders of illness experiences, proceeding mainly from the phenomenology of Heidegger, by way of the concept of "unhomelike being-in-the-world" (Svenaeus 2000). The lifeworld is usually my home territory, but in illness, this homelikeness gives way and takes on a rather *unhomelike* character, rooted in uncanny ways of being embodied. It is the mission of healthcare professionals to try to understand such unhomelike being-in-the-world and bring it back to homelikeness again, or at least closer to a home-being. This involves, but cannot be reduced to, ways of understanding and altering the physiological organism of the person who is ill. Healthcare professionals must also address matters of patients' everyday life with a phenomenological eye, addressing and trying to understand the being-in-the-world of the person's life, which has turned unhomelike in illness.[5]

A disease is a disturbance of the biological functions of the body (or something that causes such a disturbance), which can only be detected and understood from the third-person perspective of the doctor investigating the body with the aid of her hands or medical technologies. The patient can also, by way of the doctor, or by way of medical theory, or, as often happens nowadays, by way of a webpage on the Internet, adopt such a third-person perspective toward her own body and speculate about diseases responsible for her suffering. But the suffering itself is an illness experience of the person who is in a world, embodied and connected to other people around her. Illness has meaning, or, perhaps we should say instead, *disturbs* the meaning processes of being-in-the-world in which one is leading one's life on an everyday level.

Typically, when I experience illness as an uncanniness of my bodily being, my biological organism will be diseased, but there are possibilities of being ill without any detectable diseases, or of leading a homelike life, when suddenly the doctor finds a disease (for example, by way of a cancer screening). The phenomenologist would stress that the full importance and content of illness can be attained only if the doctor, in addition to being skilled in diagnosing diseases, also affords attention to the bodily experience and being-in-the-world of the patient. The life of the person (and not only the life of her biological organism) is, as a matter of fact, the reason why diseases *matter* to us as human beings—because they can make our lives miserable and even make us perish. If this were not the case, we would not *care* so much about them. It is because we want to be at home in the world and in our own bodies that we study diseases and try to find remedies for them.

The relationship between suffering illness and having a disease is in many cases far from straightforward or even clear. This is especially so in the cases of illness referred to as "mental" or "psychiatric" in contrast to somatic illness. In psychiatry, the difficulties of finding clear correlations between bodily dysfunctions (dysfunctions of the brain) and the symptoms of illness have led to the choice of the softer term "disorder" instead of disease in diagnosing illness. Nevertheless, the last thirty years have brought a heavy focus on the diagnosis of distinct disorders in psychiatry (the *DSM* movement), sadly often at the expense of any deeper phenomenological understanding of the suffering in question. Critiques talk about an increasing "medicalization" of everyday life as an undesired and even dangerous effect of the new diagnostic psychiatry (Kutchins and Kirk 1997; Horwitz and Wakefield 2007).

Mental disorders introduce many fascinating and complex issues in trying to understand illness experience from a phenomenological perspective. The complexities concern the possibilities of tracking down all forms of illness to cases of *bodily* alienation (the choice of terminology, indeed, seems to suggest that this kind of illness is exactly not bodily in nature) and the question of how the processes of alienation found in different psychiatric diagnoses should be understood and categorized. This introduces many questions regarding how the borderlines between illness and the unhappy, or, perhaps, inauthentic, life are to be mapped out, and this project in turn contains deep philosophical issues bringing us to hot spots of normative ethics and political philosophy. To avoid most of these questions, I have picked only one example of a psychiatric diagnosis to reflect upon in this chapter: anorexia nervosa.[6] This example has the advantage of introducing the experience of the *body* uncanny in a very clear manner yet doing so in ways that introduce issues of alienation that are connected to matters of identity and politics, issues that are either not present, or harder to discern, in most cases of somatic illness.

Anorexia Nervosa

Anorexia nervosa is diagnosed in *DSM-IV-TR* by four criteria: a) a refusal to maintain a minimum body weight of at least 85 percent of what would be expected for the person's age and height; b) an intense fear of gaining weight or becoming fat; c) a misperception of one's weight and shape and an overemphasis on weight or shape in self-evaluations or denial of the seriousness of low body weight; and d) cessation of menstruation, although this criterion is not applied to females below the age of puberty or to males (American Psychiatric Association 2000, 589). Two important things should be pointed out immediately regarding the diagnosis. The first one is that anorexia is categorized as an eating disorder in *DSM*, so although we do not find obsession with food and strange eating habits among the four criteria, this can more or less be taken for granted as being the case if someone has anorexia. If these eating problems include binge eating and purging, the alternate eating disorder of bulimia nervosa will be diagnosed instead of (or together with) anorexia. The body-weight-controlling behavior of the person suffering from anorexia will typically also involve intense exercise programs taken on in order to lose weight.

The second important thing to point out is that although the suffering of anorexia is not restricted to girls, it is far more common for females than for males (the ratio is about one to ten) to be diagnosed with anorexia, as it is for people living in a Western society compared to a non-Western society. Anorexia typically affects adolescents, and the prevalence of the disorder is far higher today than only about fifty years ago or so.[7] It is common that the prevalence of psychiatric disorders varies a lot over time and with gender and culture, but anorexia is nevertheless a bit extreme in this sense: it seems almost normal for a teenage girl in upper-class New York to develop a fanatical preoccupation with avoiding food for the sake of being extremely slim, whereas it would be very strange and almost unheard of for a man in his fifties living in Congo Kinshasa to do so. Many psychiatric (and somatic) diagnoses are more common in one of the sexes, in a certain age group, or in a certain ethnic population, but most other cases of diagnostic skewness do not seem to be tied to cultural norms in the strikingly clear manner that anorexia nervosa is. Nevertheless, it appears that eating disorders like anorexia are increasingly diagnosed in and suffered by women (and men) in other cultural and social groups than North American and European upper and middle classes (Bordo 2003, xv).

Is anorexia a cultural disorder in the sense that it is *created* by a society that overtly signals to young girls that their success value is tied to bodily appearance and their ability in this and other related ways to please the opposite sex? Many feminist scholars have argued that this is the case (e.g., Fallon, Katzman, and Wooley 1994; Malson 1998), but it is has also been pointed out that there is a genetic disposition to develop the disorder (Bulik 2005), and that the presence of a perfectionist personality type seems to be important to the tendency to fall ill with anorexia (Polivy and Herman 2002). In my phenomenological attempts to understand anorexia, I am not able to assess the etiology in establishing what is the most important cause of the diagnosis; rather, I attempt by following some narratives of anorexia to better understand the way the experience of the own body is involved in anorexia.[8]

Most narratives of anorexia appear to start with a scenario in which a young girl suddenly understands by way of comments or behaviors of others that she is too fat.[9] These comments can be nasty and part of bullying, but they can also be rather innocent or perhaps even self-inflicted:

> Ruth is a cheerful, lively little girl with flashing eyes and a wide, captivating grin. She's got a cheeky sense of humor and can always make her family laugh with her funny impersonations of her school teachers. Until she was ten years old, Ruth had little interest in sport or exercise. She was a real "lounge lizard" who loved eating and lazing in front of the television. All this changed when she began dance classes. Ruth looked around the class and all she could see were "skinny" girls. Although Ruth was slim and petite, she felt fat and self-conscious, particularly in the body-hugging leotard the dance class had to wear. Ruth ached to look just like all the other girls and, in an effort to recast her figure, she embarked on a fitness campaign. She began by cutting out junk food, chocolates, and the desserts that she'd always loved, and by doing a bit more exercise—nothing significant, just practicing her dance routines and riding her bike. (Halse, Honey, and Boughtwood 2008, 127)

Ruth's experience of her own body as unsatisfying is different from the way the body turns up as uncanny in somatic illnesses. It is, indeed, as Sartre has highlighted in *Being and Nothingness*, a way of being objectified by other people in being looked upon by them (1956, 345).[10] This being looked upon—the own body appearing as an in-itself for consciousness in the terminology of Sartre—is readily turned into a self-objectifying gaze, as in the case of Ruth. We can imagine her in front of the mirror (maybe a mirror present already in the ballet class) introjecting the gaze on her own body as too fat for a beautiful ballet girl in filling up her "body-hugging leotard" and resisting her efforts to display the lightness and grace of a ballet dancer in moving to the music.

But this way of being objectified as too fat by the gaze of others is just the starting point of anorexia, and the gaze in question does not seem to lead to anorexia for every person exposed to the norms of slenderness in contemporary society—not for most men, a fact that might be explained by other (bodily) ideals for men than for

women, but also not for most women, or even for most young girls
exposed to the ideals in question. There are, of course, many cases of
eating habits and slenderness among women that could be claimed to
border on the unhealthy, even if they are not diagnosed as anorexia;
however, a more common behavior regarding eating and exercise
among women *and* men today is rather to become overweight than
too thin.[11] The uncanniness of the body in anorexia is an uncanniness that resonates with cultural norms, but it does so through a
twist made by the body itself, in which our ideals of bodily beauty
are stressed to the point at which we begin to see that these bodily
ideals verge on illness. The illness of anorexia thus brings out the illness of our culture in a different way than the "fat epidemic" does.
Our disgust and fascination with the sickly thin and the sickly fat are
inverted mirror images in a culture in which food and body shape
have been made into obsessive projects tied to identity.

> Ruth pursued her fitness campaign and quickly lost her
> puppy fat. Her parents, Beth and David, were proud of her
> determination to get fit and healthy and saw this as a positive
> lifestyle move, and Ruth reveled in the flurry of compliments
> from family and friends. Even though other people thought
> she looked "just right," Ruth didn't feel as if she could relax.
> The idea of easing up and possibly losing her new slender
> shape was intolerable. She did not make a conscious decision
> to restrict her eating further or intensify her exercise routine.
> The shift crept up so gradually that no one realized what was
> happening. (Halse, Honey, and Boughtwood 2008, 127–128)

Two striking elements in all narratives of anorexia I have come
across are weak self-confidence and an urge to control one's own
(and sometimes others') life in an almost manic way. It is not strange
that self-confidence and identity are weak and searching for a firm
ground in adolescence, but in cases of anorexia this unstable selfhood
is met with strong attempts to take control of life by monitoring eating and exercise, and, by way of this, the looks of the own body. The
body that showed itself as foreign in the sense of not conforming to
an ideal of slenderness (uncanny for the girl in question) now gradually becomes uncanny to others (the family) in exhibiting a skeletal
look that the anorexic girl refuses to acknowledge as a problem. This

changed perception and loss of judgment when it comes to issues of one's weight and shape is, as noted earlier, an integral part of the diagnosis of anorexia.

> Throughout the cold winter months, Beth and David had only seen Ruth warmly rugged in layers of clothes. Their illusions were shattered when summer arrived and the family went on holidays to the beach. Beth first realized the extent of Ruth's weight loss when they went shopping for Ruth's new swimsuit. When she saw Ruth's emaciated body for the first time in the changing room, Beth was so horrified that she felt physically ill. (Halse, Honey, and Boughtwood 2008, 129)

The refusal to eat and to stop the manic exercise leads relatively quickly to a life-threatening condition:

> As soon as they returned from holidays, David took Ruth to see a pediatrician specializing in eating disorders. Ruth's weight had dropped to 32 kilos, she was clinically depressed, her ankles were purple and swollen from all the exercise, and cardiac failure looked imminent. A few days after her eleventh birthday, Ruth was admitted to a hospital where she was sedated, put on bed rest, and fed through a nasogastric tube. (Halse, Honey, and Boughtwood 2008, 130)

Ruth develops anorexia before entering into puberty. In this she is not typical but a couple of years early: most girls who develop anorexia do so after their bodies have begun to take on a more female shape and they have experienced their first menstruation (as we saw, the cessation of menstruation due to starvation is one of the criteria in *DSM* for anorexia). To experience the body changes of puberty can be an uncanny experience in itself when the body, indeed, takes on a strange life of its own that (initially at least) might feel very foreign and disgusting to the person whose body is changing. For girls with anorexia, like Carol, this seems to be particularly true:

> When I started developing I just hated it. Especially with being in ballet it was really hard because I felt really uncomfortable not wearing a bra but even having to start wearing

bras was uncomfortable. I just hated the whole changing of my body [. . . My] first period arrived when the family was travelling in the car on the way to their annual holidays. [. . .] Mom gave me this huge, thick pad and I cried the whole way to the holiday house. I cried for a whole week—just nonstop. I just couldn't handle it. I just kept thinking this is just complete hell. I don't—I can't—believe that women are putting up with this. (Halse, Honey, and Boughtwood 2008, 51–52)

Like Ruth, Carol develops an obsession with her own body, especially after having been teased at school for having breasts:

Carol concedes that the insults and taunts eroded her self-confidence. Despite being fit and slender, she became increasingly uncomfortable with the womanly shape she saw emerging in front of her eyes. She loathed her maturing body and was convinced that it was ugly. Unable to control the teasing at school, Carol's thoughts focused inward on herself and on controlling her body and what she ate. She started weighing herself regularly—often dozens of times a day—and would stand in front of the bathroom mirror for hours composing long, detailed lists of imagined physical flaws she dreamed of changing. (Halse, Honey, and Boughtwood 2008, 54)

The element of *controlling* the body through restricting food and monitoring life is even stronger in other stories:

The first obvious sign that Hannah's dieting was entangled with something more than a desire to be healthy came just before she was due to go away to camp with her school. She was anxious and agitated. What sort of food would they have at the camp? What if they didn't have the food she wanted? How would she manage? How could she stick to her current diet? The idea of varying what she ate, even for two weeks, sent her into a spin. The food at camp didn't help. It was the usual school camp fare—lots of bread, pastries, and oily, fried dinners. Confronted with this menu, Hannah either refused to eat or ate the bare minimum and ran 15 kilometers each

day to offset what she'd eaten. Her teachers were so concerned that they contacted Laura and Peter [Hannah's par-
ents] [. . .] [(Peter, collecting Hannah from camp:)] I'll be
honest, I didn't recognize her. She'd lost so much weight in
the weeks she was away. She just looked awful. And all she
talked about in the car on the way home was where she ate,
what she ate. Meal by meal. (Halse, Honey, and Boughtwood
2008, 80–81)

Maybe it is not so strange that being in control of exactly what one
is eating becomes so important if one's own body displays an alien
nature. Food is the major foreign thing that enters into your body:
if you control food you will also be able to control the body, make
it more of your own, so to speak. But this routine of surveying and
controlling eating soon develops into a pathology with a life of its
own that the person is no longer able to control:

Eventually, Hannah was surviving on little more than car-
rots and her skin turned orange from the betacarotene.
At the same time, she became increasingly suspicious. She
insisted on weighing everything before she ate it and would
carefully monitor its calories. The family had always eaten
healthy home-cooked meals together but, increasingly, Hannah refused to eat anything prepared by someone else. [. . .]
At mealtimes, she'd eat exact things at exactly the same time
and there were all these little rituals. She'd get a carrot out
of the fridge. She'd peel it. She'd top and tail it, she'd slice it.
She'd lay it out in the steamer. She'd cook it for one and a
half minutes. She'd get it out and she'd eat. And then she'd go
to the fridge and she'd get another carrot out. And she'd top
and tail it. And then she'd weigh it before it was cooked and
she'd weight it after it was cooked. Then she'd go on to the
frozen vegetables. (Halse, Honey, and Boughtwood 2008, 82)

A common strategy for dealing with anorexia, used by health professionals, parents, and, also, by patients, is to view the disorder itself
as something alien. Instead of viewing the body as something being
uncanny to the anorexic girl herself, or becoming so to others, in this
image it is not the body, but the anorexia itself as invading and taking control over the body, that is uncanny. We recognize this logic of

bodily uncanniness from the *Alien* movie and also from the idea of somatic diseases in which the body is threatened by parasites (bacteria, viruses) or cells that are dividing beyond control (cancer diseases). The idea also resonates with the old image of mental illness as demonic possession referred to by Freud in his paper on the uncanny (1959).

> The idea is that the anorexia is separate from the person with anorexia, almost like a different, distinct individual. [. . .] We said, "Hannah, we love you. We'll always love you but this person that's in you—this possessed person that's in you—we hate her. We want her gone." So we actually talked about Hannah and the other person. And when we made the definition and she made the definition, it was a lot easier to deal with. Luke (Hannah's younger brother) christened Hannah's anorexia "The Bitch." Now he could relate to his sister and he'd cuddle and console Hannah, reassuring her that "The problem isn't you, it's the anorexia." (Halse, Honey, and Boughtwood 2008, 89)

The strategy of reifying an illness by turning it into a bodily dysfunction, not having anything to do with the person's identity, is common in cases of somatic illness. It is also a strategy encouraged by contemporary medical science and practice when illness is primarily understood in terms of medical concepts and measurements: as diseases. As I pointed out earlier, this reifying strategy can develop into a problematic one if it is not kept in check by a perspective stressing the importance of illness as something that happens to persons and demands attention to lifeworld issues and habits.

The view of anorexia as something separate from the person suffering from it, which was developed by Hannah's family, is different from and more far reaching than such a medical perspective, however, since the family views the anorexia not only as another thing (a bodily dysfunction) but as another *person* in Hannah. Such a view of alienation might be present in a kind of minimal form in all cases when the body shows up as uncanny, since the body in such cases displays a kind of life of its own that is experienced as a foreign *will* by the person in question (a will is something that, strictly, only a person and not a body can have). However, when the bodily alienation turns into the image of demonic possession ("The Bitch"), we seem to be closer to the stories of *The Exorcist*, *Rosemary's Baby*, and *The Omen* than to the parasitic possession of *Alien*. "The Bitch" needs to be *exorcised* and should not be considered a result of cultural circumstances (circumstances meaning both Hannah's personal situation in her family and circle of friends and the circumstances of women in Western society and culture) that needs to be interpreted and changed.

It is tempting to consider the story of "The Bitch" as yet another move in the discursive strategies of keeping women alienated and pacified in our society. In this view, not only would our culture and society rest on ideals of success that make girls starve themselves to death, but in this starving, the illness itself would be considered an evil, female creature ("The Bitch") possessing the girl in question, a creature that must be kept under control to prevent it from taking over. But I think a feminist reading of that sort is a little too one-eyed, since no one would deny that cultural norms have a lot to do with the *onset* of anorexia. It is a nonpolitical reality, however, that illness, when it has established itself, takes on a kind of life of its own as an uncanny pattern of experiences and "musts" that are not easily dealt with and changed, no matter how politically informed the anorexic girl, her parents, or her caretakers become. Sartre, in *Being and Nothingness* (1956, 441), characterizes illness as a *melody*, in most cases a rather disharmonic one, playing itself in the embodied life-world patterns of my life beyond my control. Anorexia seems to do so too, providing the person with a style of bodily experience that is just as autonomous as the mood melody of somatic illness.

Anorexia, in most cases, is set off by cultural influences, but when the starvation and over-exercise have been brought into play, the malnourished body as a kind of self-defense inflicts moods that make its bearer strangely disembodied, increasingly apprehending the body as a thing, and a thing that is still not thin enough, despite its now uncannily thin look to others. The moods of anorexia—anxiety, irritation, hopelessness, sadness, despair, aggression—all bear witness to problems with embodiment, the anorexic person no longer being properly present in her own body, maybe even claiming that it is dead. Self-mutilation, cutting oneself in order to inflict a pain that is perceptibly *physical* in nature, in contrast to the moods making the body strangely foreign, is not uncommon, and neither is suicide (Halse, Honey, and Boughtwood 2008, 100). The stories of anorexia bear clear witness to the double experience of being plagued and depressed by the anorexia but still being unable to give it up because it provides the only security, control, and identity that there is to have. Depression and anxiety disorders are commonly codiagnosed in anorexia, but depressed, irritated, and anxious moods are always present, sometimes as a starting point and most often as an effect of the anorexia behavior (Halse, Honey, and Boughtwood 2008, 74–75).

Conclusion

I have attempted to show how being embodied is not only a basic being-at-home with one's body but also a potentially alienating and uncanny experience. The not-being-at-home with the body can make itself known at any time and it is intensified and brought to the point of being a major nuisance in various forms of illnesses. Uncanniness can be understood as a further intensified quality of the potential unhomelike-alien nature of being embodied, as compared to other ways of becoming foreign to one's life. The experience of the own-body as other is a fearful and horrifying experience because it reveals a not-being-at-home that is hidden at the very nucleus of our most intimate being-at-home: the body.

Anorexia nervosa displays several forms of being alienated from one's own body in an uncanny way. These include the ways of the body uncanny that I have identified in somatic illness, but they also concern ways of being objectified in an everyday manner in the social world by the gazes of others. However, the objectification by way of the looks of others in anorexia is not primarily a battle between consciousnesses à la Sartre, but a finding oneself in a cultural pattern of norms regarding the feminine, the healthy, the beautiful, and the successful. The gazes of the others are soon made into a self-surveying gaze by the anorexic girl, in the process of which the image of the own body is made gradually, increasingly unrealistic and self-punishing.

The different ways of becoming bodily alienated interact in anorexia in establishing an uncanniness of the body that is both conspicuous (to people around the ill person) and hard to escape (for the person herself). The diagnosis of anorexia can itself be both a relief and a shock to the patient and her family. A relief, because it defines the problem as medical and thus not personal, even if the characterization of eating disorders as mental disorders makes this depersonalization of the illness less convincing than in the cases of somatic illness. A shock, because the diagnosis means that the problems experienced with refusing to eat are serious, and, as the family will learn, potentially life threatening as well as hard to treat. Getting the diagnosis is often linked to the person's becoming hospitalized for the first time and being subjected to mistrust, surveillance, and coercion, a tough treatment regime that many find hard to accept. Treatment for anorexia may mean many more things than surveillance and coercive treatment, though, and my phenomenological analysis of the body uncanny points in the direction of giving a role to more than the acute treatment of the life-threatening starvation behavior. To focus upon the body *experience* of the anorexic person will mean to try to understand and help the person affected by anorexia with the ways she finds her body alien and uncanny, involving the prereflective experience of embodiment, in which the body may show up as absent and foreign to her, but also the ways in which the body becomes objectified by cultural and medical norms that need to be made conscious and criticized in the process of finding a personal identity possible to live and be at home with.

Notes

1. See, for instance, Guignon (2004).
2. In the case of materialism, the role of the soul as the ghost in the machine is taken over by the brain, which "does" different things by controlling its body. See Shaun Gallagher's book *How the Body Shapes the Mind* (2005) for a substantial, scientifically updated, phenomenological critique of materialistic, as well as idealistic, philosophies of mind.
3. Regarding this expression, see *At the Will of the Body* (2002), by Arthur Frank, which offers a phenomenology of illness proceeding from his own and others' experiences of being at the mercy of the body.
4. The body is thus a fundamental "vector of existence," to use the terminology of Maurice Merleau-Ponty (1962), indeed, a "fundamental existential of Dasein's being-in-the-world," in the same sense as the attunement, understanding, discourse, and entanglement doing this job in Martin Heidegger's *Being and Time* (1996). Already the founder of phenomenology, Edmund Husserl, pointed to this constitutive structure of the lived body (*Leib*) in contrast to the body that becomes the focus of attention for

consciousness (*Körper*), and this as early as 1907 in his lectures on "Ding und Raum" (Zahavi 1999, 92).

5. See here also the works by Toombs (1992) and Gadamer (1996).

6. For an attempt to address the issue of alienation in the cases of depression and anxiety disorders, see Svenaeus (2007).

7. The lifetime prevalence of anorexia for Caucasian women in Western countries is rated to be between 1.4 and 4.3 percent, which means that the lifetime prevalence in total (including women and men of all ethnic groups in all countries) for the disorder will probably be somewhere between 0.2 and 0.7 percent. Since anorexia mainly hits adolescent girls in Western countries, this still means that for this group it will be a relatively common (and potentially lethal) disorder. For information regarding anorexia, see Halse, Honey, and Boughtwood (2008), which introduces the research on anorexia and gives many examples (stories) from patients and their families living with the illness.

8. We find in Kristana Arp (1995) a sophisticated feminist analysis of bodily alienation. With the help of Simone de Beauvoir, Arp argues that although the objectification of the female body is primarily an effect of a male, oppressive culture, the embodiment of women includes features that are clearly different and distinct from men's, and this is a fact that needs to be taken into account in analyzing examples such as anorexia. See also the analysis of anorexia found in Susan Bordo (2003), which provides a phenomenology of the disorder that although Foucauldian at heart acknowledges the physical perspective of the alienation in question.

9. My main examples in this chapter are taken from Halse, Honey, and Boughtwood (2008), but there are countless stories about anorexia to be found in different books, and, above all, on the World Wide Web; see for example www.caringonline.com/feelings/byvictims/ or the videos found on www.youtube.com by entering search words like "stories of anorexia."

10. For an analysis of the outline for a phenomenology of illness found in Sartre, see Svenaeus (2009).

11. The "fat epidemic" has hit more than a fifth of the population in most developed countries (fat meaning having a BMI>30), and far more people than that, children included, are found to be overweight (meaning having a BMI>25); but this does not stop anorexic girls from comparing themselves to a bodily ideal that

is consequently becoming increasingly statistically abnormal. It seems, rather, as though the media talk of the fat epidemic has a kind of encouraging effect on anorexics in starving and exercising themselves to death, whereas the people who would benefit from cutting down on fat and sugar and trying to exercise their too-massive bodies are either unaffected or unable to profit from the message.

References

American Psychiatric Association. 2000. *DSM-IV-TR: Diagnostic and Statistical Manual of Mental Disorders*, 4th ed., text revision. Washington, DC: American Psychiatric Publishing.

Arp, Kristana. 1995. "Beauvoir's Concept of Bodily Alienation." In *Feminist Interpretations of Simone de Beauvoir*, edited by M. A. Simons, 161–177. University Park: Pennsylvania State University Press.

Bordo, Susan. 2003. *Unbearable Weight: Feminism, Western Culture and the Body*. Berkeley: University of California Press.

Bulik, Cynthia M. 2005. "Exploring the Gene-Environment Nexus in Eating Disorders." *Journal of Psychiatry & Neuroscience* 30 (5): 335–339.

Damasio, Antonio R. 1999. *The Feeling of What Happens: Body and Emotion in the Making of Consciousness*. New York: Harcourt Brace.

Fallon, Patricia, Melanie A. Katzman, and Susan C. Wooley (eds.). 1994. *Feminist Perspectives on Eating Disorders*. New York: Guilford Press.

Frank, Arthur. 2002. *At the Will of the Body: Reflections on Illness*. Boston: Houghton Mifflin.

Freud, Sigmund. [1919] 1959. "The Uncanny." In *Collected Papers*, vol. 4. New York: Basic Books.

Gadamer, Hans-Georg. [1993] 1996. *The Enigma of Health: The Art of Healing in a Scientific Age*, translated by J. Gaiger and N. Walker. Stanford, CA: Stanford University Press.

Gallagher, Shaun. 2005. *How the Body Shapes the Mind*. Oxford: Oxford University Press.

Guignon, Charles. 2004. *On Being Authentic*. London: Routledge.

Halse, Christine, Anne Honey, and Desiree Boughtwood. 2008. *Inside Anorexia: The Experiences of Girls and Their Families*. London and Philadelphia: Jessica Kingsley.

Heidegger, Martin. [1927] 1996. *Being and Time,* translated by Joan Stambaugh. Albany: State University of New York Press.

Horwitz, Allan V., and Jerome C. Wakefield. 2007. *The Loss of Sadness: How Psychiatry Transformed Normal Sorrow into Depressive Disorder.* New York: Oxford University Press.

Kutchins, Herb, and Stuart A. Kirk. 1997. *Making Us Crazy: DSM, the Psychiatric Bible and the Creation of Mental Disorders.* New York: Free Press.

Leder, Drew. 1990. *The Absent Body.* Chicago: University of Chicago Press.

Malson, Helen. 1998. *The Thin Woman: Feminism, Post-Structuralism and the Social Psychology of Anorexia Nervosa.* London: Routledge.

Merleau-Ponty, Maurice. [1945] 1962. *Phenomenology of Perception.* Translated by C. Smith. London: Routledge.

Polivy, Janet, and C. Peter Herman. 2002. "Causes of Eating Disorders." *Annual Review of Psychology* 53 (1): 187–213.

Sartre, Jean-Paul. [1943] 1956. *Being and Nothingness,* translated by H. E. Barnes. New York: Washington Square Press.

Svenaeus, Fredrik. 2000. *The Hermeneutics of Medicine and the Phenomenology of Health: Steps Towards a Philosophy of Medical Practice.* Dordrecht: Kluwer.

Svenaeus, Fredrik. 2007. "Phenomenology Listens to Prozac: Analyzing the SSRI Revolution." In *Medical Technologies and the Life World: The Social Construction of Normality,* edited by S. Olin Lauritzen and L.-C. Hydén, 164–183. London: Routledge.

Svenaeus, Fredrik. 2009. "The Phenomenology of Falling Ill: An Explication, Critique and Improvement of Sartre's Theory of Embodiment and Alienation." *Human Studies* 32 (1): 53–66.

Toombs, S. Kay. 1992. *The Meaning of Illness: A Phenomenological Account of the Different Perspectives of Physician and Patient.* Dordrecht: Kluwer.

Zahavi, Dan. 1999. *Self-Awareness and Alterity: A Phenomenological Investigation.* Evanston, IL: Northwestern University Press.

Zaner, Richard M. 1981. *The Context of Self: A Phenomenological Inquiry Using Medicine as a Clue.* Athens: Ohio University Press.

Zeiler, Kristin. 2010. "A Phenomenological Analysis of Bodily Self-Awareness in Pain and Pleasure: On Bodily Dys-appearance and Eu-appearance." *Medicine, Health Care and Philosophy* 13 (4): 333–342.

12

TOWARD A PHENOMENOLOGY OF DISFIGUREMENT

JENNY SLATMAN AND GILI YARON

> Recovering from facial injuries is, in the end, about how well you can communicate with the rest of humanity, in spite of your tarnished face.
> —James Partridge, *Changing Faces*

Introduction

Bracketing fixed beliefs and naturalized views, phenomenology aims at an unprejudiced analysis of individuals' lived experience. A phenomenology of disfigurement will thus concentrate on the way disfigured people experience their bodies. Another basic assumption of phenomenology, however, is that one needs the other (the others' gaze) to become fully conscious of one's embodied self. It is only because of one's "being for the other" (*pour autrui*) that one can be "for oneself" (*pour soi*).[1] Hence, from a phenomenological perspective, embodied self-experience and embodied agency is at once an *individual* and a *social* affair. This double view on embodiment, as we will argue, is constructive to gain both theoretical and practical insight into the meaning of disfigurement.

Our current research project, in which we explore the meaning of bodily integrity in cases of disfiguring cancer, aims to make this phenomenological approach productive in medical practices.[2] Indeed, we believe that this approach may support medical professionals in attaining a suitable and desirable attitude toward people with disfigurement. In this chapter, we will present some of our preliminary findings as well as the theoretical program that underlies and directs our research. Here, we will discuss only facial disfigurement, since this type of disfigurement, which is hard to conceal, almost always immediately affects social interaction. This focus will thus allow us to address the social as well as the individual, lived, aspects of disfigured embodiment.

Taking into account the privative meaning of the prefix *dis-*, disfigurement literally means that one's "figure" or "form" has fallen apart, that it has become formless. Hence its exclusively negative connotations: defacement, deformity, blemish, deficiency, defect—the negation of bodily wholeness and beauty. However, regardless of the obviousness of its anatomical markers, the (negative) meaning endowed to disfigured bodies cannot simply be derived from anatomical differences or deficiencies as such. As Nick Crossley (2001, 152; emphasis added) aptly argues: "Differences and deficiencies are not intrinsic properties of bodies [. . .] they are inevitably *social constructions.*"

In social (and historical) studies of science, as well as in (medical) sociology of the body and feminist philosophy, it has become virtually commonplace to think of the body in terms of "social construction." Although the usage of this term is rather disparate (Hacking 2001), generically, it refers to the idea that bodies (and their deviances) have no intrinsic (universal) meaning. Social constructivism can thus be seen as a way out of naturalistic essentialism: for its general claim is that biologically (and phenotypically) varying bodies (male, female, young, old, healthy, sick, disabled, disfigured, black, white, etc.) are not simply naturally occurring. Instead, bodily variance is ordered along social and cultural axes valorizing some qualities and rejecting others.

Although naturalistic essentialism has thus been criticized fiercely in theoretical debates, it still resonates in the dominant medical-biological view on embodiment that underpins everyday medical practices. Within this view, disfigured bodies are reduced to individualistic entities that deviate from biological norms. Consequently, medical practices aim at restoring biological intactness. Social constructivist approaches, by contrast, consider the impact and value of bodily difference against the background of prevailing social and cultural norms, thus underlining that disfigurement is more a social than an individual issue.

Despite the fact that we sympathize with the idea that the body's meaning and value should not be understood as something naturally occurring, we believe that "social constructivism" is not the most adequate answer to medical-biological reductionism in health and medicine. In its emphasis on the powerful force of social and cultural classifications, relations, and categorizations, social constructivism loses sight of the lived nature of both suffering and enjoyment: physical pain, distress, and discomfort or, conversely, pleasure, the corporeal confidence and delight derived from physical capacities, comfort, and so forth. Thus, rather than offering a sound alternative, social constructivist approaches to embodiment seem to share the same ontological premises that underlie the mainstream medical-biological view. According to phenomenological vocabulary, both presuppose the idea of the body as a thing that appears; that is, an "intentional object."[3] They both neglect the fact that the body is not only given in its capacity to be sensed but also as a "sensing thing."

As we will argue here, the meaning of disfigurement does not only concern the appearance of the disfigured body as an exposed thing or image to oneself and to others, but also how one's disfigurement is lived through, and how it may, or may not, inhibit one's bodily intentionality. To clarify and justify this double view on embodiment in disfigurement, we will present four sections in this paper. First, we will briefly discuss the gains and the limits of social constructivist approaches to embodiment. By discussing the case of disfigured war veterans in the second section, we will then show how a focus on social norms and relations can explain the positive social value attributed to some physical scars and blemishes, but, at the same time, still fails to address the body's double ontology. In the third section we will present phenomenology as an approach that amends this hiatus. In the last section, we will explore the meaning of this double body ontology in practice, by discussing the story of "Leah," a facially disfigured woman wearing a facial prosthesis.[4]

Embodiment as Social Construction: Liberating and Unsettling

As is well known, "the body" has gained enormous theoretical interest in the last two decades both in the humanities and in the social sciences. In the humanities, the most prominent examples are to be found in (medical) history and feminist philosophy. In the social sciences, a genuine "sociology of the body" has developed since the 1990s (Featherstone, Hepworth, and Turner 1991; Turner 1992, 1996; Shilling 1993; Crossley 2001; Williams 2003). Within science studies, more and more attention is paid to the way embodiment is "produced" and "manufactured" in scientific and medical practices (Hirschauer 1991; Mol 2002; Latour 2004). Typical for this interest in the body, generally speaking, is the focus on its social, cultural, and historical meaning. As this focus implies that the body's specific meaning is mainly considered in relation to others, we call it the social approach to embodiment.

To grasp the theoretical meaning and scope of this social approach to the body, we will start with a short exposition of how it was developed in feminist studies. One of the first and most famous statements about the female body's social meaning is probably Simone de Beauvoir's (1949) claim: *on ne naît pas femme, on le devient* ("one is not born but becomes a woman"). Since Beauvoir, the distinction between (biological) *sex* and (sociocultural) *gender* has become generally accepted. Accordingly, the project aiming to free women from the presumed biological fact of their womanhood has placed much emphasis on the sociality of gender (Witz 2000). The distinction between sex and gender has made it very clear that being a woman is not (only) a biological fact and that social inequalities between men and women cannot be justified on the basis of biological, anatomical features. Nevertheless, this distinction is not an uncomplicated one.

Judith Butler, for instance, argues in *Bodies That Matter (*1993) that the sex-gender distinction still presupposes a certain biological substrate on top of which gender pops up as a social construct. In her view, the idea of social construction is not useful since it suggests that "sex" is something biological that precedes construction; as such it becomes a sort of prelinguistic fantasy to which we have no access (1993, 12). Butler, therefore, rejects the idea of social constructivism and replaces it by the concept of materialization. A body is a "body that matters," that is, a body that is socially meaningful and comprehensible (as opposed to being socially abject) if it is materialized through a certain discursive practice. Inspired by Austin's idea of performativity in language and Foucault's theory on discursive power and normalization, she claims that there is no matter independent of or prior to language or to discourse in general. Sex is always already gendered (Butler 1993). Butler thus suggests that biology and biological knowledge are produced by discourses on the body. This implies that not only gender-related differentiation (such as preferred division of roles) but also "hard," "factual" biological and anatomical differences between the sexes are only intelligible against the background of social and cultural norms.[5]

Although Butler criticizes the idea of social construction and replaces it with the idea of materialization, we believe that she implicitly still endorses social constructivism at least in her early work.[6] She indeed reduces sexual markers (and the body) to a passive surface to be inscribed by social signifiers only, thus reducing materiality to signs and considering anything meaningful in our world as the outcome of social and discursive processes. Indeed, from a Butlerian perspective, the social and cultural meanings of bodies are inseparable from their material, physical manifestations. In the next section we will explore how this view on embodiment can explain the valorization of some forms of facial disfigurement.

The Social Value of Disfigurements

A visual disfigurement is a social marker. It can only be valued as a difference in relation to normal others. Indeed, a disfigured person only recognizes her own disfigurement while seeing herself through the eyes of others, while comparing herself to these others. But why are some differences valued in a negative way and some in a positive way? This question, obviously, requires a social approach.

A clear analysis of the body such as it is exposed to others—and how this exposure yields social meaning—is provided by Michel Foucault's early work. According to Foucault (1979) the body's social value is the result of normalizing power; people discipline their bodies to "normalize" them. Submitted to a constant watchful eye, whether actually present or not, modern people live in a *panopticon*—which literally means everywhere (*pan*) visible (*opticon*)—by means of which they are constantly aware of their own visible bodies and, subsequently, constantly measure and manage their visible bodies against prevailing standards and norms. According to this view, a certain physical marker can have both a positive and a negative meaning dependent on the specific situation. In a society that respects old age, an old body will be positively valued. In a society that, by contrast, adores youth, an old body becomes a "nonnormative" body.

The question is now whether this also holds for disfigurement. Is it possible to read the physical marker of disfigurement in a positive way? This question is pertinent, since, as mentioned in the introduction, disfigurement has a thoroughly privative and thus a negative meaning. From time immemorial, disfigured people have been frequently stigmatized and thus excluded from social groups. However, not all physical blemishes function as excluding social stigmas (Goffman 1963). A disfigurement or scar might even have a positive social value; a form of "physical capital" perhaps.[7]

A telling example of this is the representation of the so-called Guinea Pig Club in the United Kingdom. This club consists (consisted) of former RAF aircrew members who survived severe burn injuries during World War II. These men did not have to hide their damaged faces since they were signs of bravery; their faces expressed the honor of having served their country. In addition, these men also served medical sciences; they were real guinea pigs for the plastic surgeon Archibald McIndoe, who, at that time (rather successfully) experimented with new kinds of medical technologies (Mayhew 2004). Although his treatment could not wipe out the horrible traces of burns, he did give these men a socially faceable face. Pictures of these men show disfigured but happy and almost smiling faces.[8] One could therefore argue that the exposition of these faces to the gazes of others did not result in a social devaluation. In the context of the social value attributed to heroism, bravery, and patriotism, their marked appearance could be read as socially valuable.

Such a reading of facial disfigurement can be rather *liberating*, since it frees the person with disfigurements from the idea of being a deviant, abnormal individual, and thus from stigmatization. Yet it might be *unsettling* as well: if one interprets the meaning of one's appearance solely against the background of social norms and discourses, one fails to recognize possible personal tragedies against the background of individual and shared stories. The British Guinea Pigs may have found comfort in the positive social meaning of their disfigurements. But if their bodies are really reduced to signifiers of "bravery" and "patriotism" then these men are deprived of the possibility to express how they actually experience their being facially disfigured. Facial disfigurement, indeed, involves often more than a social valuation of visible defects. As we will discuss in the last section of this chapter, disfigurements habitually go together with a variety of disturbances in sensory perception and motor capacities. These disturbances may indeed result in a modification of one's embodied intentionality and habits.

If we frame social constructivists approaches, such as they are advocated by Foucault and Butler, in ontological terms, we can say that they, on the one hand, *liberate* the body from its being an individual, biological, and genetic entity, but on the other hand, they are *unsettling* since they share the same Cartesian ontological premises that haunted biologically essentialist accounts of the body. While biology understands the body as an object in the sense of Descartes' *res extensa* or machine, social constructivism reduces the body to a malleable thing at the mercy of certain social practices, relations, and discourses. Focusing on its visibility and its malleability, social constructivism, indeed, still endorses a Cartesian view on the body (Hacking 2007), thereby ignoring the body's own intentionality—its experienced subjectivity and agency.

Since it fails to recognize the reality of bodily experiences and embodied self-experiences, we believe that a social constructivist view on disfigurement does not offer an adequate reply to the medical-biological view on the body prevailing in current medical practices. In order to do justice to individuals' lived (embodied) experiences as they take form against the background of their lifeworld, we need to shift to a phenomenological account of embodiment.

Embodied Self-Experience:
An Individual and a Social Affair

In this section, we will clarify how the perception and experience of one's own body always takes place within a social field and simultaneously opens up such a field, while referring to some ideas of Maurice Merleau-Ponty. Although Merleau-Ponty is well known (and praised) for the idea of the lived body (*corps vécu*)—thus criticizing the Cartesian view on embodiment—we should not forget that, for him, this lived body always remains attached to its "object-side." In other words: the lived body is not just a perceiving subject, it is also a perceived object among other objects in the world. This double view on the body is most clearly articulated in Merleau-Ponty's later work, in which he replaced the notion of lived body by a double-sided "subject": a seer who is seen (*voyant-vu*) or a sensing subject who is sensed (*sentant-senti*) (Merleau-Ponty 1993; Merleau-Ponty 1968).

As the body appears to oneself, it is an intentional object. It is a *noema* that correlates with a certain intentional act or a *noese*. At first glance, we can stick to an uncomplicated phenomenological model to describe self-appearance. For, indeed, one's own body can explicitly appear as an object to which certain qualities can be attributed; one can observe, for instance, the color and texture of one's own feet while cutting one's nails. Yet, the fact that one's self-observation goes together with an explicit sense of ownership reveals that the body is not simply an intentional object. While perceiving my own body I may think "this is my body." However, the actual *experience* that this is my body involves more than an observational content. The experiential affirmation that this perceived body is *mine* is provided by nonintentional localized sensations, or "sensings." Examples include touch sensations, pain sensations, proprioception, and kinesthetic sensations. Instead of constituting an intentional object, they constitute the body as a "sensing thing."

One's own body can thus appear in two different modes: either as a thing or intentional object or as a localized lived-through experience of oneself. This double-sided experience can be explained along the lines of the Husserlian distinction between *Leib* (body as mine, based upon nonintentional sensations) and *Körper* (body as intentional object). We must stress here, however, that the phenomenological distinction in two modes of appearances does not imply a separation between two forms of embodiment. As argued elsewhere in more detail, the experience of *Leib* both presupposes and affirms the experience of *Körper* (Slatman 2005, 2008).

In his early work, Merleau-Ponty (1962) argues that the body as lived (*corps vécu* or *Leib*) forms the zero point of intentionality. As such it does not appear to oneself in the same way as everything around us appears to us but conditions that very appearance. The body as intentional object, by contrast, appears within the horizon such as it is constituted by the lived body as zero point. The double-sidedness of body appearance can thus also be explained in terms of distance: whereas the lived body is an experience of "here," the body as object appears "there" (Slatman 2009).

It is on the basis of this difference in "distance" to oneself that the social dimension within embodied self-experience comes to the fore. In the sense that my body appears as an object—for instance, in the mirror—it appears "there" and does not totally coincide with my "here" and therefore is not fully owned. As Merleau-Ponty writes: the moment I recognize my own mirror image, "I am no longer what I felt myself, immediately to be [. . .]. I am torn from myself, and the image in the mirror prepares me for another still more serious alienation, which will be the alienation by others" (Merleau-Ponty 1951, 136). It is because of one's outside, one's physical appearance, that one is delivered to (the gazes of) others, and is a social being. This phenomenological view on embodiment thus teaches us that the experience of one's own body, according to the two interdependent modes of *Leib* and *Körper*, always already involves a social dimension. Moreover, it teaches us that the social body, that is, the body as intentional object with a readable surface, is always interlaced with the body as a lived-through zero point of intentionality.

Phenomenology of Disfigurement in Practice

In order to address the double-body ontology that is at stake in facial disfigurement, we will now discuss the case of "Leah." Leah's face was severely disfigured during the treatment of cancer, which consisted in extensive radiotherapy and the amputation of the affected area (her entire nose, parts of her palate, and parts of her upper jaw). After a period of recovery, she received a silicone facial prosthesis that hides and protects her now-exposed nasal cavity. Leah's story not only illustrates the body's double-sided ontology, but also reveals that it is by no means a given, static condition. Leah does not endure her disfigure-urement passively: in relating to her condition, she develops various ways of "doing" her body anew—ways that operate both on her body as image (an intentional object or *Körper*) and on her body as lived-through (a sensing self or *Leib*).

At first sight, Leah's story underlines the major role physical appearance plays in interaction with others. Very often she has to face people in the street or in shops staring at her, commenting on her unusual appearance ("what happened to you, girl?"), giggling, and pointing. Also, some of her own friends recurrently ask to see her face without the prosthesis despite her explicit refusal. These examples underline how Leah's disfigured face appears primarily as an object of the others' gaze—an object that is labeled as strange, different, fascinating, or repulsive and receives a discursive, symbolic meaning in relation to valorized, opposing terms such as "acceptable," "normal," "common," or "attractive."

Next to these more obvious, social aspects of her disfigurement, however, Leah is also confronted with loss of and damage to several bodily functions. These changes, accessible only to Leah herself, affect both her perception of the world and of her own body. One example is her altered sense of smell. Since her treatment, there is a distinct lag in Leah's perception of scents, and sometimes she does not notice odors at all. As a result she can no longer pursue her profession: nurses must to be able to smell patients, drugs, and other scents. Radiation has also affected the functioning of Leah's tear ducts, which no longer drain her eye fluids effectively. Consequently, Leah's eyesight has become blurred, which sometimes causes her to lose her balance.

But Leah also deals with other bodily changes, changes that affect her perception of world and body and that cannot simply be labeled as "loss of function." One example is the fact that Leah can no longer expose her face to the warm water while taking a shower, as she used to do. This would result in her drowning in the water entering her unprotected windpipe. In order to cope with this very real danger, Leah has developed a new way of showering. The removal of parts of her upper jaw dictates yet other adjustments. Due to the fact that the sensitive roots of her teeth are no longer enclosed within tissue, Leah can only go outdoors when the temperature is about twelve degrees Celsius. Colder weather causes pain comparable to root-canal treatment, and the cold air entering her nasal cavity unwarmed and unfiltered often gives rise to acute colds. In a similar manner, Leah can no longer take big bites of food. This is simply too painful; it causes a sensation similar to breaking her front teeth.

Another issue in relating to her disfigurement is Leah's daily dealings with her prosthesis and bandage—dealings which come to play in both the public and the private aspects of disfigurement. A silicone "nose," for instance, is not very flexible: it does not budge when kissing someone, which is rather unpleasant for the person being kissed. This is why Leah prefers to hug her loved ones instead of kissing them. Also, the prosthesis can be quite uncomfortable: it sometimes feels quite "tight" and pressing, and the adhesive gluing it to her face irritates the much-abused skin around the cavity. At home Leah thus prefers to wear a bandage. Going out, however, she always wears the prosthesis. The bandage (she calls it her "emergency triangle") does not only generate more attention than a prosthesis, but it can also be easily blown away by the wind and gets wet in the rain. This is not to say that she has full confidence in the prosthesis remaining fixed. Leah avoids crowds for fear of having her prosthesis knocked off. She no longer goes to her favorite department store, for example.

The bodily changes caused by the radiotherapy and amputation have not only left Leah with a different exterior and numerous impairments and handicaps, however. It has also changed the way in which the world appears to her. A delayed perception of smells and diminished sight mean that Leah registers her world in an altered way: as odorless, vague, and less stable. The appearance and meaning of her world have also changed in a more subtle way, however. Eating and walking outside on a winter day have become potentially painful experiences. Showering can be lethal. As a result, sandwiches, errands, and showerheads now call for a cautious, calculating approach and cannot be handled thoughtlessly. The activities of eating, walking outside, and showering have all become cumbersome affairs. Since her amputation, Leah's world and body have become much more fragile: her world now appears as threatening and disruptive, her body as a site of pain, irritation, and hindrance. Leah's former, taken-for-granted confidence in approaching her everyday projects—projects in which world and body coincide—has thus turned into a careful, attentive attitude.

A similar point can be made with regard to Leah's relationship to her now exposed nasal cavity, her prosthesis, and the bandage. Getting rid of mucus now involves manually cleaning her nasal cavity in front of the mirror. And both the prosthesis and the bandage call for an extensive regime of caring and minding: they must be cleaned, prepared, glued to the face, and adjusted to circumstances (a windy day, for instance). Whether she wears her prosthesis or bandage or neither, Leah's altered face now appears as an object of care, calling for a careful and calculating approach. These particular regimes, based upon an explicit attentive attitude toward her own body, are not only geared toward fending off potential pain and discomfort, but also toward meeting the others' gaze. The adjustments to her body, of course, also involve changes in Leah's relationships with others (eating and shopping are often social affairs governed by strict standards regulating one's conduct and appearance). But, in this case, the caring and minding are much more obviously done not only for the sake of comfort and hygiene but also in order to present the world with an adequate, acceptable exterior.

Leah's facial disfigurement and subsequent usage of prosthesis and bandage has thus resulted in considerable changes in the way she is directed and geared toward her world, and the way she engages in her everyday projects. Some activities she undertakes in much the same way as before; other pursuits call for different doings. We could therefore say that Leah's bodily changes call for new ways of "doing" her body, in the sense that her embodied intentionality, her being engaged in projects—or her "I can" (Merleau-Ponty 1945)—goes together with the development of a host of new, embodied habits: habits that pertain to her body as image seen by others as well as to her lived body.

Intentionality and habit are constituted and inscribed in one's body, yet, at the same time, they are conditioned by the social order. This has been aptly described by Iris Marion Young in her analysis of feminine movement. Young (1990) argues that the typicality of "feminine movement" can be explained in terms of different embodied competences and self-experience in women. These are formed against prevailing social and cultural norms. Girls who are raised in a sexist society that discourages them from employing their body in the same open and expressive way as boys may develop an "inhibited intentionality"; a basic embodied attitude of "I cannot" despite their physically able bodies. The way girls (and boys) move and how they use their bodies is not simply the result of following social norms and rules. With reference to the work of Pierre Bourdieu (2000), we could call this (social) practice a *habitus*: a set of habits that are literally incorporated, that is, habits that are physically produced (in gestures, movement, expression, manners, etc.) and become part of one's body scheme. With this, they form a person's (prereflective) stance in the (social) world. Girls do not only move differently than boys. The environment and its objects appear to them differently: they literally do not inhabit the same world. A *habitus* is thus formed by given social structures but, at the same time, is inscribed throughout an individual's body and subsequently bodily experience.

The inhibitions Leah experiences originate both in the physical limitations she deals with and in incorporated, normalizing (and sometimes sexist) standards. These two, however, cannot always be seen apart. Going outside has become problematic not only due to physical constraints such as pain, discomfort, and the possibility of catching a cold: Leah avoids crowds in fear of losing her prosthesis, and favors her prosthesis over a bandage in public because of prevailing cultural ideals regarding normalcy, wholeness, and beauty—ideals that, in our society, have a much larger impact on women than on men (Grealy 1994; Shannon 2012). Likewise, Leah does not refrain from kissing her granddaughter only in order to avoid physical discomfort to both of them—she also feels very strongly about others seeing her exposed face.

Leah's story thus illustrates how the disfigured body operates not only as a symbolically charged image for the (internalized) gaze of the other but also as an experiencing agent. Both these sides to the disfigured body's ontology matter to disfigured people. Both play a major part in their altered lives. And both, rather than being static, final terms, are in fact starting points that call for new ways of "doing" the body.

Concluding Remarks

Having discussed the case of Leah against the background of a discussion on body ontology, the purpose of this chapter has been a rather theoretical one. One of our aims has been to show how the phenomenological double-sided body ontology can complement the one-sided Cartesian ontology underlying both social constructivist and medical-biological approaches. We believe, however, that this theoretical challenge of the idea of the body as an object—either as a material and readable surface of inscribed norms (social constructivism) or as a biological (and genetic) entity that can be fixed and designed (medical-biologism)—can also have its impact on medical practices. We thus hold the view that the phenomenological approach to embodiment can be applied to and implemented in the actual practice of treatment and care of people with disfigurements.

In addressing the individual, lived side to embodiment, as well as the ways it is "done," a phenomenological approach to disfigurements can help medical professionals—including ENT specialists and surgeons, prosthetic technicians and designers, speech (and swallow) therapists—to adequately adjust treatment, care, and rehabilitation programs to individual patients' ailments and subsequent needs. In their intention to help and support people with a disfigurement, medical professionals are surely guided by the idea of moral imagination or empathy, that is, the possibility of putting oneself in the place of another. Endorsing norms of biological (and social) normalcy, they naturally strive toward healing disfigurements by repairing them as much as possible.

However, moral imagination is limited as a practical guidance (Mackenzie and Scully 2007): medical professionals, like all other nondisfigured people, cannot simply presume that they know what it means to be disfigured. They may see, for instance, someone without a nose and instantly find that this defect needs to be covered up with the best lifelike prosthesis possible. This response is understandable, but it forecloses the focus on other aspects the person with disfigurement has to deal with. A person with an amputated nose may need a prosthesis to camouflage her open face, but, as Leah's case shows, such a camouflage is only a starting point for regaining one's (social) life after having acquired facial disfigurements. What medical professionals thus can learn from a phenomenological approach is that embodiment is a multilayered phenomenon that calls for multilateral attention and care. We thus suggest that medical practices could be improved if medical professionals could incorporate a wide range of questions about embodied self-experiences in their patient interviews, and if they subsequently could use patients'"body-stories" while counseling them. We hope that our currently ongoing research on facial disfigurements will result in findings that can serve as handles for medical professionals to accurately inform patients about the variety of impacts that a disfigurement can have and about the possible benefits and shortcomings of different prosthetic devices.

Acknowledgments

First of all we would like to thank all the interviewees, and especially Leah, for sharing their stories with us. Also thanks to an anonymous reviewer for providing instructive comments, to Lisa Folkmarson Käll and Kristin Zeiler for their effective suggestions, and to Dana Henning for carefully emending our text. This research is funded by the Netherlands Organization for Scientific Research—NWO (VIDI-grant 276-20-016).

Notes

1. Already in his *Ideas II*, Husserl observed that the body as *Leib* appears as "a remarkably imperfectly constituted thing" (1989, 167) See also Merleau-Ponty's (1962) remark that a cripple or

invalid man only experiences himself as a cripple or invalid "through the eyes of another."

2. Our five-year research project, Bodily Integrity in Blemished Bodies, started in the spring of 2011. In this empirical-philosophical project we examine the meaning of experiences of bodily identity or integrity in disfiguring breast, head, and neck cancer—forms of cancers that, beside the constant fear for relapses, leave manifest traces in the survivors' material bodies. Whereas head and neck disfigurements immediately disturb one's feeling of self-identification from a social perspective, disfigurement of the breast may affect self-identification more from a cultural perspective (Slatman 2012). The entire project comprises four subprojects and is carried out by four researchers. This chapter solely discusses some findings in the subproject on facial disfigurements and facial prostheses.

3. According to phenomenology the intentional object is the correlate of intentional consciousness; it is never fully given but always given in adumbrations (*Abschattungen*). For instance, if we perceive a table, the rear sides of the table are not actually present to our consciousness, but still our "consciousness of" the table also includes its rear sides and as such constitutes the table as an object. As Husserl and Merleau-Ponty have explained, and as we will underline in the third section of this chapter, one's own body can also appear to oneself in a nonintentional way. This nonintentional appearance constitutes the body as a lived body (*Leib* or *corps vécu*).

4. "Leah," a pseudonym, is one of the respondents interviewed by the second author. In the scope of her current research project, she interviewed twenty-four people who wear a facial prosthesis. All respondents were recruited through the department of facial prosthetics of the Dutch national cancer institute, Antoni van Leeuwenhoek hospital in Amsterdam. Ethical clearance for this study was provided by the ethical committee of this hospital (file number NL35486.031.11). In this study we will limit ourselves to the case of Leah and will not yet provide a systematic analysis of all the data we have collected to date.

5. A nice example of how cultural and social norms "produce" biological facts is provided by Thomas Laqueur's (1992) study on sexual embodiment and, more specifically, on female orgasm. On the basis of a meticulous analysis of historical sources (medical

textbooks, biological textbooks, etc.), he argues that during the eighteenth century a radical turn took place in the biology of sex: from a one-sex model to a two-sex model. This shift in model illustrates that the presumed plain facts of sex, sexual pleasure, and sexual difference are not universal, nor ahistorical, but rather are "contextual" and "situational" (Laqueur 1992, 16).

6. "To return to matter requires that we return to matter as a *sign* which in its redoublings and contradictions enacts an inchoate drama of sexual difference" (Butler 1993, 49; emphasis in the original). In later work, Butler shifts to a less radical position. See for instance her work on narrativity and self-narrating (Butler 2004), which, interestingly, have been positively cited by leading scholars in narrative medicine (Charon and Wyer 2008).

7. Bourdieu considers physical qualities such as fitness, strength, and stamina and aesthetic qualities as a form of cultural capital (Crossley 2001, 107). These qualities are socially valuable since they can be used to produce ends in a certain situation or in a certain social group. The Guinea Pigs' blemishes can be seen as socially valuable since they yield honorable social recognition.

8. The positive meaning attributed to the disfigured faces of the British Guinea Pigs is exceptional, mainly thanks to the extraordinary efforts McIndoe took to treat these wounded soldiers, to encourage them to still wear their military uniform, and to go to public places, as well as to encourage other "normal" people to socially interact with them in a normal way. For this see also the documentary *Guinea Pig Club: The Reconstruction of Burned Airmen in WWII* (2005). We should of course not forget that most disfigured war veterans were not treated in this way and had (and some still have) a difficult time in readjusting to society. Their disfigurements were and are hard to interpret in a positive way (see Van Ells 2001).

References

Beauvoir, Simone de. 1949. *Le deuxième sexe*. Paris: Gallimard.

Bourdieu, Pierre. 2000. *Esquisse d'une théorie de la pratique*. Paris: Seuil.

Butler, Judith. 1993. *Bodies That Matter: On the Discursive Limits of "Sex."* New York, London: Routledge.

Butler, Judith. 2004. "Giving an Account of Oneself." *diacritics* 31 (4): 22–40.

Charon, Rita, and Peter Wyer 2008. "Narrative Evidence Based Medicine." *The Lancet* 371 (9609): 296–297.

Crossley, Nick. 2001. *The Social Body: Habit, Identity and Desire.* London: Sage.

Featherstone, Mike, Mike Hepworth, and Bryan Turner (eds.). 1991. *The Body: Social Process and Cultural Theory.* London: Sage.

Foucault, Michel. 1979. *Discipline and Punish: The Birth of the Prison.* New York: Vintage Books.

Goffman, Erving. 1963. *Stigma: Notes On the Management of Spoiled Identity.* New York: Simon and Schuster.

Grealy, Lucy. 1994. *Autobiography of a Face.* New York: HarperCollins.

Hacking, Ian. 2001. *The Social Construction of What?* Cambridge, MA: Harvard University Press.

Hacking, Ian. 2007. "Our Neo-Cartesian Bodies in Parts." *Critical Inquiry* 34: 78–105.

Hirschauer, Stefan. 1991. "The Manufacture of Bodies in Surgery." *Social Studies of Science* 21 (2): 279–319.

Husserl, Edmund. 1989. *Ideas Pertaining to a Pure Phenomenology and to a Phenomenological Philosophy, Second Book [Ideas II]*, translated by Richard Rojcewicz and André Schuwer. Dordrecht, Boston, London: Kluwer.

Laqueur, Thomas W. 1992. *Making Sex: Body and Gender from the Greeks to Freud.* Cambridge, MA: Harvard University Press.

Latour, Bruno. 2004. "How to Talk about the Body? The Normative Dimension of Science Studies." *Body & Society* 10 (2–3): 205.

Mackenzie, Catriona, and Jackie Leach Scully 2007. "Moral Imagination, Disability and Embodiment." *Journal of Applied Philosophy* 24 (4): 335–351.

Mayhew, Emily. 2004. *The Reconstruction of Warriors: Archibald McIndoe, the Royal Air Force and the Guinea Pig Club.* London: Greenhill Books.

Merleau-Ponty, Maurice. [1945] 1962. *Phenomenology of Perception*, translated by Colin Smith. London, New York: Routledge.

Merleau-Ponty, Maurice. 1951. "The Child's Relations with Others." In *The Primacy of Perception*, 96–155. Evanston: Northwestern University Press.

Merleau-Ponty, Maurice. [1961] 1993. "Eye and Mind." In *The Merleau-Ponty Aesthetics Reader: Philosophy and Painting*, translation by B. Smith. Evanston: Northwestern University Press: 121–149.

Merleau-Ponty, Maurice. [1964] 1968. *The Visible and the Invisible*, translated by Alphonso Lingis. Evanston: Northwestern University Press.

Mol, Annemarie. 2002. *The Body Multiple: Ontology in Medical Practice*. Durham: Duke University Press.

Partridge, James. 1990. *Changing Faces: The Challenges of Facial Disfigurement*. Grand Rapids: Phoenix Society.

Shannon, Mary T. 2012. "Face Off: Searching for Truth and Beauty in the Clinical Encounter." *Medicine, Health Care and Philosophy* 15 (3): 329–335.

Shilling, Chris. 1993. *The Body and Social Theory*. London: Sage.

Slatman, Jenny. 2005. "The Sense of Life: Husserl and Merleau-Ponty on Touching and Being Touched." *Chiasmi International* 7: 305–325.

Slatman, Jenny. 2008. *Vreemd Lichaam: Over medisch ingrijpen en persoonlijke identiteit*. [*Our Strange Body: Philosophical Reflections on Identity and Medical Interventions*, English translation forthcoming]. Amsterdam: Ambo.

Slatman, Jenny. 2009. "A Strange Hand: On Self-Recognition and Recognition of Another." *Phenomenology and the Cognitive Sciences* 8 (3): 321–342.

Slatman, Jenny. 2012. "Phenomenology of Bodily Integrity in Disfiguring Breast Cancer." *Hypathia* 27 (2): 281–300.

Turner, Bryan. 1992. *Regulating Bodies: Essays in Medical Sociology*. London: Routledge.

Turner, Bryan. 1996. *The Body and Society*. London: Sage.

Van Ells, Mark D. 2001. *To Hear Only Thunder Again: America's World War II Veterans Come Home*. Boston: Lexington Books.

Williams, Simon Johnson. 2003. *Medicine and the Body*. London: Sage.

Witz, Anne. 2000. "Whose Body Matters? Feminist Sociology and the Corporeal Turn in Sociology and Feminism." *Body & Society* 6 (2): 1–24.

Young, Iris Marion. 1990. *"Throwing Like a Girl" and Other Essays in Feminist Philosophy and Social Theory*. Bloomington: Indiana University Press.

13

"SHE'S RESEARCH!"

*Exposure, Epistemophilia, and Ethical Perception
through Mike Nichols' Wit*

LISA FOLKMARSON KÄLL

"[W]e are *condemned to meaning*, and we cannot do or say anything without its acquiring a name in history."
—Maurice Merleau-Ponty, *Phenomenology of Perception*

Introduction

"You have cancer. Ms. Bearing, you have advanced metastatic
ovarian cancer." These are the opening lines of Mike Nichols' film *Wit* from 2001. The film, based on a Pulitzer Prize–win-
ning play by Margaret Edson, is a striking display of the exposure
and objectification (as well as self-objectification) of a human body,
and more specifically, a woman's body, for scientific purposes. The
film portrays Professor Vivian Bearing, a scholar of the seventeenth-
century metaphysical poetry of John Donne, who after being diagnosed with advanced metastatic ovarian cancer undergoes a full eight-
month treatment of aggressive experimental chemotherapy before
she finally dies. Watching over her are Professor Harvey Kelekian and
his research fellow Dr. Jason Posner, who seem blind to everything
except "raw data," and the nurse Susie Monahan who is portrayed as
representing a more humane perspective. Throughout the course of
her treatment, Vivian finds herself navigating her own dying while

literally on the stage of cutting-edge cancer research. She reluctantly leaves her role as a rigorous and uncompromising university professor and instead becomes an object for others (and herself) to study with the same uncompromising eye.

The drama of *Wit* offers a sharp eye on laboratory-based medicine and its relation to the patients that are its objects. It makes manifest a dualistic paradigm at the root of positive science and the limits of that paradigm in particular when the object of science is a living human being. The portrayal of scientific objectification and self-objectification in *Wit* brings out the phenomenological insight that all object-directed intentionality rests on and emerges from the fundamental attachment between lived embodiment and the world of which it forms part. This embodied attachment is one of intentional directedness reaching out of the self, which is at the same time exposure of existence in terms of a corporeal openness to experience and to the world impressing itself upon us.

My concern in the following is the portrayal of different dimensions of exposure in *Wit* and the way in which these bring to light the possibilities and limitations of self-objectification and of objectifying frameworks more generally. Through a reading of the film I want to suggest that our foundational attachment to the world as embodied exposure and openness is the site for an ethical relation that is not one of separation between autonomous subjects but instead opens for different modes of being between singularities in continuous becoming. An understanding of the relation of exposure as the ground for our object-directed intentionality, that is, our distancing relation to the world as an object world and to our bodies as objects detached from our minds, lays bare vulnerability and interdependence as the ground of ethical perception.

Rather than applying an ethical theory to the narrative of the film, I read it as displaying and bearing out the conditions and possibility of ethical perception as well as the limitations brought about by a reductionist objectifying gaze that transforms lived existence and its unpredictability to objects of control. I discuss the possibility of moving toward an ethics of exposure on the basis of the display in *Wit* of the failure of ethical perception within the highly controlled clinical research setting of medical science. The film does not offer any systematic ethical theory or clear principles for ethical decision-making and moral conduct. Rather, it offers a forceful encounter with an ethical dilemma that demonstrates the insufficiency of fixed frameworks and precise principles.[1]

Exposure to Epistemophilia: Exposure of Flesh

Already in the opening scene of *Wit* ("Diagnosis") where we are first introduced to Vivian and Dr. Kelekian, the stage for Vivian's exposure to medical science is set clearly. As she receives her diagnosis, there is no mention of her chances of recovery or survival. Instead the focus is on the "significant contribution to knowledge" and the furthering of research that the experimental chemotherapy of Vivian's treatment promises to bring about. In fact, Kelekian gives Vivian her cancer diagnosis as if he is presenting her with a research project and an object to study. And she readily takes on this project: eager to approach her body in an epistemophilic manner, she willingly offers it as an object for experimental medicine.[2] This is the one option she is presented with. The one challenge. The one way with no exits or crossroads. She learns that the important task at hand is for her to take the full dose of chemotherapy, and she reassures Kelekian of her resolve to withstand some of the more pernicious side effects of the treatment, that he "need not worry" and that she can indeed "be very tough." In the next scene, a bald Vivian dressed in hospital robes repeats the task she has before her: to make a "significant contribution to knowledge"; "Eight cycles of chemotherapy"; "Give me the full dose. The full dose every time."

The conversation between Kelekian and Vivian is performed in part and on the surface as one between equals, between two scholars.[3] Vivian is invited by Kelekian to participate in his scientific perspective and as a scholarly subject take part in his research project, which is the experimental treatment of her body. She is invited to approach her body in the same way, with the same detachment, scrutiny, and detail as she in her own scholarly work approaches the poetry of John Donne.[4] However, her participation is quite naturally on completely different terms. To begin with, the object of research is her own still-living body to which she and Kelekian have radically different relations. While Kelekian can treat Vivian's body as a detached object of scientific knowledge, Vivian cannot detach herself completely for the simple reason that she *is* this body and her embodiment is the very condition for her ability to distance herself and take a perspective on her own body as an object. Moreover, although Kelekian and Vivian can perhaps share the experience of pain and suffering, their bodies are morphologically sexually different and the specific cancer diagnosis Vivian receives, soaked in cultural and symbolic meaning, is a diagnosis Kelekian will never receive. There is furthermore, as Elizabeth Klaver puts it, an "epistemological coercion" attached to Vivian's gift of her body as object for experimental research in so far as it "represents the only glimmer of hope in a 'matter of life and death'" (2004, 665). Regardless of whether or not she carries any hope of curing her cancer and prolonging her life through undergoing the treatment, it makes perfect sense to her to do it in order to advance medicine and produce further knowledge. For her, the glimmer of hope is perhaps not primarily one of simply prolonging her life but of continuing the passionate project of knowledge production that is her life even as her hospitalization forces her out of her own familiar scholarly environment.

This endowment of her body to research is a way for Vivian to separate and master it as an object of science. The endowment of her body is, to put it quite crudely, the price she willingly pays for her acquisition of knowledge of that same body. This is a knowledge she desperately needs and desires in order to gain control of a situation in which she in fact has no control at all. Jackie Stacey clearly describes this predicament of epistemophilia in the face of her own cancer diagnosis:

> This desire for knowledge was clearly a bid for control at the very moment it had been taken away from me. It was also an instrumental use of the academic skills of my world and a way of making the alienating medical world, in which I had suddenly found myself, more familiar and more manageable. [. . .] Turning the disease into a research project channeled my otherwise overwhelming fear and panic. (1997, 3)

Like Stacey, Vivian is portrayed as navigating the medical world through the use of her academic skills. Her intellectual distancing from her own cancerous body and her attempts at mastery and control are a response to her experience of her body as already being other, alien, and distanced from herself. Her self-objectification is a response to her own lived embodiment and altered attachment to the world, which is brought to light as self-relational exposure. While the objectification of one's own body may take many different forms, it is perhaps most pressingly made manifest when the body is experienced as dysfunctional or alien in one way or another. In cases of, for instance, pain, injury, disease, or social ostracism, the body comes out of hiding and instead of effacing itself toward the aim of its actions, it stands out as a thematic object demanding immediate and undivided attention, making what previously was important fall into oblivion. The body in pain interrupts our everyday actions and makes itself urgently present as *dys*functional. As Drew Leder (1990) famously writes, the body in pain or distress, instead of disappearing into the background, *dys*-appears and becomes something standing between the self and the aspects of her normal life. Even though Vivian manages to ignore her pain for long before seeing her doctor, she describes how it makes itself known as an interference in her daily life as a scholar and teacher. With sharp pains and exhaustion, her body *dys*-appears to her as having a life of its own that she cannot actively control. She is exposed and subjected to the forceful passivity of her own body, the, as Paul Ricoeur puts it, "coming and going of capricious humors—impressions of content or discontent" that renders passivity "foreign and hostile" (1992, 321). The passivity of the body is here experienced as a threat and it reveals the self as exposed to herself, to her own embodiment, and left uncovered, unprotected, and vulnerable.

Through distancing and alienation, Vivian deals with her pain—at first the pain of her growing tumor and later also the pain of her treatment as well as the pain of being reduced to an object for medical science—and retains a sense of integrity in the face of exposure to what is clearly a threat to her existence. The objectification and alienation of her cancerous body, making it other to herself in important respects, offer her a way of yielding some relief. She ex-poses the threat to which she is already exposed, putting it outside of itself as an object to be understood and mastered. This objectification also serves to strengthen her role as a subject taking on a specific attitude toward her cancer and treatment, an attitude she is expected to assume not only by Kelekian and Dr. Jason Posner but also by a whole social and cultural script of fighting cancer. Throughout Vivian's treatment Kelekian appeals to her identity as a researching subject and scholar, and this identity is one of detachment and heroic conquest in the name of knowledge. The theme of heroic conquest is furthermore the propelling leitmotif of many of the socially sanctioned illness narratives in the cultural imagination of the West. As Lisa Diedrich writes, these illness narratives dwell "on the heroic overcoming of loss and failure" (2005, 136) and understandably so, since their reiteration functions in part as a strategy of survival.[5]

While Vivian shares Kelekian's perspective as a researcher and educator, she is at the same time educated by him about what is going on in her body, and he sets the terms for her participation. Ultimately she is only offered the role as research object, a role she will quite naturally fail to fully embody while still alive, even though her performance of this role throughout her treatment is outstanding. Commenting on the way she is objectified by the research fellows during grand rounds, Vivian exclaims to the viewer, "they read me like a book." While the exhibition of "subservience, hierarchies, gratuitous displays and sublimated rivalries" makes Vivian "feel completely at home," just like in a graduate seminar, in grand rounds she does not do the teaching but instead plays the part of the object being taught. This part, she tells the viewer, is much easier: all she has to do is lie still and look cancerous. Her body is, to speak with Klaver, displayed as "the specimen under observation" (2004, 659). Her body is completely exposed to interrogative eyes, hands, and comments. It is in a manner of speaking detached from and ex-posed out from Vivian as a subject. It is made manifest as a well-defined object with clearly delineated boundaries that exclude any interference of subjectivity. In its exposure her body is literally uncovered, stripped of protective sheets and gowns, and without defense against the probing examination carried out in the name of medical research intended to diminish pain and suffering. Contrary to Vivian's exposed body, the doctors surrounding her are covered in their medical profession with protective white coats, stethoscopes, and medical charts.

With the comment that she is read like a book, Vivian invokes, as Klaver notes, the postmodern figure par excellence: the body as text, governed by the repetition of regulatory norms and reified through discursive materialization.[6] This body does not precede its own discursive signification, and it becomes intelligible as a unified and recognizable body only through regulatory materialization. As Klaver argues, drawing on Michel de Certeau, Western medical research intextuates the body as an object of science through which it is constituted as an incarnation of knowledge (2004, 662). Rather than simply reading Vivian like a book, Kelekian and Jason (as well as

Vivian herself) write her like the book they read, and this writing of her body is not in any way a process taking place in the abstract but, rather, undeniably and thoroughly in the flesh. The writing of the book that is Vivian's intextuated body is characterized by a shocking and shameful paternalism and genuine indifference toward Vivian as a living being urgently in the midst of her own dying and fighting that dying. This indifference is made manifest in the emptiness of the line "How are you feeling today?" repeated throughout as a clinical requirement, and it is transformed into violent intervention as Vivian is subjected to a humiliating and quite brutal pelvic exam by Jason (who also happens to be one of her former students).[7]

Through her objectification and exposure to medical science Vivian as a person, as an individual, is eventually "silenced within the isolating spaces and hierarchical relationships of modern medicine" (Diedrich 2005, 142; see also Tauber 1999, 9, 98). However, her silencing is obscured through the appeal to her as an autonomous subject separate from but in charge of and with a right to her own body. Her silencing is also obscured by her mastery of the medical terminology used to describe her condition. Convinced that her "only defense is the acquisition of vocabulary," she wants to know what the doctors mean when they anatomize her, and she turns to the explanatory framework and language of medical science in order to be able to relate to her cancerous body and take part in the epistemophilic project of her treatment. It is through the use of precise terminology that she ex-poses her body from herself as an object of thematic reflection from which she can, to a certain extent and on a level of object-directed intentionality, detach herself.[8] But as both her body as object and her mind as subject are detached from their embodiment, from her lived embodiment, there is no longer anything to found her own expression. She is, in a manner of speaking, not simply reduced to an object for medical science but rather to a dualistic entity, to an object with a corresponding detached subject. The tidy and well-arranged correspondence between the body as object and the way it is represented in the precise form of medical terminology manages to silence Vivian's embodied self, which is irreducible to both subject and object as well as to any simple composition of the two.

The chemotherapy treatment finally eradicates Vivian's immune system more efficiently than it eradicates her cancer. As she puts it when she is placed in isolation:

In my present condition, every living thing is a health hazard to me. Particularly health care professionals. [. . .] I am not in isolation because I have cancer, because I have a tumor the size of a grapefruit. No. I am in isolation because I am being treated for cancer. My treatment imperils my health. Herein lies the paradox.

Her isolation is of course not only a protective measure to keep her alive and shielded from infection but also demonstrates and establishes her status as a controlled and controllable object exposed to medical science. Her exposure in isolation leaves her entirely unprotected from being reduced to an object while her body at the same time is closely monitored and protected from threats of infection. As she tells her viewer at another point in the film, she is no longer a person but has been reduced to a cancer. Implicating the viewer through direct address, Vivian describes her own intextuation as an object of medical science:

I don't mean to complain but I am becoming very sick. Very sick. Ultimately sick, as it were. [. . .] I have survived eight treatments of Hexamethophosphacil and Vinplatin, at the full dose, ladies and gentlemen. I have broken the record. I have become something of a celebrity. Kelekian and Jason are simply delighted. I think they see celebrity status for themselves upon the appearance of the journal article they will no doubt write about me. But I flatter myself. The article will not be about me. It will be about my ovaries. It will be about my peritoneal cavity, which, despite their best intentions, is now crawling with cancer. What we have come to think of as me is, in fact, just the specimen jar. Just the dust jacket. Just the white piece of paper that bears the little black marks.[9]

The triumph of Vivian's survival of eight full cycles of experimental chemotherapy at the full dose is somewhat ironic and bitterly tainted by the fact that her cancer has not been cured. She has been reduced to the specimen jar of her cancerous reproductive organs, to an objectified container exposed to experimental medical science and deprived of humane treatment, without the reward and relief of a cure. What is noteworthy in Vivian's testimony of her intextuation as an object for medical science is that it mirrors a long history

of scientifically defining women in terms of anatomy and reducing them to their reproductive organs. Against the background of
this history, the intextuation of Vivian's body is on the one hand an
affirmation of her womanhood, on the other hand she is intextuated as a woman who postoperatively is lacking precisely that which
(reductively) serves to identify her as woman, namely her reproductive organs.

In a warped but very demonstrative way, the spreading of Vivian's cancer cells, her unruly and unpredictable flesh, can be read as
a resistance against this reduction of her identity to the object of her
reproductive organs. Her cancer would in such a reading represent a
force kicking back against masculinized science exhibiting its limitations and failure to control the female flesh. And, her death would
effectively signal the impossibility, that many feminist philosophers
have addressed, of this female flesh to find any space to express itself
in the available language and symbolic system in which it is reduced
to muteness.

Throughout the narrative of the film, Kelekian and Jason are portrayed as being advocates of the experimental treatment as research
rather than of the treatment of the patient (Booth 2002, 10). As the
nurse Susie says, without even a glimmer of understanding in her
tone of voice, they always want to know more things. Vivian, who
can well identify with this desire for knowledge, responds that she
also always wants to know more things, thereby slightly complicating the picture of her radical objectification and exposure to experimental medicine. Right at the end of the film, when Susie interrupts
the unlawful resuscitation of Vivian, Jason enacts a final reiteration of
Vivian's exposure and intextuation as an object for medical science,
screaming over her dead body, "She's research!"

Limitations of Objectification and the Doing of Flesh

Once Vivian has received her diagnosis and committed to the epistemophilic project of Kelekian and his research fellows, she can approach
her body in pain through distancing and objectification until the
point when her suffering becomes overwhelming and uncontrollable.
She can up to a certain point ex-pose her body as an object other
to herself in order to protect herself from the exposure of her flesh
to herself. However, as seen earlier, the active ex-posure of her body

as an object rests on the exposure of her embodied self to herself, which is urgently brought to light by the experience of this exposure as threatening. Her act of taking her body as an intentional object for conscious reflection is conditioned by her lived embodiment and foundational attachment to the world. This embodied attachment is what Maurice Merleau-Ponty describes in terms of an operative or corporeal intentionality that by its own making, through its very structure, is transformed into different forms of object-directed intentionality. Although consciousness and body often fall apart into irreconcilable opposites of subject and object, which are easily given ontological status as two fundamentally different forms of existence, the phenomenon and experience of lived embodiment demand radical interrogation of any such distinctions. Belonging simultaneously "to the order of the 'object' and to the order of the 'subject,'" the lived body, writes Merleau-Ponty, "reveals to us quite unexpected relations between the two orders [and] teaches us that each calls for the other" (1968, 137). The relation of intentionality, between the knowing subject and its known object, is one of mutual co-constitution (or even co-conditioning) and as the embodied self bestows meaning on the world, the world is also given as a world of meaning.

In *Wit* we see portrayed the force of an objectifying perspective through the display of the exposure of Vivian's body as an object for medical science made intelligible through precise vocabulary. But this exposure of her body also brings to light the limitations of such an objectifying perspective. The acquisition of vocabulary that once was Vivian's defense ultimately offers her no consolation and in the face of dying, medical terminology not only falls short but also seems utterly inappropriate. Nothing, Vivian tells the viewer, would be worse than the "verbal swordplay" of "a detailed scholarly analysis and erudition, interpretation, complication." Between her experience of herself and the language she has mastered to describe her body there is what Diedrich (2005) describes in terms of a "muteness." In her reading of Gillian Rose's philosophical memoir *Love's Work*, Diedrich describes how Rose in her struggle with cancer realizes that she is in a realm beyond medicine, which the language of medicine does not recognize and which calls for other means of expression. Medicine, writes Diedrich, "does not speak of the wrong suffered by Rose; it only speaks of the capacity of one or the other consultants to properly diagnose her disease" (2005, 143). And yet, many would readily agree that the primary duty of medicine is to answer to and relieve precisely the suffering of its patients. The inability of medical language to speak of suffering is clearly displayed in the portrayal of Vivian's dying. At the very end of her struggle, before she is sedated by aggressive pain management drugs (and refused patient-controlled pain management so that she can retain her status as a controlled and controllable object), she turns to the viewer in an attempt to use her own words to share "how it feels," how she can barely stand "it," namely, being alive.

The portrayal of Vivian is thus not only of her exposure to medical objectification that also, as we have seen, serves as a protective measure in several different ways. At the moments when language fails her she is urgently faced with the ambiguity of existence and with her own dying. She is immediately exposed to her own flesh and finitude, and she finds herself falling into an abyss of anxiety that she had no way of preparing for, that she cannot escape, and where she has lost all means of control. While Vivian's body is clearly exposed as an object for medical science, there is also brought to light in the film what Klaver with reference to Richard Selzer calls a "doing of the flesh" or "an independent life of disease" (2004, 659).[10] What seeps through is the very flesh of Vivian's lived existence that resists objectification both by herself and by the medical science to which she is subjected and to which she subjects herself. The flesh is actively making its own demands, her cancer cells are multiplying and spreading throughout her body, killing her healthy cells. Her flesh, cancerous and dying, is unruly and cannot—and is finally through the DNR order not allowed to—be mastered through the control of medicine. The flesh of the dying self reveals the unpredictability and finitude of existence and brings to light a necessary, albeit excruciatingly painful, dimension of death in all of life.

Klaver discusses how the "*doing* of the flesh" that is brought out in the portrayal of Vivian's dying stands in sharp contrast to a cultural body intextuated as an object for medical research and ultimately reduced to raw data. She writes,

> no matter what the cultural constructions or medical interventions may be [. . .] we see Vivian's body succumbing to the *doing* of the flesh. And regardless of how long Western culture has struggled to change this situation [. . .], it is still the flesh, not the *body*, that is ultimately in charge. (2004, 673)

But what is the status of this flesh? While Vivian is certainly "before us in all her fleshly facticity" (672), this fleshly facticity is situated within and against the background of her whole situation. Her flesh is not any form of "pure" or underlying nature as opposed to and independently resisting the culture of medical science intextuating her body as its object. Although Vivian's flesh resists the complete control of objectifying medical discourse and practices, such discourse and practices nevertheless inform and shape her "fleshly facticity" and its expression and doings in the world. Further, the intextuation of her body is itself a process that takes place in the flesh as it were: the medical and scientific practices carried out by Kelekian and his crew are as embodied as the object of Vivian's cancerous body.[11] As said earlier, the body as text governed by discursive repetition of regulatory norms is already and always material and its intextuation is a process of materialization.

So, even if it is the flesh that is ultimately in charge, as Klaver argues, and even if mortality may still be what (in part) defines human existence, the material intextuation of the body as a scientific object contributes to forming this flesh, which in turn founds the processes of intextuation and objectification. Bioscientific advances have demonstrated and continue to demonstrate that there is no unchanging biological foundation of human subjectivity. Rather, as Margrit Shildrick puts it, "the technological possibilities of post-modern age [. . .] continually disrupt humanist certainties" (2005, 10) as they carry the potential of varying "the conditions of reproduction, of life or death, of embodiment, and indeed of human being itself" (4). This is not to say, however, that scientific knowledge, tools, and technology are completely in charge of the materially intextuated objects of knowledge. As Sarah Franklin so rightly writes, "biological knowledge, biotechniques and biology 'itself' reshape each other, and co-evolve," and this mutual impregnation and material becoming is perhaps more explicit today than ever through "the redesign of the biological in the context of bioscience, biomedicine and biotechnology" (2006, 168). What is in charge (if anything) might thus be said to be a radically altered form of foundational flesh or materiality, which incorporates the tools, techniques, and discourses of its own transformation and which due to this incorporation is unpredictable in multiple ways.

Testimony of the Body between the
Lines of Medical Description

As we have seen, the drama of *Wit* puts us face-to-face with the paradox of on the one hand demanding a rational and scientific basis for clinical practices and on the other hand insisting on empathy and compassion in the care of patients. While the film surely condemns the reductive objectification to which Vivian is subjected and the dehumanization of laboratory-based medical practices, it does not as surely assert a greater importance to compassionate treatment of patients than to the pursuit of scientific research results.[12] Rather, it recognizes the importance of both as well as the conflict between them. The film sharply portrays the paradoxical display of a concern for subjective experience that is compulsory in the clinical setting but that is present only as words empty of any intended meaning. The scripted question "How are you feeling today?" followed by the equally scripted answer "Fine" is, as Vivian tells us, the standard greeting that becomes absurd and even offensive when it is stripped of intended meaning. As she rhetorically asks her viewers: how could one possibly expect to answer the question "How are you feeling?" while "throwing up into a plastic basin" or "emerging from a four-hour operation with a tube in every orifice"? Wittily, Vivian says that she's a little sorry she will miss the moment when she is asked this question and she is dead. This type of formal consideration of the voice of the patient is also brought out with clarity when Kelekian asks a screaming Vivian if she is in pain. Her answer, directed to the viewer and not Kelekian, is "I don't believe this." In the same way that Gillian Rose becomes aware through her encounter with medicine that it has no command of a language able to speak of her suffering, Vivian experiences the failure of sophisticated descriptions and precise terminology to capture her predicament.

Even though these sophisticated medical descriptions inform the way Vivian experiences herself and her possibilities of responding to her condition, they are not what ultimately provide her with certainty of her cancer or of her suffering. When Susie eventually tells Vivian that her cancer is not being cured, Vivian responds that she already knew through reading between the lines. And what gives testimony between the lines is her own cancerous body. As is clear

from the foregoing, this cancerous body—this flesh—and the way it
is experienced cannot be divorced from its discursive articulation and
markings. The space between the lines is always read together with
the lines, and the lines are always enveloped by a between making
them stand out in different ways and with different meanings. Vivian's
experience of her own cancerous body is informed by her whole
social, cultural, historical, and personal situation in which not only
the words "ovarian cancer" but also what it means to be a woman, an
academic, single, post-menopausal, voluntarily or involuntarily child-
less is overflowing with signification. The testimony of her body is
not the testimony of some prediscursive flesh or pure pain, it is the
testimony of a lived body reaching out of and exposed to itself in its
specific situation. In *Wit*, the highly gendered dimensions of suffering
and of exposure to objectifying perception are blatantly obvious. It is
the exposure to the events of specifically female flesh that is on display; it is the intensities of sexed embodied existence that are caught
within and yet resist objectifying discourse and that are exposed to
ethical perception. The film makes manifest how the exposure to
meaning is also exposure to structures and positions of power, dominant discourses and categorizations that we cannot escape but that
nevertheless mark and form who we are as well as the possibilities
for our becoming. As stressed earlier but worth repeating, the relation
of exposure to the world (to others and to ourselves) involves the
many different and often conflicting ways in which we are objectified
and made intelligible as well as unintelligible for others. While *Wit*
brings out the exposure of lived embodiment as the very condition
of objectifying discourse and of its own intextuation, it also brings
out the impossibility and undesirability of divorcing the flesh from
the way it is situated in systems of control and objectification.

In the portrayal of Vivian's reading between the lines and the
immediate testimony of her cancerous body, there is a striking parallel to how Gail Weiss writes about Simone de Beauvoir's description
of her mother's death:

> [Madame de Beauvoir's] knowledge does not come from
> conversations with her doctors, her daughters or the nursing
> staff—it comes from her own, cancer-ridden body, which
> has become a force to be reckoned with in its own right and
> which has generated a bodily imperative that has brought

her two adult children and her grandnieces running to her bedside. (1999, 154)

Through her reading of de Beauvoir's reflective narrative, Weiss develops an embodied ethics that "works from bodily as opposed to categorical imperatives" and that can "serve as a model for how we *live*, rather than (merely) think about morality" (146). Weiss argues that our embodiment, as our capacity of being affected by the bodies of others, constitutes a necessary and sufficient condition for the generation of a bodily imperative (162). These bodily imperatives, writes Weiss, "emerge out of our intercorporeal exchanges" and continuously "transform our own body images, investing them and reinvesting them with moral significance" (149, 158).

While Madame de Beauvoir's body constitutes an ethical bodily imperative for her daughters and grandnieces, it is quite clear from Simone de Beauvoir's description that this type of ethical imperative is not present for her doctors. In the case of *Wit*, it is equally clear that Vivian's suffering does not constitute for Kelekian and his research fellows the type of ethical bodily imperative that Weiss talks about. This is also up to a certain point the case for Vivian herself. Staying in the "safe zone" of the epistemophilic project of scientific knowledge production, both Kelekian and Vivian are in a realm where embodied ethical perception is very limited, if not impossible. We might say that the situation sustaining their embodiment in a sense disembodies them both. In taking on the epistemophilic project of producing knowledge about the object at hand, namely Vivian's cancerous body, and also producing that object as the object for their knowledge, they step into and reiterate the role of disembodied subjects. At the same time however, it is crucial to recognize that this role is of course embodied in a specific way and this specific way is not divorced from the embodiment that allows for ethical perception.

Toward an Ethics of Exposure

Bringing to light the difficulty, if not impossibility, of ethical perception within the framework of laboratory-based medicine in which the patient is reduced to a diseased body and object of scientific research, *Wit* also points to the futility of attempting to resolve ethical dilemmas through formulating principles with the aim of universal validity. In the portrayal of Vivian's suffering and treatment, ethical perception is clearly made manifest in its absence as a pressing demand of the undecidable. Undecidability forces us to see clearly the difficulties of decision and the impossibility of instating systems of rules and principles to direct our decision-making (Caputo 1993, 4). Through the rejection of fixed frameworks for ethical deliberation and decision-making, facing the undecidable opens up for what we might call an ethics of exposure in which our relation to the other is one of mutual becoming. It is an ethics of a perpetual and radical openness to the unpredictable and to the ambiguity of our existence.

The point of departure for thinking the ethical relation in terms of this radical openness is neither the self nor the other as fixed entities. However, neither is the starting point the relation between the two in any simple way. The point of departure is rather relation and relata as co-constitutive of and co-conditioning one another. Such a shift away from the identity of self and other as well as any configuration of the relation between them displaces the interiority of subjectivity and brings to light the identity of the self as fundamentally relational in its exposure to the other and to its own exteriority. Interiority in this view is no longer seen as being separated from the world toward which it is intentionally directed but is rather to be found in the midst of and exposed to this world and to itself. The disclosure of the inner world of intentionality as exposure is recognition of the impossibility of pinning down subjectivity by giving it a spatial designation and locking it up on the inside of a physical body. Attempts at positing subjectivity in "the here-and-now of a palpable body," to speak with Alphonso Lingis, are bound for certain failure and will only demonstrate its absence in that body and the impossibility of making that absence present (1986, 104). Instead of being posited within the boundaries of the skin, subjectivity is everywhere present but nowhere to be grasped.

As many have emphasized in different ways, the painstaking attempts of developing universally applicable principles for moral conduct simply avoids facing the ethical issues at stake. Ethics is not primarily a matter of deliberate decision-making in relation to questions and prescriptions of what one ought to do. This type of decision-making will in fact not require much deliberation at all. Given a specific principle for how to act, the action itself does not require decision, and right or wrong becomes a matter of universal law.

Ethical decision-making demands facing the ambiguity not only of a specific situation but also of our own being as it unfolds in relation to others. As Shildrick so rightly puts it, "the task of ethics is never finally done," and no universal principle will help put an end to this task (2005, 9). While the drama of *Wit* is a scripted narrative and not in any way unexpected, it portrays beautifully an unscripted drama in Vivian's life and the tragedy of meeting this drama through the means of scripted forms and codes of ethical conduct. Instead of imposing "a decisive ethical conclusion" (Booth 2002, 10) about issues concerning life and death, "truth" and "goodness," autonomy, respect, and responsibility, the story of *Wit* in my view invites us to continuously raise such issues anew and reminds us that they cannot be solved once and for all through any decisive ethical conclusion. The drama of *Wit* shows us how any deliberate and decisive conclusion is effectively put out of play when confronted with the lived experience of ethical dilemmas. The narrative of Vivian's life, of her suffering and dying, of her passion for knowledge and need for compassion, shows us that ethics is a matter of an original exposure to others in which we must trust in order to be open to the unexpected and be able to meet all the unscripted dramas of life.

Acknowledgments

An earlier version of this essay was presented at the conference Feminist Phenomenology and Medicine, Uppsala University, Sweden, on May 20, 2011. I am grateful to the participants at the conference for comments and questions. I would especially like to thank Abby Wilkerson, Linda Fisher, Kristin Zeiler, Jenny Björklund, Ingvil Hellstrand, and Mike Lundblad for their comments.

Notes

1. Different forms of narrative, as Alfred Tauber writes, allow us to encounter ethical dilemmas and decision-making "in the full panoply of human behavior" by "tapping into collective experience" and our cultural and social imaginary (1999, xvi).
2. Originally a Freudian term, "epistemophilia" is used by Peter Brooks in his analysis of the body as object of desire in modern narrative (1993). Brooks describes how any process of knowing or symbolizing is driven by the body but also at the same time

alienates us from the body, insofar as it is made into a know-
able object. The alienation of the body further feeds itself, and
the body is turned into a deep secret to be discovered, understood, and explained. The epistemophilic project of the body is,
in Monica Rudberg's words, "propelled by bodily desire with the
ultimate aim to know the body itself" (1996, 286). With reference to the tradition of feminist science studies, Rudberg rightly
argues that the epistemophilic project traditionally has been
strongly associated with a masculine and male subject with the
goal of disclosing the inner secrets of the female body. This gendered dimension of epistemophilia is clearly displayed in *Wit* as
the film portrays the suffering and objectification of the specifically female body and the specifically female condition of ovarian
cancer.

3. However, when she receives her diagnosis, she is addressed as
Ms. Bearing while addressing him as Professor Kelekian, which
immediately signals their hierarchical and asymmetrical relation and effectively reminds her (and the audience) that she is
removed from her own professional and professorial setting.

4. As Elizabeth Klaver writes, the film puts on display how "two
humanist fields dedicated to social and individual improvement—
medicine and literature—are both guilty of yielding to a perspective that precludes compassionate treatment of human beings"
(2004, 660). That the object of Vivian's research is the metaphysical poetry of John Donne is no narrative coincidence. His poeti-
cal musings on death, life, and life everlasting form a powerful
background intertwined with Vivian's own struggle. There is no
doubt much to be said about the role played by Donne's poetry
in *Wit*, but this falls outside the scope of this chapter.

5. There are of course also other scripts of how to face and deal
with terminal cancer. In stark contrast to scripts of heroic conquest are those governed by norms of acceptance and letting go.
In *Wit* both of these conflicting cultural scripts are at play. While
Kelekian without question encourages the script of heroic conquest, the nurse Susie represents the direct opposite perspective
and comes across as condemning the medical practice carried out
by Jason and Kelekian. Susie takes on a more humane attitude
toward Vivian, but she is also portrayed as representing something of a deeper, more intuitive, or more profound knowledge
than that of medical science. Susie is represented as knowing

something about life and death that cannot be acquired through books and scholarly skills. While I do not think *Wit* asks its viewers to take any clear moral stance regarding Vivian's way of dealing with her own condition, the film does, through the character of Susie, strongly condemn the treatment and radical objectification Vivian is subjected to by Kelekian, and it invites the question whether the quest for medical knowledge can be carried out on more humane terms. It also offers a possible perspective of acceptance of death based on some kind of simple wisdom of human life and on an appeal to the course of nature. What I find highly problematic with these different scripts is the way they are often construed as complete, all encompassing, and exclusive of one another. And, this is indeed the way they are brought out in *Wit*. The script of heroic conquest leaves no room for senses of failure or the desire to just let go. The script of acceptance and letting go excludes and devalues attempts of fighting and conquering cancer as an enemy. Both scripts are equally limiting.

6. Klaver aptly compares Vivian's sense of her body as a readable narrative to "early mechanistic theories such as Descartes' comparison of the body to an automaton." She writes, "an earlier counterpart of Vivian might have complained that her doctors 'tell her like a clock'" (2004, 663).

7. The pelvic exam Jason performs is without exaggeration the equivalent of sexual assault. His callous, insensitive, even abusive, attitude is brought out again, although not in such a brutal manner, in his likening of clinicians to troglodytes and in his view of the clinical requirement as being a "colossal waste of time for researchers." Right before the examination when he remembers the "crazy clinical rule" that there has to be a woman present, he further leaves Vivian exposed in the chair with her feet in the stirrups and tells her not to move as he goes to find Susie. Peter Lewis argues that it is the trappings of the different mistreatments to which she is subjected that eventually frees or forces Vivian to "see the pretenses and errors of her own ways as a 'doctor of philosophy.'" Lewis continues, "With Jason as an impressionable undergraduate and her witness, Professor Bearing tied her students in knots with her recitations of Donne and then verbally flogged students for their lack of comprehension. [. . .] Vivian recognizes that she, in part, has fostered Jason's lack of 'bedside manner'" (2005, 397).

8. Even the soothing effect of eating a popsicle when haunted by anxiety in the middle of the night is something Vivian explains in medical terms: "The epithelial cells in my GI tract have been killed by the chemo. The cold popsicle feels good. It's something I can digest and it helps keep me hydrated. For your information." It is not without enthusiasm that Vivian takes on the project of acquiring medical vocabulary to describe her condition. Quite to the contrary. Her turn to the vocabulary of medical science may in a sense be seen as a way for her to carry on her own scholarly interest in words and their specific meaning, albeit with a different focus than that of metaphysical poetry.

9. Throughout the film Vivian implicates the viewer in the story through direct address. The viewer is placed right there with her in the hospital, at the bedside, to witness her deterioration and anxiety, to see her struggle as she becomes weaker and more pain-ridden and as she becomes objectified, as she disappears and appears through disappearance.

10. This independent life of the disease that is killing Vivian is paradoxically enough itself immortal. Jason refers to the growing of cancer cells as "immortality in culture" and describes it to Vivian with a passion and a fascination she can well recognize and identify with in her own passion for knowledge. She even provides him with the perfect word to characterize the process of the multiplication of cancer cells: awesome. A concrete case of "immortality in culture" is that of the (in)famous HeLa cell line derived from the cervical cancer cells taken from a poor black tobacco farmer by the name of Henrietta Lacks. These cells, that were taken and cultivated without her knowledge, became the first human cells to survive and grow outside of a human body, and the importance of the HeLa cell line for scientific research is difficult to exaggerate. As Rebecca Skloot has shown in her recent bestseller *The Immortal Life of Henrietta Lacks* (2010), the case of Henrietta Lacks and her immortal cell line opens up a whole can of questions concerning ethics; social, cultural, political, and economic structures of power and privilege; and meanings of autonomy and consent. The case of Henrietta Lacks raises with urgency the question Wayne Booth brings up in his reading of *Wit*: "Though almost everyone would agree that her [Vivian's] doctors have behaved immorally if they did not obtain her consent to be an experiment subject, are they genuinely to blame for

'using' her to get results that may be a blessing to many future patients?" (2002, 11). We might of course add here that informed consent to be an experiment subject is always requested and given within structures of power, privilege, and radically different conditions of knowledge. As Tauber writes, modern clinical science renders the patient "incapable of making a fully informed decision about diagnostic and therapeutic choices" (1999, 65). I would like to thank Abby Wilkerson for suggesting this connection between Jason's description of cancer as "immortality in culture" and the immortal life of Henrietta Lacks' cell line.

11. Describing scientific laboratory experiments with embryos, Sarah Franklin captures the fundamental and necessary embodiment of scientific knowledge production: "in the same way we are looking at biology when we see an embryo through the microscope, we are also using our own biological bodies to do this— to observe, to interpret, to move the focal plane up and down, coordinating our eyes with our hands, our hands with our brains, our brains with other people's brains to work out what we are seeing" (2006, 168).

12. I do not entirely agree with Wayne Booth's contention that the plot of *Wit* "depends on us taking an aggressive ethical stance" and that the power of its ending "requires us to share, without question, the author's implied judgment that humane, honest, compassionate treatment of patients is ethically far more important than the pursuit of research results" (2002, 10). In fact, I must confess that any such blatancy of the author's implied judgment in the narrative portrayal escapes me both in Edson's play and Nichols' film.

References

Booth, Wayne. 2002. "The Ethics of Medicine as Revealed in Literature." In *Stories Matter: The Role of Narrative in Medical Ethics*, edited by Rita Charon and Martha Montello, 10–20. London, New York: Routledge.

Brooks, Peter. 1993. *Body Work: Objects of Desire in Modern Narrative*. Cambridge, MA: Harvard University Press.

Caputo, John. 1993. *Against Ethics: Contributions to a Poetics of Obligation with Constant Reference to Deconstruction*. Bloomington, Indianapolis: Indiana University Press.

Diedrich, Lisa. 2005. "A Bioethics of Failure: Antiheroic Cancer Narratives." In *Ethics of the Body: Postconventional Challenges*, edited by Margrit Shildrick and Roxanne Mykitiuk, 135–152. Cambridge, MA: MIT Press.

Franklin, Sarah. 2006. "The Cyborg Embryo: Our Path to Transbiology." *Theory, Culture & Society* 23 (7–8): 167–187.

Klaver, Elizabeth. 2004. "A Mind-Body-Flesh Problem: The Case of Margaret Edson's *Wit*." *Contemporary Literature* 45 (4): 659–683.

Leder, Drew. 1990. *The Absent Body*. Chicago, London: University of Chicago Press.

Lewis, Peter. 2005. "The Wisdom of Wit in the Teaching of Medical Students and Residents." *Family Medicine* 37 (6): 396–398.

Lingis, Alphonso. 1986. *Libido: The French Existential Theories*. Bloomington: Indiana University Press.

Merleau-Ponty, Maurice. 1962. *Phenomenology of Perception*, translated by Colin Smith. London, New York: Routledge.

Merleau-Ponty, Maurice. 1968. *The Visible and the Invisible: Followed by Working Notes*, translated by Alphonso Lingis. Evanston: Northwestern University Press.

Merleau-Ponty, Maurice. 2004. *The World of Perception*, translated by Oliver Davis. London, New York: Routledge.

Nichols, Mike. 2001. *Wit*. HBO Productions.

Ricoeur, Paul. 1992. *Oneself as Another*, translated by Kathleen Blamey. Chicago, London: University of Chicago Press.

Rudberg, Monica. 1996. "The Researching Body: The Epistemophilic Project." *European Journal of Women's Studies* 3: 285–305.

Shildrick, Margrit. 2005. "Beyond the Body of Bioethics: Challenging the Conventions." In *Ethics of the Body: Postconventional Challenges*, edited by Margrit Shildrick and Roxanne Mykitiuk, 1—26. Cambridge, MA: MIT Press.

Skloot, Rebecca. 2010. *The Immortal Life of Henrietta Lacks*. New York: Crown Publishing.

Stacey, Jackie. 1997. *Teratologies: A Cultural Study of Cancer*. London, New York: Routledge.

Tauber, Alfred. 1999. *Confessions of a Medicine Man: An Essay in Popular Philosophy*. Cambridge, MA: MIT Press.

Weiss, Gail. 1999. *Body Images: Embodiment as Intercorporeality*. London, New York: Routledge.

14

ANAESTHETICS OF EXISTENCE

CRESSIDA J. HEYES

It was a question of knowing how to govern one's own life in order to give it the most beautiful form (in the eyes of others, of oneself, and of the future generations for which one might serve as an example). That is what I tried to reconstitute: the formation and development of a practice of self whose aim was to constitute oneself as the worker of the beauty of one's own life.

—Michel Foucault, "The Concern for Truth"

[T]o continue to counter the moral science of biopolitics, which links the political administration of life to a melodrama of the care of the monadic self, we need to think about agency and personhood not only in normative terms but also as activity exercised within spaces of ordinariness that does not always or even usually follow the literalizing logic of visible effectuality, bourgeois dramatics, and lifelong accumulation or fashioning.

—Lauren Berlant, "Slow Death (Sovereignty, Obesity, Lateral Agency)"

In 2006 I attended a conference on the implications of Foucault's philosophy for ethics and the body. Fogged with lack of sleep and the nervous exhaustion that comes from sitting in neon-lit rooms and listening to hours of read-aloud presentations, I repeatedly misheard one speaker talk not of "an aesthetics of existence," but rather of "anaesthetics of existence." This mishearing has turned out to be more productive than my previous reflection on the original phrase, with which I was becoming increasingly uneasy. In his final ethical work, Foucault is often said to be defending an "aesthetics of existence"—an approach to living life as art that posits the self in a certain critical relation to itself. This approach is, as Foucault himself declares, distinctive in many ways to modernity (indeed, definitive of it) and can be found in many modernist philosophical traditions, from the dandyism of Baudelaire or Wilde to Dewey's discussion of art as experience. A lot of exegetical work has tried to make sense of Foucault's "ethical" period, but I am most interested in the idea of personal transformation as a kind of aesthetic labor. In a 1982 interview with Stephen Riggins that produces quite a few revealing comments, Foucault says, in response to a question about the relation of his philosophy to the arts:

> You see, that's why I really work like a dog, and I worked like a dog all my life. I am not interested in the academic status of what I am doing because my problem is my own transformation. [. . .] This transformation of one's self by one's own knowledge is, I think, something rather close to the aesthetic experience. Why should a painter work if he is not transformed by his own painting? (1997b, 131)

I believe Foucault when he says that he worked like a dog all his life—after all, he produced such a vast amount of writing of such breadth and erudition. In the same interview he also remarks that he has "real difficulty in experiencing pleasure. [. . .] And I must say that's my dream. I would like and I hope I'll die of an overdose of pleasure of any kind [*Laughs*]" (1997b, 129). So, for Foucault personally, his practice of an aesthetics of existence is an exhausting labor, with a troubled relationship to pleasure. In other words, the work of self-transformation is *work*; the continual practice of critique is for many academics a draining rather than a replenishing activity. Giving up on this activity, zoning out, and accepting whatever particularly illuminating moments make it through the cognitive fog is a real alternative, albeit one with a complex relationship to resistance. *Anaesthetics of existence*: the routine, habitual strategies of pain-relief that we use to cope with the trials of everyday life?

In a powerful and complex essay, Susan Buck-Morss argues with Walter Benjamin that the development of the human sensorium under modernity is characterized by attempts to cope with shock (1992, 16).[1] From the battlefields of the First World War to the much more everyday public spaces of shopping arcades, factories, amusement parks, casinos, and even crowded streets, our senses are neurologically overloaded. Do we attempt consciously to process this shock experience, or do we, at a certain point, need to rely on our ability to parry the bombardment of our senses, to protect ourselves as sense-perceiving subjects from the technological overwhelm of modern experience? Under such conditions, Buck-Morss suggests, the synaesthetic system "reverses its role."[2] Its goal is to *numb* the organism, to deaden the senses, to repress memory: the cognitive system of synaesthetics has become, rather, one of *anaesthetics*" (1992, 18). "Aesthetics," she reminds us, is a term that derives from the Greek *aisthitikos*—that which is perceived by feeling. The five senses form an interface between subject and world; together, they are a physical-cognitive apparatus serving "instinctual needs—for warmth, nourishment, safety, sociability" (1992, 6). The gradual appropriation of the term into modern philosophy to mean that branch of philosophical inquiry concerned with (evaluative judgments about) sense-perception, and in particular our exercise of taste, thus represents an attempt to recommend the acculturation of our senses and transpose the focus of inquiry from sense-perception itself to objects of art. The antonym *an*aesthetic is that which deprives us of sensibility, renders us incapable of perception. Its common usages are almost always medical, and it too is usually associated with its objects—namely, anaesthetic agents (drugs that render the patient insensible or numb).

Buck-Morss points out that the aesthetic shock of modernity coincides with the development of technologies of anaesthesia. Opiates, nitrous oxide, ether, chloroform, and cocaine entered widespread and everyday use through the 1800s, developing their own economy (both within and outside formal medical practice) as tools for coping with synaesthetic overload. No longer dependent on anaesthetics as quaint as laudanum or ether frolics, we now have an amazing array of psychotropic drugs aimed at curing ubiquitous depression, anxiety, insomnia, and other synaesthetic diseases. Technologies that enhance, control, deaden, or eliminate sensation are ever more central to our lives.

In this essay I argue that tying an *ethos* to pain and pleasure, as Foucault does, demands more attention to the conditions under which contemporary synaesthetic experience is generated. Foucault's own exemplars in volumes 2 and 3 of *The History of Sexuality* predate modern anaesthetic practices, while his last comments on ethics refer to a modern attitude that is unmoored from practice altogether.

Analysis of lived experience after modernity would supplement this picture with a sense of the subject's practical relation to (an)aesthetics of existence. This is, in part, an existential phenomenological project, in the sense that a first-personal perspective on *anaesthetic* practices can supplement the speculative ethics that implicitly values an *aesthetic* subjectivity. The nature of this supplementation, however, needs explaining: both Foucault and I are interested, I take it, in what is ethically possible for subjects within the discursive terrain that both constitutes and constrains us. Foucault provides an important reading of post-Kantian autonomy and the critical attitude of modernity, but what this means for variously politically situated subjects attempting to live an aesthetic life in postmodernity remains underexplored.

Foucault was of course critical of phenomenology for the very reason that it takes as a starting point the effects of *assujettissement*, bracketing genealogical enquiry into their conditions of possibility. Yet to the extent this is a criticism of mainstream phenomenological traditions, it need not apply to feminist phenomenology, which has always insisted on both the philosophical value of the perspective of the perceiving subject *and* the cultural and historical specificity of lived experience:

> Feminist phenomenology can show how we have the bodily experiences that we do given the social and historical structures of which we partake—and how our bodies are not mere constructs, epiphenomena of ideological systems, but the encumbered and thick nexus of meaning (often implicit) through which sociality, historicity, materiality and subjectivity intertwine. Bodies (speaking, thinking, feeling, objectified subjects) are, then, more than mere objects. Bodily experience can be the ground of our awareness of social structures of oppression and the site where complicity, subversion or resistance are enacted. (Al-Saji 2010, 32–33)

Foucault's final work can also be read as a roundabout return to the more phenomenological work of his very early period—work he was quickly ambivalent about—as well as a more explicitly philosophical development of his interest in the avant-gardism of Blanchot and Bataille. He wants to come back to human existence in postdisciplinary society, to ask how we can live in the face of the political challenges his best-known work identifies. There must be a possibility of a critical relation to the subjectivities Foucault describes in his gene-alogies—indeed, it is this possibility that is a condition of Foucault's own life and work. Methodologically (if not substantively) we can say that Foucault's ethical work has much in common with feminist phenomenology.[3] To make this case in full would be a separate essay; here all I want to do is to show how, on my interpretation, Foucault's aesthetics of existence needs to be situated within a richer context, including discussion of the lived experience of self-transformation.

This discussion will be especially important for feminist analysis, as it shows how relations of power and privilege make the subjectiv-ity implicit in an aesthetics of existence more or less viable. Women and men have different subjective relations to the pleasures and pains that are part of an aesthetic ethos, and gender shapes our possibilities for living a life that is a work of art informed by practices of critique. I examine one case of a gendered relation to anaesthetics—Meredith Jones' analysis of the life and death of French celebrity and cosmetic surgery aficionada Lolo Ferrari. Ferrari embodies, I suggest, a para-doxical relation to aesthetic existence. Transforming herself by sur-rendering her agency, she is both a victim of an utterly normative femininity and a self-made woman. Taking Ferrari's love of uncon-sciousness as the most literal and extreme example of anaesthetics of existence, I briefly show how a phenomenological reading of los-ing consciousness might be one part of a new feminist ethos more attuned to the exigencies of contemporary living.

Foucault's Aesthetics of Existence

In his last writings and interviews, Foucault characterizes the aesthet-ics of existence as an ethic that contrasts with Christian asceticism and morality as obedience to a code of rules (Foucault 1996, 451). Returning to the ethical practices of antiquity, in volumes 2 and 3 of the *History of Sexuality* he is writing a new genealogy of morals (1996, 451; 1997c, 266), which will reveal "the genealogy of the subject as a subject of ethical actions" in which "we have to build our existence as a beautiful existence; it is an aesthetic mode" (1997c, 266). In his response to Kant, "What Is Enlightenment?" Foucault suggests that we think of modernity less as an *epoch* and more as an *ethos*—"a mode of relating to contemporary reality; a voluntary choice made by cer-tain people; in the end, a way of thinking and feeling; a way, too of acting and behaving that at one and the same time marks a relation of belonging and presents itself as a task" (1997a, 309). For my purposes, what is important in Foucault's characterization of this attitude is the relation to oneself to which it is tied: "to be modern is not to accept oneself as one is in the flux of the passing moments; it is to take oneself as object of a complex and difficult elaboration" (1997a, 311). From this attitude, in combination with Foucault's existing work on archaeology and genealogy, he produces a method. This method is a "critical ontology of ourselves"—a way of bringing into question the sorts of things we previously imagined ourselves to be. This ontology, he writes,

> must be considered not [...] as a theory, a doctrine, nor even as a permanent body of knowledge that is accumulating; it must be conceived as an attitude, an ethos, a philosophical life in which the critique of what we are is at one and the same time the historical analysis of the limits imposed on us and an experiment with the possibility of going beyond them. (1997a, 319)

This last work is part of a Kantian tradition solely in the sense that Foucault understands autonomy as the practice of critique of all things presented to us as necessary (including a transcendental subject) (Allen 2008, esp., 22–44).

Foucault is, of course, neither resurrecting self-sovereignty nor endorsing the disciplined subjectivity biopolitics creates—quite the contrary. One of the reasons he turns to privileged Greek and Roman men in volumes 2 and 3 of *The History of Sexuality* is to examine the practices of daily life—sex, diet, maintaining health, exercise, writing, marital relations—in a predisciplinary age, the better to contrast care of the self with the normalization that follows it. He died before he could fully articulate the connection between these historical sketches and the interviews he gave on a contemporary art of living. This leaves us with the open question of how Foucault imagined the contemporary subject would practice his aesthetics of existence. What is it *like*—as a matter of everyday life, of lived experience—to be the subject of this always-becoming, exemplary, critical, beautiful life? For Foucault himself it meant intellectual hard labor, while seeking out intense pleasures in lieu of the ordinary ones that had become inadequate: "I'm not able to give myself and others those middle-range pleasures that make up everyday life. Such pleasures are nothing for me, and I am not able to organize my life in order to make place for them" (1997b, 129).

Whatever Foucault made of the aesthetics of his own life (and I think this is an interesting question, even if many Foucault scholars are sensitive about its implications), it is not at all obvious what his work means for others.[4] Some critics have suggested that a conservative politics follows from Foucault's emphasis on the aesthetic (see, e.g., Wolin 1994 and a defense in O'Leary 1996). It is clear that Foucault was opposed to a prescriptive ethics in which he provided the rules to live by, or even to presenting his life (or his substantive ideas *about* life) as a model for others to follow. The point of a work of art is not to dictate others' experience of it but rather to open up the possibility of a novel *expérience*, of transforming oneself through a relationship to it.[5]

Even for an individual less committed to the project than Foucault it sounds like an exhausting ethical endeavor. The subject of late liberal capitalism is required to exercise his autonomy iteratively, expressing his individuality qua capacity to choose in an interminable series of self-determining moments. When presented in the language of political philosophy, we can lose sight of the lived experience of this subjectivity: it can be exhausting, ego-driven, obsessed with irrelevant choices, and abusively self-disciplining, committed to the fantasy of organizing and rationalizing a life of freedom in political contexts where freedom is systemically denied. As Lauren Berlant argues, in an essay with strong resonances with Buck-Morss' work, the "mass physical attenuation" that happens to working populations under late capitalism contrasts with the dominant account of autonomy and thereby demands a phenomenological rethinking:

> [S]overeignty described as the foundation of individual autonomy [. . .] overidentifies the similarity of self-control to sovereign performativity and state control over geographical boundaries. It thereby encourages a militaristic and melodramatic view of agency in the spectacular temporality of the event of the decision; and, in linking and inflating consciousness, intention, and decision or event, it has provided an alibi for normative governmentality and justified moralizing against inconvenient human activity. (2007, 755)[6]

In particular, she suggests, we need a better way of talking about ordinary life and its reproduction—the management of households; preparing and eating food; daily routines of traveling, working, caring for children, and so on (echoes of Foucault's *Care of the Self*). Ordinary life in the context of the pressures of disciplinary power often feels compressed, demanding, teetering on the edge of possibility, utterly draining, yet also out-of-control, micro-managed by distant institutions and individuals. The response from individuals cannot always be to sit up, pay attention, work harder, work to change ourselves—indeed, this is a mode of subjectivation that neoliberalism itself generates and exploits.[7] Sometimes, as Berlant also points out, the only possibility of resistance (or even the only viable response) might be to detach from experience, to evade pain and fatigue, to slow down, and (although she does not say this) to lose consciousness.

The elephant in the room by this point is gender: the exhaustion of ordinary life and its reproduction, set against the privileged struggle to secure existential meaning from an aesthetic attitude to life, is a gendered division of labor. Let me make a general observation that needs far more exploration and nuance. Over the last two hundred years women and men have also had different relations to anesthesia: from laudanum and patent medicines to Valium and Prozac, "feminine" drugs are more mood-leveling; they relieve anxiety, depression, disappointment, frustration, and/or provide a mild buzz while allowing one to continue to do almost everything one did before. When they are prescribed to women, as they long have been in disproportion to those prescribed to men, everyday mood-altering drugs often come with a gendered diagnosis, from neurasthenia or hysteria to female sexual dysfunction. "Masculine" drugs, by contrast, provoke big highs and lows, extreme pleasures and extreme pains: binge drinking, cocaine, LSD, amyl nitrite, crystal meth. Not without consequence, they take subjects out of the everyday, requiring periods of absence from other responsibilities, as well as (often) periods of recovery (whether a morning hangover or years in rehab) (Kandall 1996; Morris 1991, 103–124; Metzl 2003). James Miller describes some of Foucault's putative drug encounters: a road trip to Death Valley on LSD, using poppers while fist-fucking (1993, 248–251, 269). When Foucault famously says, in the context of discussing his aesthetics of existence, "we have to do *good* drugs that can produce very intense pleasure" (1997d, 165), he is participating in this gendered economy of (an)aesthetic meaning.

For most feminists this situation has provoked an immanent response: free women from the worst travails of ordinary life (or at least make them shared); make the critical ethos Foucault describes into a subjectivity for women, rather than a way of living built on our backs; maybe even embrace good drugs for all, while remaining critical of the normalizing drugs we are increasingly offered. I am not opposed to these strategies. But I think they will be meaningless if they continue to be offered at this remove from lived experience. To grasp our anaesthetics of existence as it coexists with an aesthetic ethos we need a much more fine-grained account of the ordinary lives to which both are, in their different ways, a response.

(Feminist) Anaesthetics

> Straight talk about willpower and positive thinking claims that agency is just a matter of getting on track, as if all the messy business of real selves could be left behind like a bad habit or a hangover. But things are always backfiring. Self-making projects proliferate at exactly the same rate as the epidemics of addictions and the self-help shelves at the bookstore.
> —Kathleen Stewart, *Ordinary Affects*

In her book *Skintight: An Anatomy of Cosmetic Surgery*, Meredith Jones describes how cosmetic surgery devotee Lolo Ferrari loved the oblivion of general anaesthesia and its capacity to suspend her life during a fairy-tale "enchanted sleep," allowing her to wake up transformed without any further exercise of agency (2008, 129–149). Ferrari was an ordinary middle-class French girl turned porn star and minor celebrity, who died in 2000 aged thirty-seven of a (possibly suicidal) overdose of prescription drugs, including painkillers.[8] She was best known for having the largest breast implants in the world, and at her death her chest was said to measure seventy-one inches. In her challenging analysis, Jones comments on Ferrari's avowed love of general anaesthesia:

> Like the stereotypical promiscuous woman who seeks out sex and enjoys it too much, Ferrari is too vocal about her taste for oblivion. In a culture where self-control, self-determination and self-awareness are paramount, the notion of willingly surrendering to an anaesthetic is something abhorrent, something definitely not meant to be pleasurable, but perhaps something also deeply seductive.[9]

Jones contrasts Ferrari with Orlan, the performance artist who has made having cosmetic surgeries into her art form:

> Orlan and Ferrari, two extreme practitioners of cosmetic surgery, are opposite in relation to agency. Orlan remains determinedly conscious during her operations, directing the proceedings, talking to the audience. In stark contrast Ferrari completely gives herself over to the surgeon, describing the loss of power via general anaesthetic as a joy that she "adores." (2008, 132).

As Jones implies, Orlan—who certainly considers herself transgressive and has been hailed as undermining the conformity of cosmetic surgery—is the more conventionally modern feminist. Taking control over the surgical scene, insisting on consciousness (a necessary condition of agency, we assume), and confronting the nonnormative changes to her body as they occur, she is very much a practitioner of the aesthetic rather than the anaesthetic. Ferrari, by contrast, fails one feminist test: she is passive, surrendering to her (male) doctors' ministrations, embracing and enjoying the "black hole" of general anaesthesia. Yet Ferrari could also be seen as someone who took extreme risks with her life and body, engaging in the limit-experiences of general anaesthesia and powerful narcotics, practicing self-transformation of the most dramatic kind, and making herself into a transgressive work of art.

If Foucault does not help us distinguish these divergent interpretations, it is because he relentlessly prescinds from normative content in representing his aesthetics of existence (Thacker 1993). While we may explain Foucault's lack of programmatic ethical *content*, his aesthetics of existence nonetheless seems to presuppose a certain *form* of subjectivity: he explicitly connects his ethics to pleasure, pain, and autonomy, and so his inattention to the ways we experience these in (contemporary) practice is a major lacuna. What should we make, as post-Kantian, pleasure-seeking ethical feminists, of bad habits, coping strategies, zoning out, procrastinating, drugging up, and other ways of failing to assume the mantle of self-cultivating attention? Anaesthetic practices help us to cope with ordinary sensory overload, including pain (emotional and physical), which is central to the management of postdisciplinary subjects. As Ladelle McWhorter argues, "pain is a tool that is used extensively in virtually all normalizing disciplines":

Pain and the threat of pain usually bring compliance with the dictates of a disciplinary regime; they render the subject obedient, docile. The greater and more varied the subject's capacity for pain, the wider the range of disciplinary techniques that can be used on her, and, thus, the greater her potential for directed development. Normalizing discipline uses pain, often carefully measured and graduated, as a tool for increasing the subject's productive capacities while rendering her passive and controllable; furthermore, it not only uses pain but it also develops the capacity for new kinds of pain in the subject, thus multiplying the means for maintaining the subject in near complete docility. (1999, 179)

The literal kind of anaesthetic practices Ferrari loved may have a role in shifting our relationship to these cultivated forms of political pain. In choosing to withdraw from an experience of pain, in other words—whether the psychic pain that Ferrari said had spurred her transformations or the anaesthesia she used to make them possible—we open the possibility of withdrawing from at least part of the economy of pain and pleasure that keeps disciplinary society functioning. Especially where pain is concerned, working on oneself as practitioner of critique is not the only way of exhibiting agency; withdrawing one's consent, withdrawing from the labor of being a docile body, rejecting the terms of one's own exploitation by refusing to be a subject at all—these are alternative ways of saying no. Transgression is not the only relationship one can have to a norm.

Jones' Ferrari can be read as an extreme and provocative example of the contemporary need to manage our synaesthetic systems, which coexists with (and is fueled by) competing ethical challenges to maintain a critical self-relation. Anaesthetics of existence are sensory strategies, and, as I've suggested, they are gendered. A feminist phenomenology of the anaesthetics of existence, then, could show the texture of gendered relationships to pain and pleasure; it could undertake a comparative analysis of different anaesthetic practices as they occur within a gendered cultural horizon. This essay is as much preamble to such work as it is exemplary of it, but before I conclude I want to begin to sketch one way a feminist phenomenological approach can complicate the subjectivity of the aesthetic modern man.

A Feminist Phenomenology of the
Anaesthetics of Existence?

The need to protect one's self against the sensory assault of modernity coexists with Foucault's suggestion that we engage with everyday life in an aesthetic mode and invent ourselves with a critical attitude. The case of Ferrari highlights the paradox of this demand: to survive, we use anaesthetic practices that (on one reading) prevent us living up to the ethical challenge of modernity. One conclusion (which an aesthetic ethics might demand) is that we should give up on those practices in favor of more critical, agentic ones. Yet to choose to be numbed, to withdraw from the organization of time and the economies of pain that keep us compliant—to check out—is perhaps the most literal way to passively resist disciplinary power. Significant social movements rely on shared understandings of what this means—from "drop-out culture" to Slow Food—and in other work I hope to examine this phenomenon at a more explicitly collective, political level. A phenomenological approach, however, also has something to recommend it, not at the level of prescriptive analysis but rather in service of understanding anaesthetic practices as bound by structures of consciousness. I'll start the work of outlining this approach by briefly exploring the difference between *disciplinary* and *anaesthetic* time.

In *Discipline and Punish,* Foucault himself argues—in one of his more Marxian moments—that disciplinary power invents "a new way of administrating time and making it useful" (1979, 160), "a new technique for taking charge of the time of individual existences; for regulating the relations of time, bodies and forces; for assuring an accumulation of duration; and for turning to ever-increased profit or use the movement of passing time" (1979, 157). Specifically, time is broken down into units, each of which is appointed a specific basic exercise, these exercises are cumulative and progressive, and the individual is examined on their aptitude at the end of a series before being permitted to advance. This mastery of duration, Foucault argues, allows that "power is articulated directly onto time; it assures its control and guarantees its use" (1979, 160). Typically, Foucault describes this new "linear," "evolutive" time in terms of the individuals it produces rather than in terms of how those individuals perceive it. We can see its contemporary legacy, though, in practices of "time management" that recommend, for example, breaking time down into segments, during each of which a discrete task must be completed, with the goal of completing a larger project within a set period of time and overall increasing productivity. Such strategies are often experienced as tyrannical (including when they are self-imposed) and notoriously lead to failures of "attention management," such as procrastination, deviation from the assigned task, and daydreaming. Although multitasking is more a part of postdisciplinary society than Foucault's descriptions of eighteenth-century military training allow, the increased sense of linear, protensive time urgency that discipline fosters is still very much with us, but—in the same dynamic that the quote from Stewart's book implies—it goes hand in hand with passive resistance and tacit subversion.

Recall that Foucault says "to be modern is not to accept oneself as one is in the flux of the passing moments." Yet those banal drugs—perhaps archetypally pleasurable foods (sugary things, greasy things), alcohol, and benzos[10]—that can take a while to consume or have slow, drawn-out, and relatively mild effects on one's sensorium, provide a way of gently checking out of any meta-consciousness of those "passing moments." Time drifts. Instead of the linearity of a punctuated time, a time divided into ever-smaller units, each of which must be productively used, there is a relative indifference to time passing and to the sensory demands that render our typical temporality so exhausting. The agency of eating, for example, Berlant argues, "can make interruptive episodes happen in which suspending the desire to be building toward the good life in rational ways involves cultivating a feeling of well-being that spreads out for a moment, not as a projection toward a future" (2010, 35). Time passes without our noticing—whether because we are sitting in a haze, numb, or because, more literally, we are unconscious (blacked out, sedated, asleep).

During these forms of "anaesthetic time" my intentionality slackens and shifts: I no longer have a clear object of experience, or, perhaps, my object narrows to the consumption of my favored drug and the sensations it generates. Any larger sense of myself as an agent diminishes. Both this slackening of intentionality and the changing perception of time find a limit in unconsciousness, which marks the ultimate suspension of time, and the ultimate reprieve from discipline. Sleep is the obvious example. As Nicolas de Warren interprets Husserl:

> In sleep, consciousness abstains from its own interests, and, in this sense, consciousness has retired from itself while also retiring from the world. [. . .] Falling asleep is allowing the world and myself to slip away and come to a rest. Bit by bit, particular interests and activities are let go, until [. . .] the entire "life of the will" has been let go. This "letting go" or "sinking away" ("Sinken-Lassens") is a mode of my entire life of consciousness. In other words, when I am fatigued, and falling asleep, or losing my gumption, my ego is still affected by things around me, yet the force of these affections slackens, and I no longer give myself over to these affections. I sink into an indifference in having relinquished any investment in the world. In a sense, I allow myself to become inert. (De Warren 2010, 291)

Sleep—whether drug-induced or not—can be very literally anaesthetic, as when someone who is depressed or traumatized does nothing but sleep. In the world Buck-Morss prefigures, sleep is antithetical (and antidotal) to sensory overwhelm, and also, in Foucault's terms, inimical to disciplinary time. Many of us are chronically deprived of sleep, and we use synaesthetic technologies to get into it or stave it off. Our work routines increasingly intrude on our sleep—both because for many people the raw hours we must commit to working have increased, and because technologies make us newly available to work in the hours we would otherwise sleep.[11]

Sleep is necessary to life, but somehow not a part of "lived experience." The interruption of self that sleep offers makes it hard to theorize; we tend to focus on the surrounding frame in which sleep occurs and treat actually being asleep as a philosophical blank space.[12] *Falling* asleep in particular offers an opportunity for phenomenological description. Even someone who is very tired will have a short period between wakefulness and sleep, during which breathing becomes slower and more regular, mental experience becomes lighter and less self-directed, and the muscles relax, before imperceptibly one "drifts off." To fall into sleep is to give oneself over to a netherworld in which one ceases to act; to do so requires an initial decision, a practice of letting go that has to be learned and can be resisted—deliberately or unconsciously. A baby might need a lullaby, rocking; most adults have their bedtime rituals that they need to go to sleep: a bath, a few minutes of reading, or narcotics. In his beautiful essay *The Fall of Sleep* [*Tombe de Sommeil*], Jean-Luc Nancy writes that: "whoever relinquishes vigilance relinquishes attention and intention, every kind of tension and anticipation; he enters into the unraveling of plans and aims, of expectations and calculations. It is this loosening that gathers together—actually or symbolically—the fall into sleep" (2009, 3).

I have heard Nancy's brilliant project described as providing a phenomenology of losing consciousness, but actually it only describes one way of going under. We often describe general anaesthesia as "going to sleep," which is the linguistic elision that allows Jones to describe Ferrari as being transformed by her cosmetic surgeon while she is in "enchanted sleep." On Jones' analysis, Ferrari provides a literal, living example of the fairy-tale heroine whose consciousness is suspended only for her to wake up after a difficult transition (for Sleeping Beauty, the transition from princess-girl to marriageable young woman; for Ferrari, the surgical transition from before to after). When each wakes up, it is as if no time has passed, yet each is transformed (Jones 2008, 130–136). Neither the rhetorically powerful "enchanted sleep" nor a general anaesthetic is like actually going to sleep, however, whether mythically, phenomenologically, or medically speaking. General anaesthesia is astonishingly complete and abrupt. The only time I had a general anaesthetic—for twenty minutes, in a dentist's office, for the particularly difficult extraction of an impacted wisdom tooth—I heard the anaesthetist say, after putting the needle in my arm, "here we go." Then, "you might get a metallic taste in your mouth." It was the middle of the day, I was flooded with adrenaline and completely wide awake. I remember noting the time on a wall clock directly in my field of vision. I tasted metal, and said, "oh yeah, there it is." Then a complete veil of unconsciousness descended instantly; there was no transition time at all between full alertness and nothingness. Under anaesthesia there is no dreaming. No matter how loudly the operating staff talk, or how much clatter of instrument noise or buzzing of the drill there is, I will not regain consciousness until the anaesthesiologist decides to change the drug infusion.[13] Coming around was less dramatic than going under, but still nothing like waking up from sleep. I was suddenly aware that I was conscious, and that the operation must be over, but it felt as though nothing had happened, and no time had passed. I was lying on a gurney, with partition curtains on either side of me, in a completely unfamiliar room; coincidentally, a different wall clock in my sight-line showed me that it was exactly twenty minutes later than when I had had the metallic taste. Only the light throbbing and the wad of cotton in my mouth indicated that I had been operated on.

This may be the black hole that Ferrari loved: the immediate and utterly involuntary relinquishing of vigilance; the extinguishing of self; the dramatic suspension of time; the total respite from an aesthetics of existence. Early opponents of anaesthesia were philosophically motivated: physical pain (a sensation human beings had never previously been able consistently to avoid) was understood to be part of the vital spirit that makes us human and keeps us alive, including by helping us survive the shock of surgery (Snow 2006, 23). Asleep, we dream; we trust—perhaps—that, should disaster arrive, we can rouse ourselves. But anaesthetized I am completely dependent on another to bring me round. I am absolutely vulnerable. Ferrari was unusual in loving this dependence; since anaesthesia's earliest days, prospective patients have been deeply afraid of involuntary unconsciousness (Snow 2006, 102–105). Given that being unconscious carries the risk of sexual assault, the experience is riskier for women than for men: think of all the warnings about date-rape drugs, drinking and passing out, or predatory dentists. Whatever the pains, pleasures, or risks, this sensory oblivion is not something to be recommended or rejected. Instead, it represents a limit for the anesthetics of existence; a phenomenological encounter with complete withdrawal from the exhaustion of contemporary fantasies of autonomy.

Jones' Ferrari is princess-like and playful, but Ferrari's own words are harder. She implied in interviews that her everyday life felt intolerable to her, and her anaesthetic practices seem concomitantly dramatic: "All this stuff [the cosmetic surgeries] has been because I can't stand life. But it hasn't changed anything. There are moments when I disconnect totally from reality. Then I can do anything, absolutely anything. I swallow pills. I throw myself out of windows. Dying seems very easy then." Ferrari probably was psychologically destroyed by an abusive family—she said as much.[14] There is nothing prescriptive in her story, and it is shocking that a woman would see anaesthesia as a respite from her life and troubling to note how easily Ferrari's actions can be understood through stereotypes about women's essential passivity and masochism. Her exemplary, paradoxical life, however, can also teach us something about unconsciousness as both a phenomenological and an ethical experience and about how we derive pleasure from refusals of agency as well as from the modern exercise of autonomy. As Berlant says, "the body and a life are not only projects but also sites of episodic intermission from personality, of inhabiting agency differently in small vacations from the will itself [. . .]. These pleasures can be seen as interrupting the liberal and capitalist subject called to consciousness, intentionality, and effective will" (2007, 779).

This essay has brought together vastly different registers: as we analyze the forms of subjectivity into which postdisciplinary postmodernity interpellates us, we also need (I have suggested) to keep an eye on the lived experience of that interpellation. The defense of any form of subjectivity as part of "an aesthetics of existence" needs to consider how that subjectivity will reinforce or undermine the forms that power assumes today. Foucault's "ethics of discomfort" needs to be read not as an abstract relation of the self to self but rather as a potential practice that runs into existing lived experience, including sensory experience. An ethics describing a mode of subjectivation either unattainable or in conformity with a politically damaging historical moment is no ethics at all. Foucault once said of Merleau-Ponty that his "essential philosophical task" was "never to consent to being completely comfortable with one's own presuppositions. Never to let them fall peacefully asleep" (2000b, 448). But perhaps our discomfort is such that anaesthetized peace may sometimes be a necessary solace and counterpoint to the subjectivity of an aesthetics of existence.

Acknowledgments

I would like to thank Meredith Jones, Lisa Folkmarson Käll, Robert Nichols, Lanei Rodemeyer, Chloë Taylor, and Kristin Zeiler for their helpful discussion of the ideas in this essay.

Notes

1. Buck-Morss is using the term "shock" in its psychological context rather than a medical one. That is, she appears to mean by "shock" the hyperstimulation of the sensory world as it abruptly and overwhelmingly imposes itself on the human organism, rather than an organic condition in which blood flow to crucial organs is dangerously reduced.

2. "In order to differentiate our description from the more limited, traditional conception of the human nervous system which artificially isolates human biology from its environment, we will call this aesthetic system of sense-consciousness, decentered from the classical subject, wherein external sense-perceptions come together with the internal images of memory and anticipation, the 'synaesthetic system'" (Buck-Morss, 1992, 13).

3. For more detailed discussion of Foucault's relation to phenomenology, see May 2006 and Oksala 2005, 2010.

4. Foucault himself was ambivalent about the relationship between his own experience and his work: while he said in 1978 that "I haven't written a single book that was not inspired, at least in part, by a direct personal experience" (2000a, 244), he also evaded discussion of his personal life on the grounds that it would appear prescriptive and reinstall the author-function of which he had been so philosophically and politically critical (see Foucault 1997e, 154). This ambivalence has been fueled by a secondary literature of philosophical biography: see especially James Miller's *The Passion of Michel Foucault* (1993), which agonizes over the relation between Foucault's sexuality and his philosophy, and has in turn provoked charges of sensationalism and homophobia (see, e.g., Halperin 1995, 143–152).

5. The word *expérience* in French, which Foucault uses liberally throughout his corpus, retains the double connotation of "experience" and "experiment," but is routinely translated using the former, thus emphasizing the passive undergoing of life rather than a testing or exploratory relation to it.

6. By "inconvenient human activity," I take it that Berlant is referring to the activities that contribute to the "slow death" she theorizes: overeating, in particular, but also all of the compulsive, numbing, addictive activities that render working life under neoliberalism more tolerable.

7. There is a recent but growing literature, connected to the questions I am discussing here, on whether Foucault's work on neoliberalism and governmentality is supported or contradicted by his work on care of the self. See Binkley 2009; McNay 2009; Dilts 2010.

8. Ferrari's husband and manager, Eric Vigne, was subsequently accused of her murder by suffocation, but this charge was finally

dismissed in 2007. http://www.20minutes.fr/article/140549/People-Le-mari-de-Lolo-Ferrari-blanchi.php.

9. Quote is from Meredith Jones, "Makeover Culture." Dissertation submitted for the degree of Doctor of Philosophy, University of Western Sydney, 2005, 198. An edited version of this quote appears in Jones 2008, 132.

10. Benzodiazepine drugs include Valium and Ativan and have anti-anxiety, sedative, muscle relaxing, and amnesiac effects.

11. See http://www.sleepfoundation.org/article/press-release/annual-sleep-america-poll-exploring-connections-communications-technology-use-.

12. De Warren (2010) discusses this problem in Husserl and also contrasts Jean-Luc Nancy's denial of the possibility of a phenomenology of sleep with Husserl's metaphorical use of sleep and wakefulness in his account of time-consciousness.

13. Except, of course, in those horrible cases of "anaesthetic awareness," in which patients are entirely physically immobilized but fully conscious—including conscious of pain—during an operation.

14. Quoted in Jon Henley, "Larger Than Life," *The Guardian*, Thursday, March 16, 2000. http://www.guardian.co.uk/theguardian/2000/mar/16/features11.g2.

References

Allen, Amy. 2008. *The Politics of Our Selves: Power, Autonomy, and Gender in Contemporary Critical Theory*. New York: Columbia University Press.

Al-Saji, Alia. 2010. "Bodies and Sensings: On the Uses of Husserlian Phenomenology for Feminist Theory." *Continental Philosophy Review* 43: 13–37.

Berlant, Lauren. 2010. "Risky Bigness: On Obesity, Eating, and the Ambiguity of 'Health.'" In *Against Health: How Health Became the New Morality*, edited by Jonathan Metzl and Anna Kirkland, 26–39. New York: New York University Press.

Berlant, Lauren. 2007. "Slow Death (Sovereignty, Obesity, Lateral Agency)." *Critical Inquiry* 33 (Summer): 754–780.

Binkley, Sam. 2009. "The Work of Neoliberal Governmentality: Temporality and Ethical Substance in the Tale of Two Dads." *Foucault Studies* 6: 60–78.

Buck-Morss, Susan. 1992. "Aesthetics and Anaesthetics: Walter Benjamin's Artwork Essay Reconsidered." *October* 62 (Autumn): 3–41.

De Warren, Nicolas. 2010. "The Inner Night: Towards a Phenomenology of (Dreamless) Sleep." In *On Time: New Contributions to the Husserlian Phenomenology of Time*, edited by D. Lohmar and I. Yamaguchi. Dordrecht: Springer.

Dilts, Andrew. 2010. "From 'Entrepreneur of the Self' to 'Care of the Self': Neoliberal Governmentality and Foucault's Ethics" (May 14, 2010). Western Political Science Association 2010 Annual Meeting Paper. Available at SSRN: http://ssrn.com/abstract=1580709.

Foucault, Michel. 1979 [1st American ed. 1977]. *Discipline and Punish: The Birth of the Prison*. New York: Random House.

Foucault, Michel. 1988 [1984]. "The Concern for Truth." In *Politics, Philosophy, Culture*, edited by Lawrence D. Kritzman, translated by Alan Sheridan. New York: Routledge.

Foucault, Michel. 1996 [1984]. "An Aesthetics of Existence." In *Foucault Live: Collected Interviews 1961–1984*, edited by Sylvère Lotringer. New York: Semiotext(e). [April 25, 1984, interview in French with Alessandro Fontana, trans. John Johnston.]

Foucault, Michel. 1997a. "What Is Enlightenment?" In *Ethics: Subjectivity and Truth*, edited by Paul Rabinow. New York: The New Press.

Foucault, Michel. 1997b [1982]. "An Interview by Stephen Riggins." In *Ethics: Subjectivity and Truth*, edited by Paul Rabinow. New York: The New Press. [June 22, 1982, interview in English.]

Foucault, Michel. 1997c. "On the Genealogy of Ethics: An Overview of Work in Progress." In *Ethics: Subjectivity and Truth*, edited by Paul Rabinow. New York: The New Press.

Foucault, Michel. 1997d. "Sex, Power, and the Politics of Identity." In *Ethics: Subjectivity and Truth*, edited by Paul Rabinow. New York: The New Press.

Foucault, Michel. 1997e. "Sexual Choice, Sexual Act." In *Ethics: Subjectivity and Truth*, edited by Paul Rabinow. New York: The New Press.

Foucault, Michel. 2000a [1978]. "An Interview with Michel

Foucault." In *Power*, edited by James D. Faubion and translated by Robert Hurley et al. New York: The New Press.

Foucault, Michel. 2000b [1979]. "For an Ethic of Discomfort." In *Power*, edited by James D. Faubion and translated by Robert Hurley et al. New York: The New Press.

Halperin, David. 1995. *Saint Foucault: Towards a Gay Hagiography*. New York: Oxford University Press.

Jones, Meredith. 2008. "Sleeping Beauties: Lolo Ferrari and Anaesthesia." In *Skintight: An Anatomy of Cosmetic Surgery*, 129–150. Oxford: Berg.

Kandall, Stephen R., with Jennifer Petrillo. 1996. *Substance and Shadow: Women and Addiction in the United States*. Cambridge, MA: Harvard University Press.

May, Todd. 2006. "Foucault's Relation to Phenomenology." In *The Cambridge Companion to Foucault*, edited by Gary Gutting. Cambridge: Cambridge University Press.

McNay, Lois. 2009. "Self as Enterprise: Dilemmas of Control and Resistance in Foucault's *The Birth of Biopolitics*." *Theory, Culture, and Society* 26 (6): 55–77.

McWhorter, Ladelle. 1999. *Bodies and Pleasures: Foucault and the Politics of Sexual Normalization*. Bloomington: Indiana University Press.

Metzl, Jonathan. 2003. *Prozac on the Couch: Prescribing Gender in the Era of Wonder Drugs*. Durham, NC: Duke University Press.

Miller, James. 1993. *The Passion of Michel Foucault*. New York: Doubleday.

Morris, David B. 1991. *The Culture of Pain*. Berkeley: University of California Press.

Nancy, Jean-Luc. 2009. *The Fall of Sleep*. New York: Fordham University Press.

Oksala, Johanna. 2005. *Foucault on Freedom*. Cambridge: Cambridge University Press.

Oksala, Johanna. 2010. "Sexual Experience: Foucault, Phenomenology and Feminist Theory." *Hypatia* 25 (1): 2–17.

O'Leary, Timothy. 1996. "Foucault, Politics and the Autonomy of the Aesthetic." *International Journal of Philosophical Studies* 4 (2).

Snow, Stephanie J. 2006. *Operations without Pain: The Practice and Science of Anaesthesia in Victorian Britain*. Basingstoke: Palgrave Macmillan.

Stewart, Kathleen. 2007. *Ordinary Affects*. Durham, NC: Duke University Press.

Thacker, Andrew. 1993. "Foucault's Aesthetics of Existence." *Radical Philosophy* 63: 13–21.

Wolin, Richard. 1994. "Foucault's Aesthetic Decisionism." In *Michel Foucault: Critical Assessments*, vol. 3, edited by Barry Smart, 251–271. London: Routledge.

15

WANDERING IN THE UNHOMELIKE

Chronic Depression, Inequality, and the Recovery Imperative

ABBY WILKERSON

Delmore Schwartz's poem "The Heavy Bear Who Goes With Me" is the set piece opening *Unbearable Weight*, Susan Bordo's account of the gendered nature of the mind-body dualism endemic to Western culture:

> The heavy bear who goes with me [. . .]
> Clumsy and lumbering here and there [. . .]
>
> Breathing at my side, that heavy animal,
> That heavy bear who sleeps with me,
> Howls in his sleep for a world of sugar,
> A sweetness intimate as the water's clasp,
> Howls in his sleep because the tight-rope
> Trembles and shows the darkness beneath.
> (Schwartz quoted in Bordo 1993, 1)

The "inescapable animal" walking with him, the speaker of the poem says,

> Has followed me since the black womb held,
> Moves where I move, distorting my gesture,

A caricature, a swollen shadow,
A stupid clown of the spirit's motive
Perplexes and affronts with his own darkness [. . .]
(Schwartz quoted in Bordo 1993, 1)

For Bordo, the bear suggests the burdens of physicality itself, "neither one with nor separable from" the speaking self, "vividly captur[ing] both the dualism that has been characteristic of Western philosophy and theology and its agonistic, unstable nature" (1993, 2).

Yet the poem also speaks eloquently to the lived experience of depression, suggesting Schwartz's acquaintance with the condition by age twenty-five when the poem was first published; he would later be hospitalized multiple times for depression (Storr 2005, 142). Many words and phrases capture the dull weight of depressed physicality—*heavy bear, clumsy and lumbering, dragging me with him, swollen. Heavy* is repeated four times by the beginning of the second stanza. The bear's *love* for *sleep*, that he *sleeps with me* in an indefinite ongoing present—though *howl[ing] in* [that] *sleep*—also attest to this dulled physicality. Repeated references to the bear's darkness of spirit convey the depressed mood of melancholy and futility: *the tight-rope / Trembles and shows the darkness beneath*—a darkness that for the bear, and perhaps the poem's speaker, is *his own*, as the terrified bear *Trembles to think that his quivering meat / Must finally wince to nothing at all.*

The speaker's efforts to engage with the world, and even the bear's overpowering sleep, are eclipsed by the animal's infantile yearning for *a world of sugar*, a common experience (both literally and metaphorically) in depression. The bear is not simply an unwelcome companion; his very existence seems to rob the speaker of agency: *That inescapable animal [. . .] Moves where I move, distorting my gesture, / A caricature, a swollen shadow, / A stupid clown of the spirit's motive.* Worst of all, the bear's terrible *brutish* closeness atomistically encapsulates the speaker, blocking meaningful contact with others, as the animal *Stretches to embrace the very dear / With whom I would walk without him near, / Touches her grossly, although a word / Would bare my heart and make me clear.* Ultimately, depression, read via Schwartz's "Heavy Bear," turns out to be a kind of super-dualism, the mind-body dichotomy on steroids along with all the troubles feminist philosophers and others have traced to that legacy.

If there were any question as to why the predominant approach to depression, medically and culturally, is what I will call the recovery imperative, "The Heavy Bear" makes it crystal clear. Yet the poem suggests that ditching the bear is no simple proposition. As depressions go, this one is clearly chronic, coterminous with the speaker's very existence: *That inescapable animal walks with me, / Has followed me since the black womb held.* Ongoing depression can seem so interwoven with personality and identity as to be inextricable.

For this reason and more, the imperative to recover may need some unsettling, particularly in the case of *dysthymia*, a chronic form of depression, usually defined as low moods (if less intense than in major depression) persisting for two years or more. I want to explore the burdens of the recovery demand as they interact with gender and other vectors of oppression. The World Health Organization identifies depression as both "the leading global cause of years of health lost to disease in both men and women" and "the primary cause of loss of health in middle- and high-income countries" (Daly 2009, 7). Significantly higher rates of depression are consistently reported for women than for men (Bluhm 2011, 72–73; Greden 2001; Laitinen and Ettorre 2004, 205–206).

Some variation of chronic or recurrent forms of depression may actually be typical of the condition. For major depression, "Data collected since the late 1980s [. . .] have shown that the majority of patients [. . .] will experience relapses and recurrences," with a 90 percent recurrence rate often cited (Nierenberg, Petersen, and Alpert 2003, 13; O'Brien and Fullagar 2008, 8). In Wendy O'Brien and Simone Fullagar's qualitative study of midlife women who had experienced depression, very few participants saw themselves as recovered (2008, 10) or expected that they would never "'deal with [depression] again'" (2008, 11). They spoke of "a range of gender specific reasons that they felt contributed to women's depression and impeded their recovery," including "gender inequities in the family, workplace and leisure, as well as childhood abuse and relationship difficulties" (2008, 9). Despite this awareness of contextual factors in their own depression, however, the women were deeply affected by medical and social discourses of personal responsibility for illness, expressing a need not only to comply with medical recommendations but also to control the circumstances of their lives that contributed to depression (2008, 10–11).

Dysthymia is a particularly insidious form of depression, its symptoms less severe than in other forms, rendering the condition less likely to be recognized by self and others. Thus, even more than with other forms, dysthymia may frequently be misperceived as negative personality, constitutionally poor self-esteem, and so on, exacerbating both the isolation and self-blame that are already part of the condition. Dysthymia is also thought to be more difficult to treat with medication.

Cultural studies scholar Ann Cvetkovich speaks of trauma "as part of the affective language that describes life under capitalism" (2003, 19). Extending this characterization to depression, we can think of it, like trauma, as "sign or symptom of a broader systemic problem, a moment in which abstract social systems can actually be felt or sensed" (43). Considering the interactions of social, affective, and somatic processes in chronic depression affords a more nuanced phenomenological account of the lived experience of the condition for members of oppressed groups. Phenomenology has already yielded vital tools for exploring the lived experience of dysthymia and the operations of meaning-making in this context; closer attention to social contexts can advance ongoing efforts to critique the medicalization of affect and the normalizing functions of these processes—while providing a more detailed account of the majority of cases of depression.

To that end, I draw on an "embodied cognition" account conceptualizing the somatic basis of depression through a grounding in bodily metaphors (Lindeman and Abramson, 2008). I then situate these processes in broader social power dynamics through a Marxist-influenced critical psychology analysis of the influence of social interactions on depression (Cromby 2004). Finally, I consider the implications for dysthymia of disability studies critiques of bodily norms in order to indicate the limitations of the powerful cultural imperative toward recovery.

Phenomenology, Depression, and the Self

Because phenomenology addresses meaning "at the level of the life-world" and contextualizes this lived experience in the interactions of "embodiment and culture," it opens up a critical space for assessing the life impact of medicalization through attention both to how normality and its boundaries are defined and to the nature of subsequent interventions into departures from normality (Svenaeus 2007, 155). Fredrik Svenaeus identifies three elements of the standard diagnostic criteria for depression that reflect its phenomenological significance. The first is "altered embodiment," including changes in body weight, altered sleep patterns, "psychomotor agitation or retardation," and "fatigue or loss of energy" (2007, 156)—just the conditions illustrated by "The Heavy Bear." Second is "estranged engagement with the world," including "diminished ability to think or concentrate" and "a loss of interest or pleasure" (2007, 156)—just as the bear is a heavy presence inserting itself between the poem's speaker and his world. Third, these and other alterations are characterized by "painful feelings" that are not "directly caused by medication or bereavement," such as "feelings of worthlessness or excessive or inappropriate guilt" and "recurrent thoughts of death," constituting "clinically significant distress or impairment in social, occupational, or other important areas of functioning" (2007, 156)—as in the "darkness" shadowing the speaker in the form of the bear and his impaired ability to connect with his "very dear."

Svenaeus situates such feelings in the context of moods, specifically a Heideggerian notion of moods as "world-constitutive phenomena" (2007, 157). In contrast to emotions, which "have an object and are based upon beliefs," moods "lack a distinct object" and instead "color the way in which things appear to the subject in general [. . .] determin[ing] what kinds of thoughts the thinker will be able to entertain" (2007, 157). Svenaeus also takes up Heidegger's concept of being-in-the-world, in which objects' meanings depend on their role in human projects of all kinds. This "meaningfulness [. . .] has a characteristic tune," an attunement or mood-state (2007, 158). Moods shape or alter "the possibility of being in the world [. . .] of engaging with things and other human beings in a way that makes sense to us" (2007, 158). In other words, moods "connect the self to the world, thereby making being-in-the-world possible" (2007, 158).

Heidegger focuses particularly on boredom and anxiety, which, as Svenaeus points out, can be characteristic of depression. Heidegger characterizes them as "*unhomelike* phenomena" (quoted in Svenaeus 2007, 158). According to Svenaeus these "make settling in the world and being at home in the world impossible, since [in such cases] the world resists meaningfulness" (2007, 158). Melancholy, I would add, renders the world unhomelike and may be more characteristic of the general tone of dysthymia than boredom or anxiety, which fail to capture all cases of dysthymia. For Heidegger, unhomelikeness is a necessary tool in the quest for authenticity; however, as Svenaeus notes, when it is not "balanced by homelikeness [. . .] we fall into a bottomless pit of darkness" (2007, 158). In depression, unhomelikeness suffuses embodiment, illustrated well by the bear, lumbering and slow yet always capable of annihilation, a creature whose presence would seem to render home itself unhomelike.

The lived body "makes it possible for us to have a world," yet "still retains a certain thing-like quality" that depression exacerbates (2007, 160). Here Svenaeus takes up Fuchs' account of the lived body as a "physical resonance chamber for free-floating moods" (2007, 160). Depression is thus a "loss of bodily resonance [. . .] that renders the sufferer unresponsive to the calls of the world and thus leads to a failure of transcendence," a state of "being locked-in"—like the "withness" of the "heavy bear" "inescapabl[y] distorting my gesture [. . .] with his own darkness."

For Svenaeus, then, there is a spectrum of resonance or attunement from normal to pathological. Physical alterations can alter attunement and "thus the person's being-in-the-world"—but the world affects attunement too (2007, 161). The unhomelikeness engendered by depression is "rooted in an embodiment that is out of tune," linked to the profound loss not only "of the world, but also a loss of oneself" (2007, 161). Thus, in depression, grief and guilt become directed against the self (2007, 161). Though Svenaeus expresses certain cautions and reservations regarding antidepressants, for him their potential value "can be thought of in terms of alterations of bodily resonance—alterations that make new forms of transcendence to the world possible" (2007, 162).

Meaning-Making, Bodily Metaphors, and the Lived Body

One context for conceptualizing bodily resonance and the heavy bear's alterations to it is the emotional, physiological, and meaning-making processes within individuals. Lisa Lindeman and Lyn Abramson situate their analysis of depression within an "embodiment paradigm" of cognition (2008, 229). For some time, cognitive theories of depression have attributed "slowed motor movements and lethargy," and more specifically, "deficits in response initiation," to the "expectations of powerlessness and hopelessness" associated with depression (2008, 229). Lindeman and Abramson "present a theoretical model describing the *causal* mechanisms that link these cognitive and somatic elements of depression" (2008, 228; emphasis added). This model may partially explain the mechanics of the phenomeno- logical state of bodily resonance within the individual, with implica- tions for alleviating depression as well.

Lindeman and Abramson contend that "[h]opelessness leads to a cluster of bodily symptoms that include low energy, retarded ini- tiation of voluntary responses, and psychomotor retardation" (2008, 228). Researchers working within "the embodiment paradigm" of cognition have found that "concepts, rather than consisting of arbi- trary symbols for things in the world, involve mental simulations of perceptions and actions using many of the same neurons as actual perception and action" (2008, 229). When we encounter a word asso- ciated with a particular physical action, such as "kick" or "throw," the corresponding area of the sensorimotor cortices is activated (2008, 229). Embodied cognition research indicates that "cognitive schemas activated during episodes of depression are multisensory memories of past events stored as a unitary concept" (2008, 229).

Lindeman and Abramson discuss how abstract concepts as well as action-based concepts involve "sensorimotor simulation": for exam- ple, "the idea of grasping, whether it be grasping a mug or grasping the meaning of a joke, is instantiated by mentally simulating the motor action of grasping physical objects" (2008, 30). One study "found that this simulation is accompanied by weak motor impulses to the hands" (2008, 230). Such a process involves "conceptual metaphors" acquired through early experience associating "an abstract domain of experi- ence (e.g., knowledge, time, affection)" with "a sensorimotor experi- ence (e.g., sight, traversing a landscape, warmth)" (2008, 230). Because "the two are associated with the same experience" (2008, 230), they are mentally "conflated" in a way that becomes crystallized through metaphor, a process that tends to be automatic rather than conscious (2008, 231).

Research on mental imagery confirms that "the sensorimotor simulations in embodied cognition" trigger motor responses such as neural activity in areas of the body associated with an image. Such effects have been demonstrated for positive imagery (imagining per- forming a certain action) as well as for negative imagery (imagining suppressing an action or being unable to perform it), and here too, the process can occur unconsciously (2008, 231).

Lindeman and Abramson begin to trace the implications for depression: "some emotions are mental simulations or reenactments of bodily experiences (e.g., falling, smothering, carrying a heavy weight) that result when one conceptualizes the abstract, personal meaning of a situation or event (e.g., financial loss, a restrictive relationship, social pressures) metaphorically in terms of that experience" (2008, 232). These simulations in turn lead to physiological effects associated with emotion such as "muscle tension [or] changes in body temperature and breathing patterns" (2008, 232).

A depressed person's difficulty in engaging with the world or accomplishing desired projects is, according to Lindeman and Abramson, "conceptualized metaphorically" by that person "as motor incapacity" (2008, 232). This conceptualization involves motor simulation, which "leads to subjective feelings of immobility and lethargy as well as corresponding peripheral physiological changes, namely, low energy and psychomotor retardation" (2008, 232). Lindeman and Abramson note the ubiquity in everyday speech of physical metaphors for incapacity of all kinds, through expressions such as, "*I cannot* lift *my grade. All my hard work is* getting me nowhere. *My dreams are* out of reach. *My goal is* too far away. *My hands are* tied" (2008, 232). They contend that such language is only a surface reflection of deeper experiential learning processes, noting further that research confirms the origins of depression not simply in loss but in loss involving "entrapment (e.g., blocked escape) or defeat (e.g., a put-down)" (2008, 233).

They also cite a number of studies confirming the association of powerlessness with "being down or low" in the sense of spatial positioning as well as slumped posture, which were shown to result in reduced performance and learned helplessness (2008, 234–235). Lindeman and Abramson emphasize the experiential basis of such metaphors: "Physical powerlessness resulting from low physical energy or being overwhelmed by a physical force (e.g., a multitude of objects, ocean waves, physical burdens, or opponents in a fight)"—or being dragged by a very heavy bear, we might add—"typically causes the body to occupy a low position in space in a painful or uncomfortable manner" (2008, 235). They identify past experiences of this physical positioning as the basis for mental simulations of powerlessness (2008, 235).

A central component of depression, of course, is negative views of the self, a feature that Lindeman and Abramson's model accounts for as well, through experiences of rejection by others, which are then internalized in a process of bodily simulation based on metaphor:

"Being humiliated by negative social judgments [. . .] can be conceptualized as being put down or cut down, reduced in size, or taken down a level. People *look down on* those who are of *low* status. [. . .] Worthlessness and rejection [. . .] are associated with being low (e.g., low self-esteem, low regard, lowly servant)" (2008, 235). Due to such metaphors, "social rejection and the belief that one is worthless may cause a person to feel subjectively low [. . .] they may [even] infer that they are worthless or deficient, because they *feel* low" (2008, 236).

Lindeman and Abramson's account of the interplay of learned experience and its translation through metaphor into depressed embodiment emphasizes cognitive-physiological loops internal to the individual. From a phenomenological perspective, however, as Svenaeus puts it, "there exists no private world, apart from other people, in which we can exist" (2007, 159). Thus, Lindeman and Abramson's useful picture of cognitive-physiological processes in the altered bodily resonance of depression must be supplemented with a more detailed account of the *social* aspects of these processes.

Public Processes and Bodily Resonance

While depressed people may, like the speaker of "The Heavy Bear," *feel* encapsulated, shut off from the social world, they are nonetheless always enmeshed within it. In a recent Finnish study, Irmeli Laitinen and Elizabeth Ettorre conclude that "[d]epressed women [. . .] may experience private distress shaped by public processes, structural relations and gender inequalities" (2004, 218). Thus, I turn now to John Cromby's work in order to develop an understanding of social power dynamics as they influence bodily resonance in depression. If Cromby's analysis is correct, the social environment's influence on depression is strong in a significant proportion of cases, exerting itself to some degree in any instance.

Cromby provides a critical psychology perspective on the "social and neural processes" linking depression and social inequality, addressing social bases for the negative views of self that predominate in depression (2004, 13). Where Lindeman and Abramson's account illuminates processes within the individual, Cromby offers a social constructionist analysis of depression via German Critical Psychology, taking up Marxist accounts of social power structures to conceptualize possibilities for social change. On this view, "subjective possibility space" is "the range of options available to an individual, the sum total of things they can anticipate [. . .]. Because material resources are unevenly distributed, there will be variation in the subjective possibility spaces of individuals" (Cromby 2004, 6). Cromby draws on neurobiologist Antonio Damasio's work on "somatic markers," feelings that are "bodily states [based on previous experiences] called out within streams of interaction and used to weigh alternatives and provide a guide to action" (2004, 8). Cromby uses the concept of somatic markers to theorize "a thoroughly embodied subjectivity that is simultaneously both relational (located in and formed through ongoing relationships) and material (structured and informed by the material resources available to the person)" (2004, 9). This is a "hybrid" notion of subjectivity: "discursive, material and embodied [. . .] processes work together to *co-constitute* subjectivity" (2004, 9).

Cromby draws on the concept of "transactional patterns" advanced in earlier research on "discursively structured variation in social practices within Western culture" (2004, 9). This work identifies "three social transactional scripts (Helpless-Helpful, Powerless-Powerful and Worthy-Worthless) that, if they predominate during socialisation, might generate three distinctive ways of being in the world that psychiatrists would categorise uniformly as depression" (2004, 9). The Helpless-Helpful script refers to "experiences wherein individuals gain recognition and reward for positioning or describing themselves as inferior and incapable" (2004, 9–10). Powerless-Powerful involves "experiences where individuals are rewarded for placating others and ingratiating themselves" (2004, 10). Worthy-Worthless describes "experiences where individuals gain rewards for apologising and deploying self-deprecating discourses" (2004, 10). All three result in impaired decision-making ability, with different effects depending on the pattern (2004, 10); this impairment is a significant feature of all forms of depression, and its impact on agency speaks for itself.

The transactional patterns expressed in these scripts are pervasive discursive features in social contexts of inequality, where "legitimated discourses will consistently invite persons to understand themselves as helpless, worthless or powerless, and consistently make germane dimensions of efficacy, power and self-worth. Alongside these discourses, and reinforcing devalued subject positions within them, will be affective flows or repertoires of feelings" (Cromby 2004, 10). The resulting transactions "will generate corresponding patterns of somatic markers," which in turn "may influence subsequent activity by attaching negative or low values to options sensitively intertwined with self-image, or by making choices which would affirm personal worth, power or efficacy *feel* impossible" (2004, 10). These transactions influence self-conceptions, which seem to take on legitimacy through repeated exposure. The resulting negative views of self, the "associated somatic markers" and social settings "where discourses of power, efficacy or self-worth are deployed" offer powerful mutual reinforcement (2004, 10).

Moreover, the ongoing nature of these ("sometimes covert") processes, according to Cromby,

> helps explain the relative intransigence of unhappiness and shows how the experience of powerlessness, for example, is much more than just a discursive construction. Alongside its discursive aspect, powerlessness acquires an embodied, feelingful character composed of facial expression, posture, gaze direction and duration, breathing, head inclination, muscle tone, and less visible characteristics such as visceral and blood vessel activity. (2004, 10)

These "somatic markers" in turn "could potentiate further trajectories of social transaction wherein power becomes salient. People who construct and display themselves as powerless (however unwittingly) may invite responses from others that accord with their self-construction" (2004, 10). Thus, once one of the three scripts is activated and repeated, each aspect of the process reinforces the others in a vicious circle.

Cromby's account of a key feature of the social context is useful in understanding depression's interactions with oppression. For example, in the United States, research verifies a greater vulnerability to depression among Native Americans, Pacific Islanders, and Alaska Natives (Page and Blau 2006, 107); poor people and recipients of public benefits (Page and Blau 2006, 105); people experiencing discrimination based on race or sexual orientation (Carten 2006, 130; Mays and Cochran 2001); and, from adolescence on, girls and women (Nolen-Hoeksema and Girgus 1994). World Psychiatric Association president Pedro Ruiz links women's higher rates of depression to single parenthood burdens (Daly 7). Overall, as Robyn Bluhm succinctly states, "greater rates of mental disorders [are associated] with a lack of social power" (2011, 78)—an effect we can assume is compounded when multiple vectors of oppression are experienced simultaneously, as is the case for many women.

A study of Filipino Americans found an association between internalized oppression and depression symptoms (David 2008)—clearly illustrating how social transaction scripts involving differential social worth, power, and efficacy influence depression, as Cromby suggests. In O'Brien and Fullagar's qualitative research with women recovering from depression, some participants expressed "a dawning recognition that the gender expectations they lived out as women may have contributed to their situation (self sacrificing, pleasing others, motherhood guilt, responsibility for others wellbeing [*sic*] and/or perfectionism, over achievement, being superwoman)" (2008, 9). Such expectations, far from neurotic patterns within individuals, constitute gendered forms of the Helpless-Helpful, Powerless-Powerful, and Worthy-Worthless transactional scripts that Cromby identifies as structural features of contemporary social contexts.

The Trouble with Normal

As I noted earlier, it is abundantly clear why depression—its chronic forms especially—is seen as something to get over (another spatial metaphor asserting itself). Yet the recovery imperative is particularly fraught for members of oppressed groups, who face depressogenic social transactions regularly; such experiences are among the hallmarks of oppression. Thus, oppressed people are not only more vulnerable to depression as a result, but if they do become depressed, the ongoing nature of such transactions imposes obstacles to recovery. Moreover, when society fails to address depression among members of oppressed groups (for example, through differential access to health care or obstacles to utilization), their oppression is further compounded.

The recovery imperative, however, is something more, and more complicated, than the goal to eliminate suffering. A host of critics have pointed out the increasingly influential social tendency to redefine normalcy in terms of the ideal, and the corresponding imperative to bring individuals into conformity. Disability scholar Robert McRuer offers a notion of "compulsory able-bodiedness," the normative apparatus that includes aesthetic ideals, cultural narratives, and medical norms and practices (2006). It includes, for example, neoliberal expectations of more or less consistent and continuous productivity and emotional functioning, as well as cultural stigmas against illness that are particularly strong in the case of mental illness. While these norms and stigmas are likely to hold intensified power in the lives of members of oppressed groups, given the interactions of ableism with other vectors of oppression, they factor into any instance of depression. Given this broad social context, what does the recovery imperative mean in the lives of oppressed people with dysthymia?

An emphasis on recovery is meant to promote agency. However, as feminist and other critics are wont to point out, medical and social understandings of agency are all too often couched in terms of adjustment to the social context as it stands, reinforcing inequality, for what else is meant by promoting health through individual "adjustment" to a public domain characterized by capitalist norms of productivity, with privatization rapidly diminishing whatever social safety nets still exist? Or promoting individual adjustment to the private world of the home where traditional gender-based divisions of labor and power differentials are still not eradicated, heteronormativity is far from unsettled, and increasing wealth differentials and immigration controls allow some unions far greater economic and legal stability than others?

Thus, the mental health goal of "adjustment" implicated in the recovery imperative creates direct conflicts for oppressed people. The discourse of adjustment, along with the biochemical reductionism that answers the call of distress with an antidepressant prescription, is ineluctably bound up with notions of individual responsibility that only compound the injustices faced by members of oppressed groups. As O'Brien and Fullagar note, "Recovering individuals are positioned as responsible for seeking and adhering to expert advice from physicians to ensure that, as virtuous neo-liberal citizens, they recover their autonomy and ability to be economically and socially productive" (2008, 8). Such positioning introduces burdensome expectations for many people with depression, especially its chronic forms, and especially so for those who are members of oppressed groups. Grounding mental health promotion efforts in a social justice analysis can help reduce the possibility of compounding social incursions on self-regard and agency.

Talk therapy and other approaches, including physical activity, improved nutrition, and alternative treatments such as yoga and acupuncture, have been shown to benefit people with chronic or short-term depression and therefore should be supported. However, these alternatives may be inaccessible to members of oppressed groups, so they are hardly a panacea and, in any case, are far from being established as any kind of definitive cure.

No wonder, then, that SSRIs are used by so many, despite concerns of safety as well as efficacy, given the research demonstrating that they are outperformed by placebos. Surely any relief SSRIs provide is of value. If their potential for providing relief and enhancing agency is to be realized, however, the considerations explored here suggest that this can only happen in a context significantly different than the present one: a context in which serious efforts are made to see that all individuals have access to a full range of health care, including effective alternative treatments, and that health care is informed by a social justice analysis—but most importantly, that the social bases of well-being are more equitably distributed.

Questing Together, Accompanied by Bear

This chapter is aligned with the view that depression research must be situated within analysis of social power differentials to conceptualize depression accurately and be of use in people's lives. Lindeman and Abramson posit therapeutic value for spatial metaphors of "overcoming" and physical activity embodying these metaphors, such as climbing, moving ahead, and the like (2008, 238–241). This idea speaks powerfully to the phenomenological notion of bodily resonance and its disturbance in depression. Yet inattention to the ongoing nature of oppressive social transactions, the conditions that crush and overwhelm us, limits the value of these metaphorical interventions.

Feminist action research suggests promising possibilities. Irmeli Laitinen and Elizabeth Ettorre's ethnographic study found that Finnish women participating in guided self-help groups with other depressed women came to see their experiences "through the lens of a collectivist [. . .] rather than individualistic model of health" (2004, 217). The collective process of meaning-making in the groups and the resulting sense of solidarity "allowed depressed women's voices to become audible. By constructing gender-sensitive understandings, women who had traditionally been dealt with as objects of treatment were more able to become active subjects in healing their depression"

(2004, 217). Like the feminist consciousness-raising groups that preceded them, the guided self-help groups enabled the women to move from a sense of their struggles as strictly personal to a new understanding of the larger social problems they were tied to, alleviating the burden of self-blame. In Cromby's terminology, this indicates that the women's work together may have helped them to recognize oppressive social transactions that undermined their agency and their mental health. Clearly, the process of the guided self-help groups suggests possibilities that could not be duplicated by medication nor within the bounds of individual talk therapy.

The concept of "healing" articulated by the Finnish study participants suggests an emerging alternative to biochemical notions of treatment, one that includes developing life skills that their circumstances as women seem to have interfered with—greater self-trust, improved relationships, "hav[ing] energy again to fight for things that are important" to them, and increased general "effective[ness] in their lives" (Laitinen and Ettorre 2004, 216). Exercising agency, it would seem, is healing. The women also expressed a concern with "dealing with [their own] femaleness" as part of healing (2004, 209). Overall, "the future picture was a woman who is self-focused [. . .] with a relative amount of female authority [and] more choices" (2004, 216). Laitinen and Ettorre cite other feminist research indicating that "members of a women's group are aware that the group generates a series of choices for members and these choices run in parallel to personal coping strategies, including anticipating the future" (2004, 216).

This notion of choice and its association with "female authority" resonates with Cromby's concept of subjective possibility space cited earlier, which he understands as "the range of options available to an individual, the sum total of things they can anticipate" (2004, 6) and part and parcel of the experience of depression. One's sense of possibility is strongly linked, in his view, to the material resources available to him or her. The depression group findings also suggest that the group process of building solidarity may help to open up a previously foreclosed subjective possibility space. Indeed, in these experiences a collective impetus toward social change may be a crucial component of the "personal coping strategies" they foster.

In their conclusion, Laitinen and Ettorre acknowledge that "while depression may be shaped by gender, cultural stereotypes, space and climate may take their toll" (2004, 218). Generally, however, they tend to rely on a unitary concept of women, specifying "social characteristics of respondents" only in terms of "age, employment, education, training, [and] living situation" (2004, 207). Thus, their results require cautious assessment. The project arose from a feminist mental health context that emphasized "becom[ing] a *sisukas nainen*, meaning a strong Finnish woman" (2004, 205); the level of collective identification emerging in the project—which the authors identify as central to its positive results—may not obtain as readily in more ethnically and culturally diverse contexts. Moreover, therapeutic emphasis on "femaleness" unmodified, even in feminist contexts, is of limited value—potentially damaging even—insofar as it fails to address the complex situations of women experiencing additional vectors of oppression beyond "female" identity or the complexities of feminine and woman-based identities themselves.

In medical sociologist Arthur Frank's analysis of illness narratives, illness and its disruptions to "normal" life present the opportunity for a quest of meaning-making and social critique—possibilities shut off by culturally sanctioned "restitution" narratives involving a return to an idealized past prior to illness. Such a quest promotes healing that "may not cure the body, but it does remedy the loss of body-self intactness" imposed by suffering (1995, 183). Frank could be speaking of the Finnish participants and their notion of healing when he writes, "The sufferer is made whole in hearing the other's story that is also hers, and in having her own story, not just be listened to but heard as if it were the listener's own, which it is" (1995, 183).

The figure of the inescapable heavy bear between self and world vividly illustrates the moods of depression and how they render the world unhomelike. The Western social project in regard to depression, an uneasy marriage of the human desire to alleviate suffering and the transnational capitalist drive to maximize productivity and profit by medicating as many conditions as possible, posits the unhomelikeness of depression as only something to be overcome. Yet the evidence reviewed here indicates that the unhomelikeness and altered bodily resonance of dysthymia may fluctuate with no endpoint that can be anticipated. However, feminist research—in part by foregrounding oppressive social conditions and power differentials—offers hope for alleviating suffering without imposing recovery as an expectation that only increases the self-blame so deeply woven into the experience of dysthymia.

Schwartz's bear figures chronic depression as external to the self (if closely though involuntarily linked), nonhuman even, animal, utterly alien—a form of projection that is as problematic as it is moving and expressive. The recovery imperative, like the poet's disavowal of the bear/body, seeks to transcend the suffering of depression precisely because of its alien, unhomelike quality. Rather than grasping for a cure or cursing its elusiveness, feminist research allies with Frank's vision of narrative, leading us to quest with the bear, a project best imagined collectively, together finding our way and seeking new meanings both from and against the overwhelm of this heavy embrace.

Schwartz's speaker closes the poem with the bear

> Dragging me with him in his mouthing care,
> Amid the hundred million of his kind,
> The scrimmage of appetite everywhere.
> (Quoted in Bordo 1993, 2)

If any hope is to be found in Schwartz's poem, it lies in its recognition that the speaker, despite his (?) sense of isolation, is far from the only one accompanied by "his kind," and its marking of troublesome desires as "appetite"—a force vital for survival and well-being. Reading these lines through the disability rights insistence that disability is central to the human condition, rather than a departure from it (Wendell 1996), the bear reminds us we are situated with others and must work together for justice in our workplaces, in our communities, and in our homes.

Acknowledgments

The author wishes to thank Lisa Folkmarson Käll, Kristin Zeiler, and an anonymous reader of an earlier draft of this essay, for their invaluable guidance. The attendees of the Feminist Phenomenology and Medicine conference at Uppsala University, as well as Cathy Eisenhower, provided spirited conversation that informed this work in many ways. Pam Presser, Karen Sosnoski, and Pat McGann responded thoughtfully and perceptively to this project at multiple stages in the process.

References

Bluhm, Robyn. 2011. "Gender Differences in Depression." *The International Journal of Feminist Approaches to Bioethics* 4 (1): 69–88.

Bordo, Susan. 1993. *Unbearable Weight: Feminism, Western Culture and the Body*. Berkeley: University of California Press.

Carten, Alma J. 2006. "African-Americans and Mental Health." In *Community Mental Health: Challenges for the 21st Century*, edited by Jessica Rosenberg and Samuel Rosenberg, 125–140. New York: Routledge.

Cromby, John. 2004. "Depression: Embodying Social Inequality." *Journal of Critical Psychology, Counselling and Psychotherapy* 4 (3): 176–187.http://www-staff.lboro.ac.uk/~hujc4/Depression%20 embodying%20social%20inequality%20PUBLISHED.pdf,p~8

Cvetkovich, Ann. 2003. *An Archive of Feelings: Trauma, Sexuality, and Lesbian Public Cultures*. Durham: Duke University Press.

Daly, Rich. 2009. "Depression Biggest Contributor to Global Disease Burden." *Psychiatric News* 44 (1): 7. http://pn.psychiatryonline. org/content/44/1/7.1.full.

David, Eric John Ramos. 2008. "A Colonial Mentality Model of Depression for Filipino Americans." *Cultural Diversity and Ethnic Minority Psychology* 14 (2): 118–127.

Frank, Arthur. 1995. *The Wounded Storyteller: Body, Illness, and Ethics*. Chicago: University of Chicago Press.

Fuchs, Thomas. 2005. "Corporealized and Disembodied Minds: A Phenomenological View of the Body in Melancholia and Schizophrenia." *Philosophy, Psychiatry & Psychology* 12 (2): 95–107.

Greden, John F. 2001. "The Burden of Disease for Treatment-Resistant Depression." *Journal of Clinical Psychiatry* 62 (Supplement 16): 16–31.

Laitinen, Irmeli, and Elizabeth Ettorre. 2004. "The Women and Depression Project: Feminist Action Research and Guided Self-Help Groups Emerging from the Finnish Women's Movement." *Women's Studies International Forum* 27: 203–221.

Lindeman, Lisa M., and Lyn Y. Abramson. 2008. "The Mental Simulation of Motor Incapacity in Depression." *Journal of Cognitive Psychotherapy* 22 (3): 228–249.

Mays, Vickie M., and Susan D. Cochran. 2001. "Mental Health Correlates of Perceived Discrimination among Lesbian, Gay, and

Bisexual Adults in the United States." *American Journal of Public Health* 91 (11): 1869–1876.

McRuer, Robert. 2006. *Crip Theory: Cultural Signs of Queerness and Disability*. New York: New York University Press.

Mollow, Anna. 2006. "'When *Black* Women Start Going on Prozac . . .': The Politics of Race, Gender, and Emotional Distress in Meri Nana-Ama Danquah's *Willow Weep for Me*." In *The Disability Studies Reader*, 2nd ed., edited by Lennard J. Davis, 283–299. New York: Routledge.

Nierenberg, Andrew A., MD; Petersen, Timothy J., PhD; Alpert, Jonathan E., MD. 2003. "Prevention of Relapse and Recurrence in Depression: The Role of Long-Term Pharmacotherapy and Psychotherapy." *Journal of Clinical Psychiatry* 64 (Supplement 15): 13–17.

Nolen-Hoeksema, Susan, Girgus, Joan S. 1994. "The Emergence of Gender Differences in Depression during Adolescence." *Psychological Bulletin* 115 (3): 424–443.

O'Brien, Wendy, and Simone Fullagar. 2008. "Rethinking the Relapse Cycle of Depression and Recovery: A Qualitative Investigation of Women's Experiences." *Social Alternatives* 27 (4): 6–13.

Page, Jaimie, and Joel Blau. 2006. "Public Mental Health Systems: Breaking the Impasse in the Treatment of Oppressed Groups." In *Community Mental Health: Challenges for the 21st Century*, edited by Jessica Rosenberg and Samuel Rosenberg, 103–116. New York: Routledge.

Storr, Anthony. 1988. *Solitude: A Return to the Self*. New York: Free Press.

Svenaeus, Fredrik. 2007. "Do Antidepressants Affect the Self? A Phenomenological Approach." *Medicine, Health Care and Philosophy* 10: 153–166.

Wendell, Susan. 1996. *The Rejected Body: Feminist Philosophical Reflections on Disability*. New York: Routledge.

CONTRIBUTORS

Sᴀʀᴀʜ LᴀCʜᴀɴᴄᴇ Aᴅᴀᴍs is Assistant Professor of Philosophy at the University of Wisconsin–Superior. She is the author of *The Ethics of Ambivalence: Mad Mothers, Bad Mothers, and What a Good Mother Would Do* (forthcoming), which concerns the ethical and intersubjective implications of maternal ambivalence and filicide. She is the coeditor of an anthology entitled *Coming to Life: Philosophies of Pregnancy, Childbirth, and Mothering* (2013). Her current research project is on erotic love.

Pᴀᴜʟ Bᴜʀᴄʜᴇʀ is Assistant Professor of the Alden March Bioethics Institute at Albany Medical College. He has recently completed a dissertation in philosophy at University of Oregon entitled *The Doctor-Patient Relationship: A Physician's Philosophical Perspective.* In it he argues that a responsive model of care in all aspects of the clinical encounter needs to be taught and encouraged as a way of improving patient care. He is a practicing obstetrician/gynecologist who has worked recently with a medical anthropologist to explore ways of improving collaboration between homebirth midwives and obstetricians as a way of improving patient safety. Burcher graduated at University of Arizona Medical College and completed his residency in OB/GYN at University of Rochester. Recent publications include "The Just Distance: A New Biomedical Principle," in *The Journal of Clinical Ethics*, and "The Noncompliant Patient: A Kantian and Levinasian Response," in *The Journal of Medicine and Philosophy* 37 (1) (2012): 74–89.

ELLEN K. FEDER is Associate Professor of Philosophy at American University in Washington, DC. She is author of *Family Bonds: Genealogies of Race and Gender* (2007) and coeditor of *A Passion for Wisdom: Readings in Western Philosophy on Love and Desire* (2004) as well as *The Subject of Care: Feminist Perspectives on Dependency* (2002). Her book *Making Sense of Intersex: Changing Ethical Perspectives in Biomedicine* (2014) examines the ethical questions raised by the medical management of children born with atypical sex anatomies.

LINDA FISHER is Associate Professor in the Department of Gender Studies at Central European University, Budapest. Her research areas include contemporary Continental philosophy, phenomenology, hermeneutics, feminist philosophy and gender studies, philosophy and literature, and aesthetics. Her current work in feminist phenomenology explores the intersections of temporality, intersubjectivity, difference, and embodiment, with a particular focus on developing a phenomenology of gendered experience. She is coeditor of *Feminist Phenomenology* (2000) and *Feministische Phänomenologie und Hermeneutik* (2005). Recent publications include "Feminist Phenomenological Voices," *Continental Philosophy Review* 43 (1) (2010): 83–95 and "Gendering Embodied Memory," in *Time in Feminist Phenomenology* (2011).

LISA GUNTRAM is a PhD candidate at the Division of Health and Society, Linköping University. In her ongoing PhD project she combines a qualitative empirical approach with her interest in feminist phenomenology, the phenomenology of the body, and gender theoretical perspectives on sexuality. Guntram more specifically aims to examine norms and beliefs concerning female embodiment and sexuality, particularly through explorations of young women's narratives and experiences of atypical sex development in their teens. She is also one of the authors of Kristin Zeiler, Lisa Guntram, and Annette Lennerling, "Moral Tales of Parental Live Kidney Donation: A Parenthood Moral Imperative and Its Relevance for Parental Living Kidney Donors' Decision-Making," *Medicine, Health Care and Philosophy* 13 (3) (2010): 225–236.

CRESSIDA J. HEYES is Professor of Political Science and Philosophy and Canada Research Chair in Philosophy of Gender and Sexuality at the University of Alberta. She writes and teaches in feminist theory, contemporary social and political thought, and philosophy of the body. She is the author of *Self-Transformations: Foucault, Ethics, and Normalized Bodies* (2007) and *Line Drawings: Defining Women through Feminist Practice* (2000); the editor of *Critical Concepts: Gender and Philosophy* (2011); and the coeditor (with Meredith Jones) of *Cosmetic Surgery: A Feminist Primer* (2009).

LISA FOLKMARSON KÄLL is Associate Professor (Docent) of Theoretical Philosophy and Research Associate in Philosophy of Medicine and Medical Ethics at the Centre for Dementia Research, Department of Medical and Health Sciences, Linköping University. Her work brings together phenomenology with current gender research and feminist theory to inquire into questions concerning embodied subjectivity, bodily constitution of sexual difference and sexual identity, intersubjectivity, and the relation between selfhood and otherness. She is currently working on a project on intercorporeal sharing and alterations of self-experience in dementia. Käll is editor of *Dimensions of Pain* (2013) and coeditor with Ulrika Björk of *Stil, Kön, Andrahet: Tolv essäer i feministisk filosofi* (Style, sex, otherness: twelve essays in feminist philosophy) (2010).

ERIK MALMQVIST is Lecturer at the Department of Medical and Health Sciences, Linköping University. His research explores ethical and philosophical issues raised by biotechnology and medical practice and research. Recent publications include "Are Bans on Kidney Sales Unjustifiably Paternalistic?" *Bioethics* 2012: DOI: 10.1111/j.1467-8519.2012.01984.x; "Reprogenetics and the 'Parents Have Always Done It' Argument," *Hastings Center Report* 41 (1) (2011): 43–49; and (with Kristin Zeiler) "Cultural Norms, the Phenomenology of Incorporation, and the Experience of Having a Child Born with Ambiguous Sex," *Social Theory and Practice* 36 (1) (2010): 133–156.

LANEI M. RODEMEYER, Associate Professor of Philosophy at Duquesne University, works primarily in the areas of Husserlian phenomenology, continental philosophy, the philosophy of time, and feminist/gender philosophy of the body. In her book on Husserl's phenomenology of inner time-consciousness, *Intersubjective Temporality* (2006), she argues that this apparently solipsistic structure is actually integrated with an open intersubjective structure. In her articles, she takes up questions of the body through pregnancy, eating disorders, and transsexuality, and she also examines the phenomenological body as temporal.

Margrit Shildrick is Professor of Gender and Knowledge Production at Linköping University and Adjunct Professor of Critical Disability Studies at York University, Toronto. Her research covers postmodern feminist and cultural theory, bioethics, critical disability studies, and body theory. Her books include *Dangerous Discourses of Disability, Subjectivity and Sexuality* (2009), *Embodying the Monster* (2002), and *Leaky Bodies and Boundaries* (1997), as well as several recent journal publications on organ transplantation.

Jenny Slatman is Associate Professor of Philosophy at the research institute CAPHRI, Department of Health, Ethics and Society, Maastricht University, and project leader of the NWO-VIDI project Bodily Integrity in Blemished Bodies. Her publications include various journal articles and book chapters on the phenomenology of the body; a monograph on *L'expression au-delà de la représentation: Sur l'aisthêsis et l'esthétique chez Merleau-Ponty* (2003); and a book-length study, *Our Strange Body: Philosophical Reflections on Identity and Medical Interventions* (forthcoming). Her current research involves philosophical and ethical analyses of bodily identity and integrity in reconstructive medicine, oncology, and public health interventions.

Nikki Sullivan is Associate Professor at the Department of Media, Music, Communication and Cultural Studies at Macquarie University. Sullivan's research focuses primarily on modificatory practices (e.g., tattooing, intersex surgeries, genital modifications, elective amputation, cosmetic surgeries) and the (soma)technologies in and through which such practices are regulated, shaped, lived, and experienced. She is the author of *Tattooed Bodies: Subjectivity, Textuality, Ethics and Pleasure* (2001) and *A Critical Introduction to Queer Theory* (2003); coeditor (with Samantha Murray) of *Somatechnics: Queering the Technologisation of Bodies* (2009); and coeditor (with Jane Simon) of the *Somatechnics* journal. She is currently working on a coedited (with Lisa Downing and Iain Morland) book on the work of John Money, *Fuckology: Critical Essays on John Money's Diagnostic Concepts* (forthcoming 2014).

FREDRIK SVENAEUS is Professor at the Centre for Studies in Practical Knowledge, Södertörn University. His main research areas are philosophy of medicine, bioethics, medical humanities, and philosophical anthropology. He has published a considerable number of articles and books on these subjects, most often from a phenomenological point of view. Two recent examples are "The Body as Gift, Resource, or Commodity: Heidegger and the Ethics of Organ Transplantation," *Journal of Bioethical Inquiry* 7 (2) (2010): 163–172 and "Illness as Unhomelike Being-in-the-World: Heidegger and the Phenomenology of Medicine," *Medicine, Health Care and Philosophy* 14 (3) (2011): 333–343.

GAIL WEISS is Chair of the Department of Philosophy and Professor of Philosophy and Human Sciences at The George Washington University, Washington, DC. She is the author of *Refiguring the Ordinary* (2008) and *Body Images: Embodiment as Intercorporeality* (1999), the editor of *Intertwinings: Interdisciplinary Encounters with Merleau-Ponty* (2008), and coeditor (with Debra Bergoffen) of the Summer 2011 Special Issue of *Hypatia: A Journal of Feminist Philosophy* on "The Ethics of Embodiment," 26 (3). She is also the coeditor of three anthologies: *Feminist Interpretations of Maurice Merleau-Ponty* (2006), *Thinking the Limits of the Body* (2003), and *Perspectives on Embodiment: The Intersections of Nature and Culture* (1999). Her publications include journal articles and book chapters on philosophical and feminist issues related to human embodiment.

ABBY WILKERSON is Associate Professor of University Writing at George Washington University in Washington, DC. As a philosopher in an interdisciplinary writing program her work focuses on embodied agency and social movements, particularly in the contexts of food, disability, health, and sexuality. Her publications include *The Thin Contract: Social Justice and the Political Rhetoric of Obesity* (forthcoming); *Diagnosis: Difference: The Moral Authority of Medicine*; "Refusing Diagnosis: Mother-Daughter Agency in Confronting Psychiatric Rhetoric," *Disability and Mothering*, edited by Cynthia Lewiecki-Wilson and Jen Cellio; and other articles in anthologies and journals. She coedited (with Robert McRuer) the award-winning "Desiring Disability: Queer Theory Meets Disability Studies," a special issue of *GLQ: A Journal of Lesbian and Gay Studies*.

Gili Yaron is a PhD candidate at the research institute CAPHRI, Department of Health, Ethics and Society, Maastricht University. Her research project aims to examine the meaning of bodily identity in people with a different face by using qualitative empirical methods (interpretative phenomenological analysis of in-depth interviews with facially disfigured people). Her award-winning essay "Tussen vreemdheid en eigenheid: werken aan een gaaf gelaat" (Between strangeness and ownness: working on a flawless face) appears in a compilation volume (2012) on the current state of affairs of Disability Studies in the Netherlands.

Kristin Zeiler is Associate Professor of Medical Ethics at the Department of Medical and Health Sciences, Linköping University and Pro Futura Scientia Fellow at the Swedish Collegium for Advanced Study, Uppsala. Her research areas include medical ethics, philosophy of medicine, and feminist philosophy. She has published a number of articles examining ethical aspects of organ donation, IVF-related practices and intersex treatment, as well as phenomenological analysis of pain and pleasure. Among her publications, see Kristin Zeiler, "A Phenomenology of Excorporation, Bodily Alienation and Resistance: Rethinking Sexed and Racialized Embodiment," *Hypatia: A Journal of Feminist Philosophy* 28 (1) (2013): 69–84 and Kristin Zeiler, "A Philosophical Defense of the Idea That We Can Hold Each Other in Personhood: Intercorporeal Personhood in Dementia Care, Medicine, Health Care and Philosophy (2013, Early Online View).

INDEX